Corticospinal Neurones

MONOGRAPHS OF THE PHYSIOLOGICAL SOCIETY

Published by EDWARD ARNOLD

1 *H. Barcroft and H. J. C. Swan*
Sympathetic Control of Human Blood Vessels, 1953*

2 *A. C. Burton and O. G. Edholm*
Man in a Cold Environment, 1955*

3 *G. W. Harris*
Neural Control of the Pituitary Gland, 1955*

4 *A. H. James*
Physiology of Gastric Digestion, 1957*

5 *B. Delisle Burns*
The Mammalian Cerebral Cortex, 1958*

6 *G. S. Brindley*
Physiology of the Retina and Visual Pathway, 1960 (2nd edition, 1970)

7 *D. A. McDonald*
Blood Flow in Arteries, 1960*

8 *A. S. V. Burgen and N. G. Emmelin*
Physiology of the Salivary Glands, 1961

9 *Audrey U. Smith*
Biological Effects of Freezing and Supercooling, 1961

10 *W. J. O'Connor*
Renal Function, 1962*

11 *R. A. Gregory*
Secretory Mechanisms of the Gastro-Intestinal Tract, 1962*

12 *C. A. Keele and Desiree Armstrong*
Substances Producing Pain and Itch, 1964*

13 *R. Whittam*
Transport and Diffusion in Red Blood Cells, 1964

14 *J. Grayson and D. Mendel*
Physiology of the Splanchnic Circulation, 1965*

15 *B. T. Donovan and J. J. van der Werff ten Bosch.*
Physiology of Puberty, 1965

16 *I. de Burgh Daly and Catherine Hebb*
Pulmonory and Bronchial Vascular Systems, 1966*

17 *I. C. Whitfield*
The Auditory Pathway, 1967*

18 *L. E. Mount*
The Climatic Physiology of the Pig, 1968*

19 *J. I. Hubbard, R. Llinás and D. Quastel*
Electrophysiological Analysis of Synaptic Transmission, 1969

20 *S. E. Dicker*
Mechanisms of Urine Concentration and Dilution in Mammals, 1970

21 *G. Kahlson and Elsa Rosengren*
Biogenesis and Physiology of Histamine, 1971*

22 *A. T. Cowie and J. S. Tindal*
The Physiology of Lactation, 1971*

23 *Peter B. C. Matthews*
Mammalian Muscle Receptors and their Central Actions, 1972

24 *C. R. House*
Water Transport in Cells and Tissues, 1974

25 *P. P. Newman*
Visceral Afferent Functions of the Nervous System, 1974

Published by CAMBRIDGE UNIVERSITY PRESS

28 *M. J. Purves*
The Physiology of the Cerebral Circulation, 1972

29 *D. McK. Kerslake*
The Stress of Hot Environments, 1972

30 *M. R. Bennett*
Autonomic Neuromuscular Transmission, 1972

31 *A. G. Macdonald*
Physiological Aspects of Deep Sea Biology, 1975

32 *M. Peaker and J. L. Linzell*
Salt Glands in Birds and Reptiles, 1975

33 *J. A. Barrowman*
Physiology of the Gastro-intestinal Lymphatic System, 1978

Published by ACADEMIC PRESS

34 *C. G. Phillips and R. Porter*
Corticospinal Neurones: Their Role in Movement, 1977

Volumes marked * are now out of print

Monographs of the Physiological Society No. 34

Corticospinal Neurones

Their Role in Movement

C. G. PHILLIPS, FRS
Dr Lee's Professor of Anatomy
University of Oxford, England

and

R. PORTER, FAA
Professor of Physiology
Monash University, Australia

1977

ACADEMIC PRESS
LONDON NEW YORK SAN FRANCISCO
A Subsidiary of Harcourt Brace Jovanovich, Publishers

Academic Press Inc. (London) Ltd
24–28 Oval Road
London NW1

US edition published by
Academic Press Inc.
111 Fifth Avenue,
New York, New York 10003

Library of Congress Catalog Card Number: 77-71834
ISBN: 0-12-553950-9

Printed in Great Britain by
Cox & Wyman Ltd,
London, Fakenham and Reading

Preface

Non-neurophysiological readers of neurophysiological research papers might be forgiven if they believed that the writers were not much interested in fitting their contributions into any general framework of facts and ideas. Lengthy introductions and discussions are out of fashion. If, however, the neurophysiologist writers are also university teachers, they will certainly have discussed with their students the contemporary status of their field, the history of its cultivation by their forerunners, and the prospects for future harvests. We have always tried to do this, and have been glad of the opportunity to get some of it down on paper. We have not wished to be encyclopaedic, but rather to describe and discuss the results of relatively few and clear-cut observations and experiments. Above all, we have tried to address ourselves to the general readership to which the Physiological Society's Monographs are dedicated, and to avoid talking in undertones to our fellow specialists and to one another.

Our narrative tells of the growth of modern ideas of the control of movement by the brain from their first discernible origins in the mid-nineteenth century. Clinical study of focal convulsions and paralysis in man, and experimental stimulations and ablations in other mammals, established the fact of localized motor outflow from the fore-brain. Micro-anatomical research soon discovered the corticofugal neurones and began the laborious task of tracing their axons to their targets throughout the neuraxis: first, to the motor nuclei of the spinal cord; much later, to the 'relay' nuclei of the somaesthetic system and to the nuclei of the sub-cortical and cerebellar motor systems. Microanatomical research is still gathering pace, drawing on new methods of visualizing connexions by injecting radioactive amino acids or horseradish peroxidase and utilizing their incorporation into and transport along neuronal processes.

Electroanatomical research has also moved forward rapidly in the last thirty years, from the crude electrical stimulations of the nineteenth-century physiologists to the refinements of the modern microelectrode era. Electroanatomy adds details of the distribution of cortically mediated synaptic excitation and inhibition to the purely microanatomical account. Specification of the sources of excitatory and inhibitory inputs to the corticofugal neurones came last, and aroused fresh interest in these neurones regarding their role as projectors of the integrated output of the elemental input–output modules of which the cerebral cortex is built up. The corticofugal outputs are 'commanded' by higher hierarchical levels of the fore-brain. The discharges of the cortical neurones in response to 'commands' can be monitored electrophysiologically while trained monkeys are performing specific movements. The same neurones are also responsive to the afferent inflow from the muscles, joints and skin of the moving limb.

In our electroanatomical and electrophysiological chapters we draw extensively on the results of our own experiments. We have attempted to describe our individual and joint observations in the context of accumulated knowledge about corticospinal neurones and the control of movement. It has been possible to re-examine results we reported before more modern techniques of microanatomy and microphysiology were in general use, and this has allowed the complementary contribution of different techniques to be evaluated and a general account to be provided of our state of knowledge. In our final chapter we try to interpret some of the facts of motor control and perception of movement in man in the light of the structure and properties of the corticospinal projection in monkeys.

We have avoided the use of 'small print' for material which the more general reader might skip. Instead, we have writen somewhat lengthy legends to most of the illustrations. The text is meant to be intelligible without mastering everything we have relegated to these legends, and they can be neglected, and the illustrations simply treated pictorially, by readers who do not wish to work through them in detail.

Because our subject is advancing rapidly, we know that parts of our book will have been overtaken by the time they appear in print, and we have simply had to give up worrying about this, and to comfort ourselves with the hope that our attempt to picture the field as we saw it in 1976, and to trace its origins in the work and thought of the last hundred years, may retain some interest when today's granary of facts has been enlarged and today's concepts revised almost beyond recognition. Our medical orientation will be obvious and it is our view that our readers may also be concerned to understand what functions corticospinal neurones subserve in man and how the interruption of their axons by disease may produce the signs and symptoms which are manifest. Our debt to countless informal discussions with colleagues at home and overseas we acknowledge gratefully. We ask for the understanding of friends whose work we admire but have not had room to describe in full; we have however been to special trouble to cite papers whose bibliographies will guide our readers to it.

We wish to thank the Royal Society, The Wellcome Trust and the Ramaciotti Foundation for making it financially possible for us to work together at our writing for several weeks in Oxford in 1973 and at Monash in 1975–6. When writing the first drafts of some of his contributions, one of us (C.G.P.) was grateful to Professors G. Moruzzi and V. Capelletti for allowing him to expand some material from his article in 'Enciclopedia Italiana' (Pyramidal Tract, Physiology of, to be published by Istituto della Enciclopedia Italiana, Rome). Successive drafts of text and legends were typed by Mary Cutcliffe, Glynis Clayton, Josephine Champkin, Jane Ballinger, and Lynne Hepburn; the illustrations were prepared by Christine Court, Gill Smith and Jill Maplesden, and were photographed by Diana Harrison, the late Sandy Austin, Penny Paterson, Lawrence Waters, Brian Archer and Jacqueline Brazier; the bibliography was checked by Gaby Fodor, Molly Collen and Glynis Clayton. The patience and kindness of all our helpers were inexhaustible, and we thank them most warmly. Lastly we thank Alfreda Wilkinson of the Society of Indexers for putting the Index we had compiled into professional form, and Dorothy Sharp of Academic Press for her help in producing the book.

September 1976   C. G. PHILLIPS

R. PORTER

Contents

1
Evolutionary Status of the Pyramidal Tract

1.1 The physiological position and dominance of the brain

In his ninth Silliman Lecture, 'The Physiological Position and Dominance of the Brain', Sherrington (1906) said: 'By a high spinal transection the splendid motor machinery of the vertebrate is practically as a whole and at one stroke severed from all the universe except its own microcosm and an environmental film some millimetres thick immediately next its body.' This book is concerned with one only of several descending nerve paths whose simultaneous severance disconnects the spinal segments from the brain and so destroys the organism's ability to explore its environment and to respond to complex features and changes in it. This is the pyramidal tract (Fig. 1.1), a structure found only in mammals, whose corticospinal component is best developed in primates and reaches its greatest development in man.

Thus disconnected from the brain, the neural segments of neck, trunk and limbs cannot generate 'total posture' and 'total locomotion' or any other elaborate behaviour of the animal as a whole. Local stimuli may elicit local reflexes, scratching or withdrawal, for example, or local fragments of postural or locomotor behaviour.

Sherrington saw that the 'total posture' and 'total locomotion' of the intact vertebrate depend on motion-sensitive, gravitational and 'distance receptors' located in the head, whose reflexes dominate and 'integrate' those of the trunk and limbs. Limbs, trunk and neck then cooperate in holding the head upright, and function as a 'motor train' which propels it forward into the environment 'at the behest of the distance-receptor organs in front'. The 'higher' the vertebrate, the greater its 'receptive range'. The corresponding enrichment of behaviour is related less to improvements in the distance-receptors themselves than to increases in the size, complexity and synaptic connectivity of the fore-brain. With these increases, and with their 'untold potentialities for redistribution of so-to-say stored stimuli by associative recall', an enlarging range of distant objects can be discriminated as neutral, as to be avoided or escaped, or as inviting tactile exploration or capture. Appropriately steered loco-motion can then avoid obstacles, remove the animal from danger, or bring it into contact with an attractive object. 'Nothing, it would seem, could tend to select more potently the individuals taking the right course than the success which crowns that course, since the consummatory acts led up to are such—e.g. the seizure of prey, escape from enemies, attainment of sexual conjugation, etc.—as involve the very existence of the individual and the species.'

Most mammals use their muzzles for tactile exploration of the environ-ment and for taking hold of objects. 'Many postures and movements of the organism are advantageous or disadvantageous to the animal's existence mainly inasmuch as they improve or disimprove the position or attitude of the mouth in relation to objects in the external world.' (Sherrington, 1906.) The elephant's trunk is an extreme case of the exploitation of facial musculature in tactile exploration and skilled performance. In other mammals it is the forelimbs which have come to be more important for prehension and exploration, and which have been brought under greater cerebral control. The terrestrial carnivores, helped by stereoscopic vision, can strike and grasp their prey with their forelimbs before their muzzles get to it. But skilled use and stereoscopic and stereognostic guidance of the forelimb have reached their greatest degrees of refinement in the primates. It is natural for man to view his own skilled performances as supreme examples of the 'physiological position and dominance' that the brain has come to hold over the muscles: over those which work his hands, in shaping and building, writing and playing instruments, as well as over those which work his voice, in speech and song.

Primates, more than any other mammals, have depended for success in the struggle for existence on the behavioural adaptability conferred by big brains. Their behaviour is less stimulus-bound than that of lower forms: more marked by learning, internal trial and error and prediction. They have evolved 'under selection that mental extension of the present backward into the past and forward into the future which in the highest animals forms the prerogative of more developed mind'. Sherrington's (1906) recapitulation of their major evolutionary landmarks could be endorsed by any primatologist today. 'The parallelism of the ocular axes and the overlapping of the uniocular fields of photoreception which in mammals has gradually reached its acme in the monkey and in man . . . together with promotion of the forelimb from a simple locomotor prop to a delicate explorer of space in manifold directions, together also with the organization of mimetic movements to express thoughts by sounds, have, with the developments of central nervous function which they connote and promote, probably been the chief factors in man's outstripping other competitors in progress towards that aim which seems the universal goal of animal behaviour, namely to dominate more completely the environment.'

The fore-brain and its distance receptors gain their controlling access to the neural networks of the spinal segments, and to the motoneurones which constitute the 'final common path' which leads to the muscles, by way of 'extensive internuncial paths'—'mesencephalospinal' and 'pyramidal or other palliospinal' (Sherrington, 1906). He saw the pyramidal tract (PT) as 'a path of internuncial character common to certain arcs that have arisen indirectly from various receptors . . . and are knitted together in the cerebral hemisphere'.

1.2   Categories of movement elaborated by the brain

It is helpful, if we do not try to press the distinction too far, to follow Hughlings Jackson (1897; 1932, p. 437) in distinguishing between 'more automatic' and 'less automatic' performances. Originally he had graded performances on a scale of hierarchical levels ranging from 'most voluntary' to 'most automatic', until he remembered that he was a dualist and ought not to be mixing psychological and physiological language.

The practical usefulness of such a distinction can be made clear by a few examples. The rhythmic alternation of inspiration and expiration is a highly automatic performance. It persists under anaesthesia deep enough to obliterate all other movements, all postures, and all segmental reflexes other than the monosynaptic tendon jerks. But in the waking individual the muscles it employs are shared by postural mechanisms of trunk and shoulder girdle which form part of Sherrington's 'total posture' (less automatic) and also by speech and song (least automatic).

Exploratory, prehensile and manipulative performances would be graded as 'less automatic' than those of 'total posture' and 'total locomotion'. Prehension, however, has 'more automatic' postural and locomotor as well as 'less automatic' exploratory and manipulative functions, particularly in arboreal animals. These functions are differentially vulnerable to lesions of the fore-brain and its projection pathways. Thus, a monkey may cling, climb or clutch for support with a hand which has been rendered useless for tactile exploration and manipulation and skilled performance in general. Again, different classes of movements of the head and eyes are selectively vulnerable to fore-brain injury: the 'more automatic' pursuit of moving objects by the visual axes may survive loss of the 'less automatic' exploratory steering of the gaze.

There are signs that present-day thinking about the organization of movement may be hardening divisively between those who hold that movements are controlled by *programmes* within the central nervous system and those who hold that their organization is wholly *reflex* (cf. Massion, 1973). We wish in this book to maintain an eclectic position. It has long been appreciated that the rhythmic alternating movements of stepping, scratching and rhythmic respiration can continue in the absence of afferent inputs, but that they are normally modifiable by such inputs. The patterning of these movements depends on central nervous organizations (e.g. Graham Brown's 'paired half-centres'), that is, on programmes, which can be switched on and off, and modified, reflexly. This interaction between programmes and reflexes is supported by the fine work on locomotion in the decerebrate and decorticate cat by the schools of Lundberg and of Orlovskii, Severin and Shik. We think therefore that over-insistence on programmes to the exclusion of reflexes (as an over-reaction against an earlier insistence on stimulus-response theories of behaviour) is more likely to hinder progress than to advance it. The programmes of 'most automatic' reflex performances are likely to depend on 'inherited structure in the nervous system and not on individual experience' (Marshall Hall: cf. Creed, 1934). 'Least automatic' performances would depend on patterns (programmes) built up by learning processes ('involving the redistribution of so-to-say stored stimuli by associative recall', in Sherrington's quaint phraseology of long ago). We shall assume for the present, and shall discuss the evidence later, that the outputs of central programmes are normally subject to correction (whether continuous or intermittent) by feedback from the moving parts and by feedback of *results* from the environment.

Skilled ('least automatic') performances may be expressed in virtually any field of musculature. Those born without arms can perform astonishingly with their feet. 'Study of tiqueurs and "muscle developers" soon convinces one that practically any movement can become "voluntary".' (Denny-Brown, 1950.) Skilled ('least automatic') performances may sometimes seem to engage the musculature practically as a whole, as in performing seals, dolphins and ballet dancers, or to be narrowed to more local fields of musculature, mouths, hands or feet, brought into position by 'more automatic' movements and held there by 'more automatic' postures.

If there is still general agreement that the fore-brain subserves 'least automatic' behaviour, there is now less consensus than formerly about the status of the PT as the major efferent pathway available to decision making and movement planning regions of the brain. Our task is to try to reassess its status, (1) as a 'common' or 'internuncial path' projecting the commands of the central programmes and subroutines towards the target muscles; (2) as a source of internal feedback (*efference copy, corollary discharge*) to the central programme, informing it of the progress of the subroutines of performance; (3) as a controller of the gain and discrimination of afferent systems supplying information to the fore-brain and cerebellum; and (4) as the efferent limb of transcortical reflex arcs whose afferent limbs may provide feedback control of the subroutines.

1.3 Classical and modern views of the 'motor' cortex and the pyramidal tract

It is not difficult to imagine how the 'motor' cortex and the PT came to occupy the forefront of neurological thinking about the control of movement by the brain. Fritsch and Hitzig's (1870) discovery of the electrical excitability of the dog's frontal cortex had a certain dramatic quality. Not only did electrical stimulation establish the fact of cortical *localization*, it seemed also to bring cerebral *function* within the experimenter's grasp. But what function? The battle was soon joined over whether the excitable area was a 'motor' or a 'sensorimotor' centre, or a centre for 'memories of movements' or tactile memories. To avoid these controversies, Sherrington (1885) proposed the term 'cord area' to denote merely 'all this region of the cortex cerebri which is so directly connected with the spinal cord that lesions in the former induce degeneration in the latter'. François-Franck (1887) concluded that the areas were 'points de départ et non des centres de mouvement'. 'The motor bundle gathers up the voluntary motor commands from the surface of the brain and transmits them to the effector apparatus of the brainstem and spinal cord. From the standpoint of anatomy, this bundle is a crossed corticobulbar and corticospinal tract; from the standpoint of physiology, it is a system which is *afferent* to the motor cells of the brainstem and cord. In this respect it is comparable to the dorsal roots; but these, instead of bringing voluntary commands to the motor cells, elaborated in the brain, bring crude stimuli from the periphery which excite them in purely reflex fashion.' (Our translation.)*

The motor bundle was already synonymous with the PT. This owed its name to the medullary pyramid (Fig. 1.1), well known to gross anatomy as a protuberance on the ventral aspect of the hind-brain, adjacent to the midline. The crossing-over of the paired pyramids at their entry to the spinal cord had been discovered by Mistichelli and by Pourfour du Petit early in the eighteenth century (Liddell, 1960). At this level the PT appears

---

* 'Le faisceau moteur recueillant à la surface du cerveau les incitations motrices volontaires, les transmet aux organes d'exécution bulbo-médullaires: ce faisceau constitue donc, au point de vue anatomique, une commissure croisée cortico-bulbo-médullaire et, au point de vue physiologique, un système *afférent* aux cellules motrices du bulbe et de la moelle. Il est en cela comparable aux fibres médullaires afférentes des faisceaux postérieurs de la moelle, lesquelles, au lieu d'apporter aux cellules motrices des incitations volontaires, élaborées dans le cerveau, leur apportent des incitations brutes, de provenance périphérique, qui les sollicitent à l'action par la voie réflexe pure.'

in transverse section as a fibre-bundle as compact as any to be found in
the brain, for example, as the optic or olfactory tract. Its origin from the
fore-brain was first determined by gross dissection, which led to the erroneous conclusion that it arose from the corpus striatum (Jefferson, 1953).
The discovery of the cortical origin of the PT was reviewed by Dejerine
(1901). Gudden showed in puppies, and Vulpian confirmed in adult dogs,
that the PT and its continuation, the contralateral corticospinal tract,
degenerated when the excitable sigmoid gyri were ablated. Charcot and

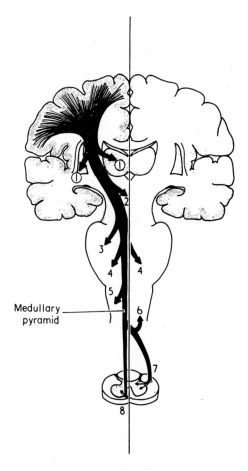

Fig. 1.1. Stylized diagram showing the components of the pyramidal tract. These components are unequally developed in different mammals. 1, Corticostriatal and corticothalamic; 2, cortico-rubro-spinal; 3, cortico-ponto-cerebellar; 4, cortico-reticulo-spinal; 5,
cortico-olivo-cerebellar; 6, corticocuneate and corticogracile; 7, crossed corticospinal; 8,
uncrossed corticospinal. See text. Connexions 1 to 6 are partly made by collateral and
terminal branches of PT axons and partly by parapyramidal axons (for definitions see
Chapter 4).

Dejerine, studying degenerations secondary to cortical disease, traced the very prominent human PT from the Rolandic cortex through the internal capsule, cerebral peduncle and pyramidal decussation and down the spinal cord. Thus, the excitable cortex was shown to be connected by a major, apparently single cable to the spinal segments. Other cortical areas gave no obvious responses to stimulation, and the then available anatomical techniques, which could trace only dense pathways containing thick myelinated axons, found no compact outflows from those areas. The existence of corticostriatal connexions, for example, was denied by some (Wilson, 1914), but affirmed by others (Dejerine, 1901). It was natural that the pioneers should set the excitability of the cortex in animals beside the severity of the paralysis caused by haemorrhagic destruction of the internal capsule in man, and should regard the motor cortex and the PT as the main, if not the only motor system of the fore-brain, uniquely responsible for the initiation and execution of voluntary movement.

In the case of the dog, however, it was soon found that the PT was not the only outflow, even from the motor cortex itself, for Wertheimer and Lepage discovered that the responses to cortical stimulation were not prevented by cutting the pyramidal tracts (Schäfer, 1900). Schäfer concluded that there was probably 'another path of communication between the motor cortex and the nuclei of the motor nerves', with interruptions in the substantia nigra and nuclei pontis. The pioneers were also surprised when Starlinger in 1895 found no permanent paralysis following bilateral pyramidotomy in the dog (Schäfer, 1900). Regarding the PT as the main motor outflow from the brain, they had, perhaps, expected effects as disabling as those of human hemiplegia, and they found it remarkable that such a dog could not only walk, run, and jump, but could even be taught simple tricks like 'giving a paw' (Marquis, cited by Fulton, 1943).

That generalizations were dangerous and species differences important was, perhaps, insufficiently appreciated. Neglect of species differences led even to denial of the fact of cortical localization: thus Goltz, who ablated cortical areas in dogs, denied localization, whereas Ferrier and Yeo, who used monkeys, affirmed it. The debate reached its climax at the Seventh International Medical Congress in 1881. 'This was a battle of the giants, Goltz and Ferrier. . . . The long verbatim report seems not to have lost a word of the discussion and to transmit the high temperatures then engendered, even to the reader of today.' (Liddell, 1960.) It is surprising that when biologists had so recently been set thinking about evolution, there should have been relatively little interest in the probable importance of differences in structure and function in the brains of different mammals in relation to their various modes of posture, locomotion and prehension.

Modern work with refined microscopical and electroanatomical techniques has revealed some of the elements missing from the classical story:

the 'parapyramidal' projections from the motor cortex itself (e.g. cortico-callosal, corticostriatal, corticothalamic), whose cells of origin are inter-spersed among the cells of the origin of the PT within the same cortical area; the cortico-reticulo-spinal and cortico-rubro-spinal connexions of the PT; the 'supplementary' motor area; and the 'extrapyramidal' projections from other cortical areas to the striatum, pontine nuclei and cerebellum. All this work has rescued the PT from its former isolation and set it in a truer perspective: as an 'internuncial' pathway 'common' to the whole of the fore-brain and the cerebellum (Fig. 1.2).

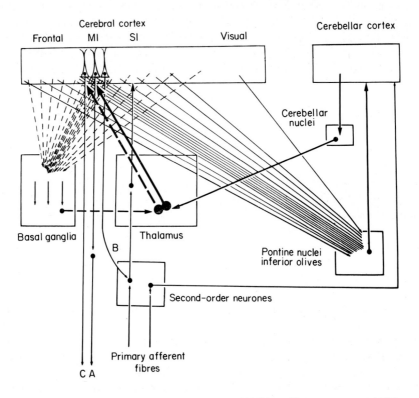

FIG. 1.2. Diagram (based on Kemp and Powell, 1971b) to illustrate status of PT as a major common outflow from fore-brain and cerebellum. S1, Somaesthetic receiving area; M1, motor area; A, cortico-reticulo-spinal projection; B, projection controlling inputs to central nervous system (primary afferent fibres and second-order neurones in spinal cord, nuclei of dorsal columns, trigeminal nucleus, etc); C, corticospinal projection to spinal interneurones and (in primates) to motoneurones. See text.

Figure 1.2 is a much oversimplified scheme based on experiments on cats and monkeys. It emphasizes the central position of the motor cortex (Fig. 1.2, M1) as the target and common output of two sets of neural networks. Of these, one originates from most areas of the cortex (least from the visual areas) and converges on the motor cortex by way of basal ganglia and ventrolateral thalamus (Kemp and Powell, 1971b). The other network has a similar cortical origin, and converges on the motor cortex by way of pontine nuclei (Fig. 1.1, 3; Fig. 1.2), inferior olive (Fig. 1.1, 5; Fig. 1.2), cerebellum, red nucleus (omitted from Fig. 1.2) and ventro-lateral thalamus (Eccles *et al.*, 1967).

Hughlings Jackson (1897; 1932, p. 422) generalized his clinical studies of disordered movement by the theory that cerebral function is organized in hierarchical levels of control. 'Least automatic' behaviour was controlled by the 'highest level', 'most automatic' by the 'lowest level'. He sought to cor-relate these functional levels with anatomical structures. He tentatively localized the 'highest level' in the 'pre-frontal lobe' (region in front of the precentral sulcus) but admitted that 'this part of my scheme is very hypothetical'. The 'middle level' he placed in the sensorimotor cortex (Fig. 1.2, M1 and S1). Ferrier (1886), who had discovered the electrical excitability of this area in monkeys, rejected Jackson's idea of a separate localization for the 'highest level'. 'This hypothesis receives no confirma-tion from the facts of experiment. It seems more reasonable to suppose that there may be higher and lower degrees of complexity or evolution in the same centres' (those of Jackson's 'middle level') 'than to assume the separate existence of more highly evolved centres.' Later experiments, however, have found that the monkey's motor cortex is not the repository, or at any rate is not the sole repository, of the engrams of learned perform-ances (Lashley, 1950). It is plausible therefore to think that it may norm-ally be 'instructed' from topographically separated 'higher' levels. But it may not seem useful, in the present state of knowledge, to try to localize Jackson's 'highest level' in the prefrontal cortex or in any other part of the complex networks that are outlined in Fig. 1.2, for example, in the 'centrencephalic' parts (Penfield, 1954); and better to retain it, for the time being, as a purely functional concept. Electrical sampling of the discharges of single neurones in the brains of monkeys performing learned move-ments for reward has detected prior activity in ventrolateral thalamus (Evarts, 1970), cerebellar cortex (Thach, 1970b), cerebellar nuclei (Thach, 1970a) and basal ganglia (De Long, 1971), as well as in the motor cortex (Evarts, 1968—see also Chapter 7). There are no grounds at present for ascribing initiation of movement to any one of these loci rather than to any other. It is clear from Fig. 1.2 that the motor cortex lies furthest down-stream, that is, that it is interposed between the other fore-brain structures and the cranial and spinal segments in which Jackson uncontroversially localized his 'lowest level'. It is remarkable that bilateral integrity of the corticospinal pathways is of no avail to patients rendered akinetic by lesions of the basal ganglia (Denny–Brown, 1962).

Figure 1.2 stresses the role of structures lying *upstream* of the motor cortex in the programming and initiation of 'least automatic' movements. The part of the cerebellum which lies thus *upstream* forms the lateral lobes, whose bulk has increased *pari passu* with the bulk of the fore-brain, and forms the main mass of the cerebellum in man. Its cortex is associated with the large, laterally placed dentate nucleus (included in *cerebellar nuclei* in Fig. 1.2). Another, smaller part of the cerebellar cortex is interposed between the lateral lobes and the median part of the vermis. This part lies functionally *downstream* of the motor cortex, and receives its main input from it. In Fig. 1.2 this input is represented by the most closely spaced of the arrows which run from the motor cortex to the pontine nuclei and inferior olives. In the cat, on which most of the work on cerebro-cerebellar interactions has been done, the output from this intermediate zone of the cerebellar cortex exerts its recurrent influence on the motor cortex by way of the nucleus interpositus (included in cerebellar nuclei in Fig. 1.2). This downstream cerebro-cerebello-cerebral network will be considered in detail in Chapter 4 (cf. Fig. 4.8, p. 118). It would be involved in the automatic governing of the movements that are programmed and initiated in the structures lying upstream of the motor cortex (Allen and Tsukahara, 1974).

Figure 1.2 gives no idea of the sheer profusion of the connexions it summarizes. For example, there are about 20 million corticopontine axons in each cerebral hemisphere in man (Brodal, 1973) and about one million axons in each human PT (Lassek, 1948).

Figure 1.2 divides the descending projections from the sensorimotor cortex of cat or monkey to the 'lowest level' into three main functional groups. Axons of the first group (Fig. 1.1, 6 and uppermost arrow of 7; Fig. 1.2, B) are distributed to the sites of termination of primary afferent axons—in nucleus proprius of dorsal horn, spinal trigeminal nucleus, dorsal column nuclei, etc. (Chapter 4), where they would be in a position to control the inputs from the body surface, muscles, tendons and joints to the cerebellum, thalamus and cortex. Some at least of these descending axons travel in the medullary pyramid and are therefore, by definition, components of the PT. Axons of the second group (Fig. 1.1, 1, 2, 4; Fig. 1.2, A) project towards the 'lowest level' by interrupted pathways involving the striopallidum (Fig. 1.1, 1), red nucleus (Fig. 1.1, 2), and reticular formation (Fig. 1.1, 4). The probable projections from the pallidum to the reticular formation and thence to the spinal cord are not included in Fig. 1.2. All these projections are in a position to control the bilateral motor output from the reticular formation to the spinal cord. Axons of the third group (Fig. 1.1, 7, 8; Fig. 1.2, C) are corticobulbar and corticospinal axons, which connect the motor cortex directly to the motor apparatus of the cranial and spinal segments.

1.4 Pyramidal tracts: comparative morphology and behaviour

Axons of all three functional groups are present in the corticobulbar as well as in the corticospinal projections from the fore-brain. In this book we shall largely neglect the control of facial musculature, although this is to ignore its great importance in the life of most mammals, but in Chapter 7 we shall have something to say about the control of movements of the eyes and jaw. We shall concentrate on control of movements of limbs and trunk, and especially of the forelimbs, by the PTs (Fig. 1.1). These are more compact than the corticobulbar pathways, and, especially in their course through the paired medullary pyramids, are more conveniently accessible to the experimenter. The PTs are classically defined as axons composing the medullary pyramids. Such a merely morphological definition may have tended to encourage the *a priori* assumption that because we are dealing with a compact tract, we are also dealing with a single neural *system* with a single *function*, and that this function is the same in all species of mammals. We may well be grateful for the experimental convenience entailed by the morphological compactness, but our task is to try to identify axon groups with different cortical origins and different types of subcortical destination, and to associate these *structural components* with distinguishable *functional systems*. To investigate the relation of the PT to the 'least automatic' functions of the limbs, in those mammals in which these are highly developed, may be technically less daunting than to investigate the corresponding functions in other mammals in which their expression is pre-eminently in the face.

We have seen that the cells of origin of PT axons are located in and near the area of cortex from which electrical stimulation excites muscular responses from the limbs and trunk of the opposite side of the body at lowest threshold. In all of the limited range of mammals that have been studied many axons establish connexions from the cortex to the nuclei of the dorsal columns (Fig. 1.1, 6) and to the reticular formation of the hind-brain (Fig. 1.1, 4).

To these projections has been added a relatively insignificant prolongation of corticofugal axons into the first few segments only of the spinal cord (e.g. goat, rabbit) or a more extensive prolongation along its whole length (rat, cat, primates). This is the corticospinal component of the pyramidal tract. In infant cat and human, Ramón y Cajal (1909, p. 970) described how in longitudinal sections of the pons, the thick pyramidal tract fibres can be seen to end elaborately in relation to cells of the reticular formation, and to give off thin branches (which Cajal regarded as collaterals rather than terminals) which descend towards the spinal cord. Of the corticospinal component Sherrington (1900a) remarked: 'There is no other system which shows such increase in relative size as traced from lower to higher mammalian types. Hardly perceptible as a spinal tract in the rabbit, it in the monkey is much larger than in other laboratory forms, and in man is larger still.' Elsewhere he noted: 'I believe that the step from the dog and cat to the macaque is hardly greater than from the macaque to man, for the latter passage is really so wide.' (Liddell, 1960.) The PT, expanded by an enlarged corticospinal component, bulks largest in those mammals with the largest repertories of 'skilled' performance involving limbs and trunk: and largest of all in the higher primates with the largest repertories of 'least automatic' performances of the hand.

The relative paucity of comparative studies of the PT is therefore disappointing. We shall see that much work has been done on cats, less on primates and much less on other mammals. Primates have not evolved from carnivores, but from presumed common ancestry; thus any resemblances between the smaller projection in cats and the much larger projection in monkeys would be the result of parallel or convergent evolution. Similarities and differences in a wider range of mammals should be looked for and should ultimately be related to different modes of life— arboreal, terrestrial, aquatic; to domination of behaviour by vision, hearing, smell, or touch; to different modes of posture, locomotion and prehension. Comparative studies ought eventually to lead to some understanding of the evolutionary advantages that PTs have conferred on different mammals, and to some suggestion as to which advantage or disadvantages are shared by all species which possess PTs. In the meantime, the advisability of avoiding dogmatic generalizations about the PT and its 'functions' (or nonfunctions) should be obvious (cf. Towe, 1973).

The corticospinal tract (CST) differs, as between different mammals, not only in its bulk and in the length of its prolongation along the spinal cord, but also in its funicular location (Schoen, 1964). In monotremes, insectivores and the elephant it occupies the ventral funiculus (Fig. 1.3). In the hedgehog, very few corticospinal axons enter the cord. In the elephant, uncrossed axons run in the ventral funiculus for the length of the cervical cord, and crossed and uncrossed axons run in the intercommissural bundles (within the ventral grey commissure) as far as the mid-thoracic level. In ungulates (goat, sheep, cow, horse) the medullary pyramids are small, their decussation is inconspicuous, and the corticospinal axons travel in the crossed dorsolateral funiculus and in the crossed and uncrossed intercommissural bundles and ventral funiculi (Fig. 1.2), ending within the cervical segments. In marsupials, edentates, rodents, (mouse, rat, guinea-pig) and tree shrews the CST is crossed and runs in the dorsal funiculus, ending in the cervical and thoracic segments in tree shrew and marsupial phalanger, but reaching the lumbar segments in the rat. The rabbit's CST runs in the crossed dorsolateral funiculus, ending at C_3. Carnivores have a large pyramidal decussation, leading the majority of the pyramidal axons of each side into the well-marked lateral corticospinal

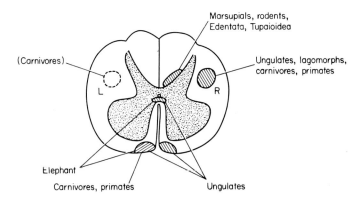

FIG. 1.3. Cross-sectional areas of cervical spinal cord which contain corticospinal axons originating from the left cerebral hemisphere in different orders of mammals. L, left; R, right. Data from Schoen (1964). See text.

tract in the crossed dorsolateral funiculus: relatively few axons travel in the uncrossed dorsolateral and in the ventral funiculi. Most axons end in the cervical enlargement, but a large contingent reaches the lumbosacral segments. The seal, an aquatic carnivore which lacks 'hands' but does not lack the ability to learn skills, has a PT comparable in bulk to a chimpanzee's; unfortunately its CST was not investigated (Lassek and Karlsberg, 1956). The massive CST of monkeys, apes and man are distributed mainly through the crossed dorsolateral funiculi; the ventral tracts are apt to show individual variation in apes and man.

Preponderantly contralateral projections are the rule in mammals whose behaviour is dominated by vision; thus, the input from the right half of visual space, and the somaesthetic input from the right half of the body, are projected predominantly to the left fore-brain, whose motor output is projected predominantly back to the right side of brainstem and spinal cord. Thus, related tactile, visual and motor activities would be integrated in the same cerebral hemisphere. In other mammals (e.g. goat), smell may be more important than sight in exploratory behaviour. The olfactory input from each half of the nose is projected to the fore-brain of the same side. Electrical stimulation of the fore-brain elicits motor responses of the exploratory and prehensile lips of the same side (Bell and Lawn, 1956), and mechanical stimulation of the lips evokes electrical activity in the fore-brain of the same side (Adrian, 1943). Thus, these tactile, olfactory and motor activities would be integrated in the same hemisphere.

In the spinal segments, the CST axons are distributed in a fashion which corresponds in general with the distribution of PT axons in the brainstem. In the dorsal horn they are related to primary afferent axons and second-order neurones. Here they could control the somaesthetic inputs from trunk and limbs to the spinal reflex arcs and to the cerebellum, thalamus and cerebral cortex. This is equivalent to the distribution of PT axons to the trigeminal nucleus and the dorsal column nuclei. More ventrally, in the intermediate region and, in primates, in the ventral horn, they come more directly into relation with the segmental outputs, especially those to the limbs.

The CST finds its greatest development in primates, whose evolution has been essentially 'cerebral' and 'behavioural' rather than muscular and skeletal. On the details of the evolution of brain structure the fossil record is of course silent, although it is eloquent on the increase in brain size: man's has grown by 50 per cent in 0.5 million years (Le Gros Clark, 1962a). But the skulls and teeth of living primates tend to correspond with those of fossil series (Napier, 1961) so it is natural to look to the living series for clues to the course of the neurophysiological and behavioural evolution. Primatologists (e.g. Schultz, 1968) agree that an increasingly refined cerebral control of the hand has played a central role in a story which began in Eurasia and North America, about sixty million years ago. Elliot-Smith (1924) speculated that the acquisition of skilled movements and the correlation of these with vision had been essential features: that arboreal habits had 'tended to develop the motor cortex itself, trained the tactile and kinaesthetic senses, and linked up their cortical areas in bonds of more intimate associations with the visual cortex'. In the forelimbs, arboreal selection pressures led to the retention of an 'ancient simplicity of structure and function' (Le Gros Clark, 1962a) with free mobility at shoulder and separate ulna and radius allowing pronation and supination of the hand. There was also an actual but advantageous retrogression: the sharp, hollow claws of primitive vertebrates have degenerated into flattened nails, which support the finger-pads and allow prehension 'to be adapted with much more precision to surfaces of varying shape, size and texture . . . in arboreal acrobatics'. The progressive trends have all been neural: richer innervation of the finger-pads and enlargement of their cerebral representation, and an increasingly refined cerebral motor control. For an extreme morphological contrast one has only to look at the forelimb of the horse, in which selection pressures for high-speed quadrupedal locomotion have led to limitation of shoulder movement to fore and aft, fusion of ulnar and radius, and loss of digits.

Comparative neurological studies are still relatively few. Prosimians use their hands in a stereotyped prehensile pattern, the digits all extending together as the hand approaches its target and closing together over it; there is no independent movement of individual fingers (Bishop, 1964) and no opposition of the thumb. They do not explore surfaces with their finger-pads. The PT of a prosimian, the slow loris (*Nycticebus coucang*), contributes synaptic endings to the crossed dorsal column nuclei, and is prolonged as a crossed dorsolateral corticospinal tract which reaches the sacral segments. A few uncrossed dorsolateral axons reach thoracic segments. There are no ventral tracts. Most axons end in the cervical and lumbar enlargements, at the base of the dorsal horn and in the zona intermedia, but a few end in relation to the cell-bodies of motoneurones lying dorsolaterally in the ventral horn (Campbell *et al.*, 1966). These are an early indication of an important component of the CST which is virtually exclusive to primates: the corticomotoneuronal component, which increases in bulk as one ascends the scale of living primates, and correlates with their increasingly versatile use of their hands (Phillips, 1971). Electrical stimulation of the cortex in a potto (*Perodicticus potto*), whose brain resembles that of nycticebus, elicited extension of thumb as an isolated response, and also extension of all digits; stimulation of a bush-baby's cortex (*Galago demidovii*) elicited finger responses only in combination with responses of elbow and shoulder (Zuckerman and Fulton, 1941).

In the Anthropoidea, precision patterns and grips are added to the 'whole-arm control' of prosimians (Bishop, 1964). The New World monkeys have pseudo-opposable thumbs. Some use 'whole-arm control', and one of these, 'a pet *Aotes*, will feel over one's face with its touch pads' (Bishop, 1964). Others show precision activity: the capuchin (*Cebus*) grips small objects between the sides of thumb and first finger or of first and second finger, or flexes the thumb round the object. Spider monkeys (*Ateles*) have no external thumbs, but can pick up small objects between the sides of adjacent fingers, or curl the radialmost digit round the object. Bishop (1964) cites these as precision patterns which have not evolved in relation to the thumb. Spider monkeys and woolly monkeys (*Lagothrix*) can also pick up small objects with the glabrous-skinned tips of their prehensile tails. In *Cebus*, *Ateles* and *Lagothrix*, Petras (1968) showed that the spinal motoneurones supplying fingers, toes and also, in *Ateles* and *Lagothrix*, the prehensile tail, receive abundant corticomotoneuronal connexions.

In the Old World monkeys, apes, and man, the thumb is rotated through 90 degrees in embryonic life, and is truly opposable. Napier (1956) differentiates the 'power grip' of the whole hand from the 'precision grip' of thumb and index. 'With thumb and index finger any baboon can extract the sting from a scorpion, and every chimpanzee a thorn out of its skin— and this more dextrously than most of us.' (Schultz, 1961.) Independent movement of other fingers is seen in Orang-utan (Tuttle, 1969). It reaches its fullest development in man. There has been a corresponding increase in the corticomotoneuronal component of the PT (Kuypers, 1964; Liu and Chambers, 1964). Petras (1966) records the impression that the corticomotoneuronal projection in gibbon and chimpanzee forms a 'distinctively greater part of the total corticospinal projection than is the case with the spider and rhesus monkeys', and that these axons 'appear somewhat comparable in number to the overlying fibres in the zona intermedia and external basilar region of the dorsal horn'. The connexion is not present at birth: in 4-day-old rhesus monkeys there are virtually no endings on motoneurones, but these are present in adult profusion by 8 months, though the axons are still thinner than in the fully adult (Kuypers, 1964).

The corticomotoneuronal component of the CST is not absolutely exclusive to primates, although nothing approaching its bulk has been found in other mammals. In the rat, its presence has been claimed in intra-cellular recordings of EPSPs from forelimb motoneurones (Elger *et al.*, 1974) but not from hindlimb motoneurones (Elger *et al.*, 1974; Shapovalov, 1975). Bannister and Porter (1967), however, found possible traces of it in records from hindlimb motoneurones. But the problems of detecting small monosynaptic effects, especially if produced by activity in slowly conduct-ing corticospinal fibres or if exerted on distal dendrites, affect this con-clusion. Moreover, other pathways in addition to the CST were still intact in many of these experiments. In the raccoon, a semi-arboreal carnivore with relatively unspecialized digits, corticospinal axons have been detected in the ventral horn in relation to motoneurones (Petras and Lehman, 1966; Buxton and Goodman, 1967; Wirth *et al.*, 1974). More comparative studies are called for. A description of the components of the seal's CST would be of special interest.

1.5 Summary

The 'motor' cortex and the pyramidal tract form a major 'common path' projecting from the fore-brain to the spinal segments, common to the whole of the cerebral cortex which is connected to the motor cortex by complex networks passing through the basal ganglia, cerebellum and thalamus. The pyramidal tract is found only in the brains of mammals. In all forms, it arises near the somaesthetic cortical receiving area, and projects to the dorsal column nuclei and to the trigeminal nucleus, where it would provide for centrifugal control of somaesthetic and proprioceptive inputs to the fore-brain and cerebellum. It projects also to the reticular formation of the hind-brain, which supplies bilateral motor control to trunk and limbs. Some thin collaterals of the corticoreticular axons extend downwards for a few segments into the spinal cord in most mammals; but in carnivores, and especially in primates, the corticospinal projection is strongly developed and includes, in primates, a corticomotoneuronal component which connects the fore-brain directly to the motoneurones, especially to those controlling the muscles of the hand. The corticospinal component bulks larger as one ascends the scale of living primates and is the major component of the PT in man.

Most research on the PT has been done on cats and monkeys, and a wider extension of studies is needed to discover the relative preponderance of the PT and of other, less direct, descending pathways in the control of various categories of movements in different mammals, most of which use their muzzles, rather than their forelimbs, for tactile exploration, prehension and manipulation of objects.

The movements controlled by the PT are probably mainly those in the 'less automatic', i.e. more 'skilled', categories rather than in the 'more automatic' categories of posture and locomotion, though these cannot really be separated since, for example, 'less automatic' performances of the hand must always be supported by 'more automatic' postural fixations of the trunk and limbs.

Only by an extension of comparative studies will it be possible to relate the evolution of the PT to the various modes of posture, locomotion, prehension and reactions to contact in tactile exploration of the environment; to see what evolutionary advantages it may have conferred on different mammals, and to see if any of these are common to all mammals and could therefore be regarded as expressions of any particular function or functions of the fore-brain.

1.6 Prospect

It has been hard to decide how best to present the material we have chosen for this book. A logical arrangement (Fig. 1.4) has the advantage that it provides a model into which many (though not all) details can be satisfyingly fitted, and without which they remain fragmentary and uninteresting; but it fails to convey the sense of the advance of knowledge by discovery. Discoveries have been determined in complex ways, not only by the intuition of individuals against a background of developing fashions in ideas, but also by the invention of new techniques, which removed obstacles to progress. Thus the discoveries were not necessarily pieced together into logical frameworks in the order in which they were made, and did not necessarily set out to answer questions that anyone would be asking today. The overriding disadvantage of presentation in terms of a particular model, however, is that it may seem to claim finality for something which is in essence provisional. The models that might have been built up at various times during the past 100 years would have differed from the present model, just as this will differ from those that will supersede it.

The presentation will therefore be mainly historical. We shall follow four streams:

1. Effects of electrical stimulation of the brain.

2. The mapping of neural connexions by Wallerian and retrograde degeneration and by analogous electroanatomical techniques. Recently these classical techniques have been enhanced by new methods of tracing connexions of individual neurones by incorporation into them of radio-active amino acids or horseradish peroxidase.

3. The electrical recording of neural activity during specific perform-ances.

4. Description and analysis of normal performance and of the effects of central and peripheral disturbances upon it.

Each chapter will usually span more than one stream. Each stream has nourished the others and been nourished by them: each has thrown up questions calling for simultaneous investigations in parallel. But in follow-ing the streams, it will be helpful to keep the model of Fig. 1.4 always in mind.

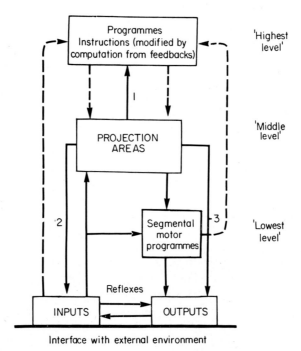

FIG. 1.4. Levels of motor control. Explanation in text.

In principle, structure and function are inseparable, but we happen to know more about structure. The centre of the model is occupied by the motor cortex ('middle level'), which is built up of many areas giving pro-jection to many sites. Of these projection areas we shall consider only those which project through the PT. These form a set of outputs (clusters of corticofugal neurones) that are available for excitatory selection or inhibitory suppression by the 'programmes' ('instructions') of the 'highest level'. We shall be concerned with their architectonics, and whether the clusters are intermingled or sharply sequestered from one another; with the radial and horizontal arrangement of their excitatory and inhibitory inputs from the highest and lowest levels; and with the activities of single neurones and aggregates of neurones in specific performances. We shall be concerned with these single neurones or aggregates as samples of inputs (from where?) and as samples of outputs (to what?). We have glimpsed already that the outputs that can be sampled are complex: to intrinsic cerebral and cerebellar networks (Fig. 1.4, 1); to input pathways (2); to segmental motor patterns; and, by-passing these, to the motor output of Sherrington's 'final common path' (3).

Behavioural study of different categories of motor performance includes accurate description and timing of the movements, and 'black-box' theorizing about their central organization: ballistic movements may be pre-programmed; other movements may also be totally specified in this way or they may be subject to continuous or intermittent correction by internal feedback from serially ordered 'boxes', by feedback from the moving parts, and by knowledge of results. Attempts can be made to relate the black boxes to known structures in the model. One can study the effects on performance of disconnexion of the segments from the CST; of disconnexion of the projection areas from specific inputs (visual, skin, muscle, joint); and of the nature of deviations brought about by abnormal quantities and patterns of input (as by vibrating the muscle to stimulate the muscle spindles). The timing of the response of motoneurones (recorded electromyographically) to sudden perturbations of movements in progress provides evidence of the activity of 'lowest level' and 'middle level' feedback loops. Finally, in man, the correct execution of perception of positions and movements can be disturbed by interference with parts represented in the model.

Each chapter, therefore, will generally develop its themes historically, and its conclusion will summarize its contribution to the model.

2

The discovery of localized motor outflow from the cerebral cortex: electrical stimulation I

2.1 Introduction

In the first half of the nineteenth century it was generally believed that 'there was no localization of particular functions in particular parts, that the cortex must act for each and all of its functions as a whole' (Schäfer, 1900). This belief was, in part, a reaction against the once influential phrenologists who had taught that particular mental faculties were localized in particular 'organs' of the human brain, which gave rise to identifiable 'bumps' on the overlying skull. Critical reaction was not confined to the scientific community. Of the Vienna physician F. J. Gall (1757–1828), the leading exponent of phrenology, Napoleon I remarked: 'He ascribes to certain prominences, propensities and crimes which do not exist in nature but are the growth of society and are merely conventional. What would the organ of theft effect, if there were no property, the organ of drunkenness if there were no spirituous liquors, or the organ of ambition if there were no society?' Müller, who quoted this passage, pointed out that Gall's system did not include an 'organ of drunkenness' (Liddell, 1960). The scientific community's denial of cerebral localization was based mainly on Flourens' crude experiments on rabbit and dog in which pricking the spinal cord caused convulsive movements whereas pricking the cortex was without visible effect.

2.2 'Discharging lesions' in man

During the eighteen-sixties, J. Hughlings Jackson's clinical researches convinced him that different activities are localized in different parts of the brain (see Phillips, 1973). His evidence was derived from a very detailed description of focal convulsions ('convulsions beginning unilaterally') due to localized 'discharging lesions'. He saw, in 'convulsions beginning unilaterally', not only 'a symptom of disease of the brain', but also 'an experiment made on the brain by disease' (1931, p. 37). 'Of course a coarse lesion of a nervous centre, or a sudden discharge of one, is not a very neat experiment.' (1931, p. 75.) Jackson was interested in establishing the fact of localization, as well as in formulating concepts of cerebral function (see Chapter 1, sections 1.2 and 1.3; Chapter 8). This chapter will be primarily concerned with the fact of localization: with cortical areas as 'points of departure' and not as 'centres for movement' (see Chapter 1, section 1.3). His ideas about function will be deferred to Chapter 8.

'The fact that the symptoms are local implies, I hold,' (wrote Jackson) 'that there *is* of necessity a *local* lesion . . . where the fits always start on one side and always in the very same fingers, it is simply incredible that there is no persistent local lesion.' (1931, p. 24.) And even if, in many cases, no changes were to be found postmortem, 'I should still believe in their existence . . . even in those cases where we *do* find a lump in the brain, we do not discover the *very* changes on which the discharge depends. The lump does not discharge, but some ("softened") part of the brain near it—which part cannot be destroyed or it would not discharge at all, but which part must be diseased or it would not discharge so much, nor in so disorderly a manner, nor on slight provocation.' (1931, p. 25.)

Jackson's brilliant speculations about the explosive, paroxysmal discharges of nerve cells in epileptic foci have been fully supported by modern electrophysiological studies.

'The important matter, with a view to localization, being the starting-point of the spasm, our clinical study of it must be minute and precise.' (Jackson, 1931, p. 332.) But his early attempts to correlate the accurately observed sites of onset of convulsion with the sites of the lesions were usually disappointing. In one patient, whose fits always began in his left thumb, there was found, after death, 'a tubercle the size of a hazel nut in the hinder part of his third right frontal convolution' (1931, p. 68). More often, however, 'The cases I have recorded have for the most part been cases of tumour, and the disease has been too often so wide that most of them are not of much beyond clinical value.' (1931, p. 339.) It is not surprising, therefore, that his first attempts to localize the 'discharging lesions' should have led to some confusion. From 1864 he 'believed the corpus striatum to be the part discharged in *convulsions* beginning unilaterally', although in 1868, 'and several years before I believed the convolutions also to contain processes representing movements' (1931, p. 38). He therefore welcomed the discovery of the electrical excitability of the cerebral cortex in the dog by Fritsch and Hitzig (1870) and in the monkey by Ferrier (1875), as likely to 'help this investigation to an extent difficult to overestimate; for I most willingly admit that the method I uphold has made very little way. From their researches we shall learn where to look for the minute changes which constitute the discharging lesions.' (1931, p. 202.) By 1881 he could write unequivocally: 'The evidence from morbid anatomy, agreeing with that of the physiological experiments . . . is that there is in these cases cortical disease, and that the part of the cortex affected is within the mid-region of the brain—of convolutions bordering the fissure of Rolando.' (1931, p. 331.)

2.3 Demarcation of the projection area by electrical stimulation

Fritsch and Hitzig's (1870) discovery was made by applying galvanic currents to the cortex through a pair of fine, blunted platinum wires which were generally 2–3 mm apart, at an intensity just sufficient to evoke a sensation when applied to the experimenter's tongue. Figure 2.1 reproduces their drawing of the dog's brain and presents the whole of their evidence. The five symbols mark the 'centres' from which they evoked twitches of five different peripheries on the opposite side of the body. Their paper made no reference to Jackson's work.

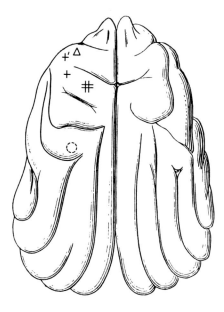

FIG. 2.1. Fritsch and Hitzig's (1870) historic map of galvanic stimulation of the dog's brain. Δ, 'Centre for the neck muscles'; +′, 'centre for the extensors and adductors of the forelimb'; +, 'centres for the flexion and rotation of the limb'; #, 'centre for the hind leg'; ◌, 'facial'. 'We did not always succeed in setting the neck muscles in action. . . . The muscles of the back, tail and abdomen we have often enough excited to contraction from points lying between those marked, but no circumscribed point from which they could be individually stimulated could be satisfactorily determined. The whole of the convexity lying behind the facial centre we found absolutely unexcitable, even with altogether disproportionate intensity of current.' (David Ferrier's translation.)

David Ferrier, however, had already been excited by Jackson's clinical discoveries when he first heard of Hitzig's experiments. Early in 1873 he discussed these experiments with his friend James Crichton-Browne, the Medical Director of what was then known as the West Riding Lunatic Asylum. Crichton-Browne placed a laboratory at his disposal. Ferrier (1873) confirmed Hitzig's results, and soon extended them to monkeys (1875). His declared intention was 'to put to experimental proof the views entertained by Dr. Hughlings Jackson on the pathology of Epilepsy, Chorea and Hemiplegia, by imitating artificially the "destroying" and "discharging" lesions of disease, which his writings have defined and differentiated' (Ferrier, 1873). 'The phenomena of localized and unilateral convulsive movements, depending, as Hughlings Jackson shows, on vital irritation of certain regions of the cortex, are essentially of the same nature as those caused by electrisation of the same regions' (Ferrier, 1876). Although Jackson had 'furnished many arguments in favour of his hypothesis, since verified', his views had been 'regarded merely as ingenious speculations, and devoid of any actual proof that the grey matter of the convolutions was really excitable' (Ferrier, 1886). Ferrier preferred faradic stimulation (pulses at 30–40 Hz from an induction coil with an interrupter in the primary circuit) to the galvanic stimulation used by Fritsch and Hitzig, which 'causes only a sudden contraction in certain groups of muscles, but fails to call forth the definite purposive combination of muscular contractions, which is the very essence of the reaction, and key to its interpretation'. We shall return to this aspect in section 2.5.

Ferrier's (1875) map of motor responses from the monkey's brain is reproduced in Fig. 2.2A. In 1876, he transferred the centres to an outline of the human brain, (Fig. 2.2C), and described the relations between brain fissures and bony landmarks (craniocerebral topography). In 1883, he proposed that localized cortical lesions should be excised by the surgeon.

FIG. 2.2. A. David Ferrier's historic map of faradic stimulation of the monkey's brain (1875). 1, 'The opposite hind limb is advanced as in walking. . . .' 2, 'Flexion with outward rotation of the thigh, rotation inwards of the leg, with flexion of the toes—the action being such as is seen when a monkey makes a grasping movement, or scratches its chest or abdomen with its foot. . . . The action is similar to that caused by stimulation of the sixth lumbar root of the crural plexus. . . .' 3, As for 1 and 2—'In some cases also the tail is moved. I have not been able to dissociate the movements of the tail from those of the trunk and hind limb.' 4, 'The opposite arm is adducted, extended, and retracted, the hand pronated . . . almost exactly in the same way as occurs on stimulation of the seventh cervical root of the brachial plexus . . . if the hand were the fixed point . . . would . . . raise the body upwards and forwards, as in climbing a trapeze.' 5, 'Extension forwards of the opposite arm, as if the animal tried to reach or touch something in front'. a, b, c, d, 'Clenching of the fist. With slight stimulation the action begins in the thumb and index finger, followed on longer stimulation by flexion of all the fingers and firm clenching of the fist. With the closure of the fist is associated the synergic action of the extensors of the wrist and fingers, but centres for the individual flexors and extensors could not be differentiated.' 6, 'Flexion and supination of the forearm—the completed action bringing the hand up to the mouth. The movement is essentially the same as that which occurs on

In 1888 he recalled with amusement that *The Lancet* had demurred. But his monkey experiments had shown that the brain could be handled and incised without fatal consequences; and on 25 November, 1884, Jackson and Ferrier saw Rickman Godlee remove a tumour of the size of a walnut from a patient's ascending parietal convolution through an opening

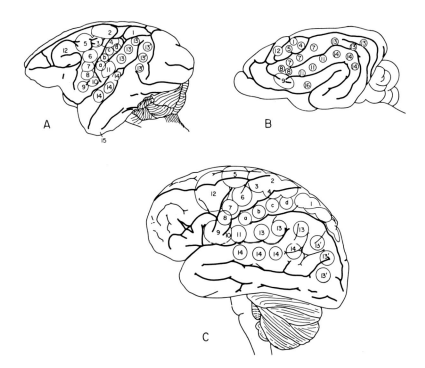

stimulation of the sixth cervical root of the brachial plexus.' 7, 'Retraction and elevation of the angle of the mouth.' 8, 'Elevation of the ala of the nose and upper lip.' 9 and 10, 'Opening of the mouth, with protrusion (9) and retraction (10) of the tongue.' 11, 'Retraction of the angle of the mouth.' 12, 'The eyes open widely, the pupils dilate, and head and eyes turn to the opposite side.' 13 and 13', 'The eyes move to opposite side, with an upward' (13) 'or downward deviation' (13') . . . 'Sometimes the head turns with the eyes.' 14, 'Pricking of the opposite ear, head and eyes turn to the opposite side, pupils dilate widely.' 15, 'On the anterior and inner aspect of the uncinate gyrus . . . Torsion of the lip and semiclosure of the nostril on the same side, as when the interior of the nostril is irritated by some pungent odour.' At lower extremity of middle temporosphenoidal convolution: 'movements of the tongue, cheek pouches and jaws . . . very like those which are characteristic of tasting'.

B. Ferrier's map of the dog's brain. The numbers refers to responses resembling those recorded by the same numbers in the monkey map. 'They do not pretend to indicate more than approximate physiological homologies, certain individual peculiarities being observable in different animals which scarcely admit of strict comparison with each other.' (Ferrier, 1876.)

C. Ferrier's (1876) transfer of his monkey centres to an outline of the human brain.

exactly overlying it and but little larger than itself. This was a triumph of cerebral localization and of the now-forgotten science of craniocerebral topography. The tumour had first declared its presence by local convulsions of the face and tongue and hand and arm of the opposite side, later by weakness of hand, arm and leg. 'The immediate effect of the operation was wholly satisfactory. There was a slight increase of the hemiplegic weakness but all the other symptoms were relieved and the intelligence was fully retained. It had been proved for the first time that without the least external abnormality of the skull to point the way, a local lesion of the brain substance could be found and could be removed by operation leaving the general functions of the brain unimpaired.' Sadly, 'a slow infection of the wound occurred, and after four miserable weeks of disappointed hopes the patient died of meningitis.' (Trotter, 1934.)

In his Lumleian Lectures in 1890 Jackson could therefore reiterate the need for detailed clinical study of focal convulsions on diagnostic as well as on physiological grounds. 'It is in epileptiform seizures that operations have been done by Macewen, Godlee, Horsley, Barker and others. Hence, very precise study of fits of this kind is necessary.' (Jackson, 1931, p. 424.)

Ferrier did not believe that all the centres he had marked with circles (Fig. 2.2) were 'truly motor, in the sense of being due to irritation of a part in direct connexion with the motor strands of the crus cerebri and spinal cord' (1886, p. 268). 'We cannot conclude from the mere occurrence of movement on the electrical stimulation that the regions are truly motor; for the stimulation of a sensory centre may give rise to reflex or associated movement.' (1886, p. 347.) Thus, he presumed that the response from Centre 14 (Fig. 2.2A)—'pricking of the opposite ear, head and eyes turn to the opposite side'—was equivalent to the response given by a normal monkey when he whistled loudly and unexpectedly, close to its ear (1886, p. 306). Bilateral ablations which included Centre 14 resulted in nonresponsiveness to explosion of a percussion cap in a monkey which was exhibited at the International Medical Congress in 1881. Since this monkey was not paralysed at any stage of recovery, Ferrier concluded that Centre 14 was not a 'truly motor' centre.

Although it is not relevant to the subject of this book, the temptation to refer to another of Ferrier's 'sensory centres' (Fig. 2.2A, 15) is irresistible. From 1875 onwards, Hughlings Jackson was studying cases of 'dreamy state' and defining what we now know as 'temporal lobe epilepsy'. In one of his patients, Dr Z, the spells of unconscious, automatic behaviour were sometimes accompanied by 'tasting movements'. 'In one he stopped talking to me, remained standing, and made slight, very slight, just audible smacking movements of his lips.' The patient died from an overdose of chloral. 'I begged Dr Colman to call on me before he went to make the necropsy on Z, in order to ask him to search the taste region of Ferrier on each half of the brain very carefully. Dr Colman found a very small focus of softening in that region (in the uncinate gyrus) of the left half of the brain.' (1931, p. 461.)

In contrast to the 'sensory centres', ablations of pre- and postcentral gyri did cause paralysis, associated with scarring and loss of nerve fibres along the course of the pyramidal and crossed corticospinal tracts of monkeys which had survived for several months (Ferrier, 1884). Ferrier was sure that his 'truly motor' centres had nothing to do with sensation. Against him, in the inconclusive polemics of those days, Hitzig held that the 'centres' were those of 'muscle sense', and Schiff, those of tactile sensibility (François-Franck, 1887).

Ferrier regarded the postcentral gyrus, as well as the precentral, as 'truly motor'. Thus his 'centres' for the fingers (Fig. 2.2A, a, b, c, d) were placed in the ascending parietal convolution. Later workers were to find the lowest threshold for the fingers in the precentral gyrus. From the first, there had been controversy about the exact locus of the structures stimulated and the possible extent of spread of electrical stimuli: to more or less remote areas of the cortex, to the subcortical white matter, even to the corpus striatum (see Ferrier, 1886; Schäfer, 1900). In the 1870s there was no reliable way of measuring the spread. One ingenious attempt to do this made use of the so-called 'physiological rheoscope': the nerve of a frog's nerve muscle preparation was laid across the posterior part of the brain and the anterior part was stimulated by paired electrodes. The frog's muscle twitched, proving that the flow of current was not confined to the interpolar region (Dupuy, cited by Ferrier, 1886). In another experiment, a galvanometer was used to detect the extrapolar spread (Carville and Duret, cited by Ferrier, 1886). Accepting this, Ferrier rightly insisted that 'under the degree of narcotisation necessary to eliminate all spontaneous movements . . . the great and significant feature of the reactions produced by electrical excitation of the cortex is that they are definite and predictable, and vary with position of the electrodes.'

Victor Horsley, who, alone of the surgeons listed by Jackson as having operated for focal epilepsy, deserves to be regarded as the first specialist neurosurgeon, was also an indefatigable experimentalist. His monkey maps, produced in collaboration with C. E. Beevor and with E. A. Schäfer (later Sharpey–Schäfer), confirmed Ferrier's 'in all essentials' but were 'worked out with more elaborate detail and minuteness' (Ferrier, 1890). Figure 2.3 shows that they, too, included postcentral cortex. This map clearly includes what is now known as the supplementary motor area on the medial surface of the hemisphere (Woolsey, 1964; see Fig. 2.6C); but Horsley and Schäfer's results (1888), on which this part of the map is based, were less detailed than Woolsey's, and were regarded as the mere medialward extension of the dorsolateral map. Beevor and Horsley (1890) were the first to stimulate the brain of an ape—a single orang-utan. Their map showed postcentral excitable foci. At the turn of the century Grünbaum and Sherrington began their studies of chimpanzee (Fig. 2.4), orang-utan and gorilla, which were not published *in extenso* for several years (Leyton and Sherrington, 1917). Grünbaum (=Leyton) and Sherrington, who had deliberately restricted themselves to minimal faradization with a focal stigmatic electrode (the other electrode was of large area, on an 'indifferent' part of the body), found that the excitable foci were all precentral. 'We have not found that the free surface of the postcentral convolution belongs to the motor cortex. Brodmann (1903) and Campbell (1904) have since called attention to marked structural differences between the cortex respectively behind and in front of the central sulcus. The arrangement of the fibres and the character of the cells is different. Ramón y Cajal (1890), using the Golgi method, and Flechsig (1904) following the myelinization, had also previously drawn distinction between the structure of the two convolutions divided by this great fissure; and observations by Mott, A. Tschermak, and others had indicated an especially close connexion of the postcentral gyrus with ascending, presumably afferent, paths. Evidence of this last by excitation methods is of course difficult to obtain. . . .' (Sherrington, 1906). It was first obtained by Cushing (1909) in two patients undergoing surgery under local anaesthesia.

Horsley (1909) accepted Sherrington's restriction of 'motor' cortex to the precentral gyrus. He had come to believe that the electrical elicitability of motor responses from the postcentral cortex diminishes as one ascends the primate scale. The thumb and finger movements he had found with Beevor in monkeys had been 'restricted and feeble' or unobtainable. He had never been able to evoke motor reactions from postcentral cortex in human patients at operation. Woolsey (1958), however, regards the higher-threshold responses evoked from postcentral cortex in monkeys as valid evidence of motor outflow from cortex which is mainly somaesthetic. He designates this cortex as 'Sensori-motor' (SmI) and designates the precentral cortex as 'Motor-sensory' (MsI) (Fig. 2.6C: Woolsey, 1964).

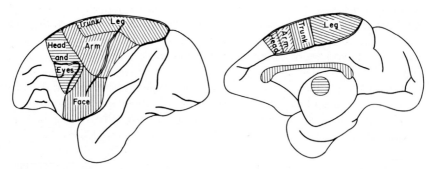

Fɪɢ. 2.3. 'Motor zone' of monkey's brain: dorsolateral aspect (left) and medial aspect (right), based on the experiments of Victor Horsley with C. E. Beevor and E. A. Schäfer (Schäfer, 1900).

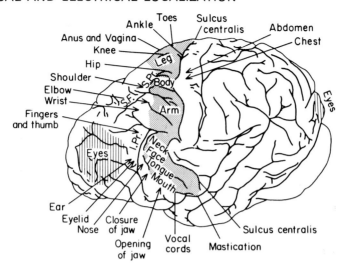

FIG. 2.4. Dorsolateral aspect of left hemisphere of chimpanzee; motor area indicated by stippling. Much of it is buried in sulci. This is a pictorial summary of the results in a whole series of experiments (see Fig. 2.5). (Sherrington, 1906.)

2.4 Clinical and electrical investigation of localization within the motor cortex

Although Hughlings Jackson was primarily interested in the localization of what he variously called 'sensorimotor processes', 'processes representing movements', and 'processes for movements' (Phillips, 1973), he was also greatly interested in the facts of localization and interconnexion: thus his own Hughlings Jackson Lecture was entitled 'Relations of different divisions of the central nervous system to one another and to parts of the body' (1897; 1932, p. 422).

Two extreme opinions have been held about localization within the cortical projection area: one, that the outputs to the different peripheries are sharply marked off from one another, like the stones of a mosaic[1]; the other, that these outputs, although arranged in finely detailed patterns, overlap one another partially or even completely. Jackson used his own terminology for these extremes: for the first, 'abrupt localization' (which he rejected); for the second, 'minute localization' (in which he believed). Discussion of his ideas about 'processes for movements' will be deferred to Chapter 8; our immediate task is to try to disentangle his contribution to knowledge of the localization of outputs within the projection area.

---

[1] An early user of the works *mosaic* was C. K. Mills (1888): 'Wonderful indeed is this motor zone of the cerebrum, a marvellous mosaic of centres of function . . . a mosaic to each block, angle and jointure of which the neurologist can point the surgeon and say "cut here or there, or touch not this or that." '

To this knowledge, Jackson's own factual contribution was rather small because, by the time of a patient's death, the (presumably) initially circumscribed lesions had usually become 'ill-defined, coarse and widespread. I have very little to say on the exact relation of the particular convulsive movements to the seat of disease.' (1875.) 'Clinical knowledge is not yet precise enough for minute localization.' (1886.)

In the case of 'convulsions beginning unilaterally', he wrote in 1873, 'the discharge being of the grey matter of processes for *movements*, there is caused by it a development of movements in the related and connected external regions' (1931, p. 66). These may be in any part, for example, the shoulder or thigh (1931, p. 262), but begin most commonly in the hand, face or foot. 'In each of these varieties there must be some difference in the situation of the grey matter exploded. In one part the movements of the hand have the leading representation. . . . I say *leading* representation because spasm of the hand, etc. is only the *beginning* of the seizure.' (1931, p. 68.) He goes on to describe how it spreads up the arm, into the face, then down the leg (the March of Spasm). The spasm of the hand continues, and increases in intensity, as the seizure spreads up the arm (1932, p. 30). Jackson believed that the sequence of involvement is related to the normal combination of movements in the natural use of the arm. 'For example, if a fit begins in the thumb and index finger, there will probably be developed as the spasm spreads that series of movements which in health serves subordinately when the thumb and index finger are used.' (1931, p. 69.) Since their normal use requires fixation of the wrist, and of other parts 'according to the force required, we should *a priori* be sure that the centre discharged, although it might represent movements in which the thumb had the leading part, must represent also certain other movements of the forearm, upper arm, etc. which serve subordinately'.

From 1876 onwards, Jackson had clearly wished to see *all* parts of the body included within *any* area of 'Hitzig and Ferrier's region'. 'Thus, to take an arbitrary and limited illustration, supposing one centre . . . to represent specially the hand, another specially the face, another the foot, I should believe that each one of them represented all the movements of the chest.' (1931, p. 144.)

Although this is all couched in terms of the *functional* concept of 'movements' as intracerebral *processes* (Phillips, 1966), it is clear that Jackson believed, as a corollary, in overlapping *structural* projections issuing from every part of the arm area. Thus, in 1890 (1931, p. 444) he cited Sherrington's (1889) description of fibres descending from the monkey's arm area as far as the lumbo-sacral enlargement of the spinal cord, admitting, however, that Sherrington suspected their function to be visceral. Repetition of this experiment has always given the same result

(Leyton and Sherrington, 1917; Glees and Cole, 1950; Barnard and Woolsey, 1956). Chapter 4, section 4.4, cites electroanatomical evidence of axons which arise in the cat's forelimb area and branch to supply the lumbar as well as the cervical enlargement (Asanuma *et al.*, 1976b).

Jackson believed that the successive involvement of different parts of the body in his famous March of Spasm was due to intensification of convulsive activity within the area of cortex that was 'exploded' initially, without need for horizontal spread of excitation beyond the limits of that area. As Walshe (1943) has pointed out, this idea was never discussed by the experimentalists. By 1900, 'abrupt localization' of the areas for arm, face, leg, trunk and head and eyes had become the textbook story, and the Jacksonian March was explained in terms of horizontal spread from each area to the next, as 'apparently dependent in each case upon the relative propinquity of the several centres in the motor region of the cortex, and when they are equally close, upon their relative excitability' (Schäfer, 1900). This explanation also came to be accepted by clinical neurologists. 'As the motor points are arranged in the cortex in a manner corresponding with the anatomical relations of the parts in which they initiate movement, a stimulus that spreads over the cortex excites a sequence of movements which spread or march in a more or less constant and regular manner from the segment of the body that is first convulsed. This is the essential feature of a Jacksonian attack; any chart of the motor representation of the cortex explains the march of the convulsions.' (Holmes, 1927.)

Discussing a case in which a fit began in the left toes, spread up the leg, and then involved, 'slightly', the left arm, Jackson (1890; 1931, p. 444) wrote: 'The current hypothesis would be that, in causing this part of the fit, the discharge spread from the leg centre to the arm centre. This I cannot disprove. Yet I think it an equally legitimate hypothesis that the discharge causing the slight movements of the arm in this case was of those elements of the "leg centre" representing subordinate movements of the arm. No doubt, of course, in a severer fit other centres of the motor region would be discharged.'

It is interesting that Jackson does not seem to have gone into any detailed discussion or criticism of the procedures or the results of the experimentalists. He says simply: 'I do not accept the current doctrine of localization. The minute investigations of the monkey's cortex by Horsley and Beevor go strongly against it.' Elsewhere (1888; 1932, p. 385) he invoked their experiments, 'without, of course, committing these able observers to any hypothesis of mine', as seeming 'to be in great disaccord with the current doctrine of localization'. But in what respects he does not say. Was he, perhaps, thinking of their finding of primary movements of thumb over the upper two-thirds of the face area (of which Schäfer wrote in his Textbook: 'There must have been some unrecognized source of error in this observation')? Or of their finding that 'the hallux is frequently represented all over the area for movements of the lower limb'?

We may distinguish between 'abrupt' inter-areal localization—between the areas for arm, face, leg, trunk and head and eyes—and 'abrupt' intra-areal localization within each of these main subdivisions of the projection area. Reviewing his own pioneering experiment on monkeys, and those of Horsley, Beevor and Schäfer, Ferrier (1890) wrote: 'So far as the excitation method is concerned, we are entitled to say that, whether the individual segments of a limb are separately localized, or are represented, more or less, throughout a common area, the areas as a whole . . . are as completely differentiated from each other as the limbs themselves. . . . We have seen, however, in respect to the individual movements of a limb, that though one particular movement can frequently be isolated by minimal stimulation of a definite point within the general area, yet the same movement may occur along with others when another part of the area is under stimulation. This may be interpreted either on the supposition that the particular movement, say of the thumb, is represented throughout the arm area, or that it is only a case of diffusion of the stimulus from one part to another. It is difficult to decide which of these views is the correct one, and it may be that neither accurately represents the whole truth.'

Thus, in the case of spread from arm into face and then down the leg, there was no experimental support for Jackson's hypothesis of increasing activity confined within an arm area which contained also elements of face and leg. But in the case of the march within a single limb, for example from thumb and index to fingers, wrist, elbow and shoulder, the experiments did not rule it out, but, rather, encouraged it. Writing of Beevor and Horsley's 'intra-areal localizations', Schäfer noted: 'In some individuals even minimal stimulation of what has been termed the hallux centre produced movements, not only of the hallux but also of other toes, and even of the foot and leg; and stimulation of the ascending parietal [sic!] may cause not only flexion of the fingers but also extension of the wrist. Such movements may succeed one another, or they may be simultaneous.' It has been usual to speak of the movement which is most often or most readily obtained on excitation of a particular localized area, as the 'primary' movement, and the others as 'secondary'. Horsley (1909), to whose experiments Jackson had turned for support, stated that 'a minimal stimulus may only be adequate for one item of several represented in one portion of the cortex'.

Leyton and Sherrington's (1917) experiments, in which they deliberately restricted themselves to minimal unifocal faradization, and to periods of stimulation limited to '1 or 2 s or little more', found a much greater differentiation of intra-areal responses within the arm, face and leg areas of their great apes than Beevor and Horsley had found in their intra-areal studies in monkeys. Here was a fresh profusion of 'minute' localization; was it also 'abrupt'? The responses evoked by minimal stimulation were not always confined to a single joint. Isolated extension of index finger was common. Adjacent 'points' were apt to give similar responses grading into one another (Fig. 2.5). Stronger and more prolonged faradism evoked characteristic sequences of primary, secondary and tertiary responses at the same or at additional joints: 'not only a considerable "march" or sequence of responsive movement, but also, as is well known, an epileptiform convulsion'. To explain such responses, as well as to explain minimal responses which involved more than one joint, the advocates of 'abrupt' localization could always invoke 'diffusion of the stimulus from one part to another'. Quantitative experimental refutation of the diffusion hypothesis would have been impossible with the methods then available.

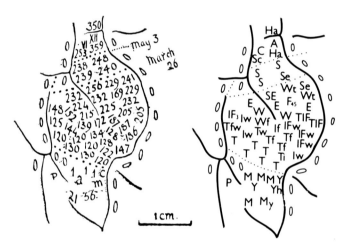

FIG. 2.5. *Left*: detailed map of motor responses to stimulation of arm area of left hemisphere of an individual chimpanzee. O, no response. Other numbers refer to cumulative list of responses in whole series of experiments (from Leyton and Sherrington, 1917). *Right*: same points have been lettered to indicate responding parts of contralateral forelimb. *Capital letters* signify primary responses, *small letters* secondary responses. Thus point 147 (left of figure) gave prompt extension of index finger (primary response) and delayed supination of wrist (secondary response). Where the numbers differ, but the letters are the same, the responses of the same parts were different; thus point 152 and 144 are both marked Iw, but 152 gave primary flexion of index and secondary flexion of wrist, and 144 gave primary extension of index and secondary extension of wrist. H, hip; A,a, abdomen; C,c, chest; M, angle of mouth; Y,y, eyelid; P, pinna; h, face turned to opposite side; S, shoulder; E,e, elbow; W,w, wrist; I,i, index finger; F,f, all fingers except index; F_3, third finger; F_{45}, fourth and fifth fingers; T,t, thumb.

Points 1, 238, 239, 240, 248 gave same responses when re-stimulated five weeks after excision of area enclosed between lower dotted line and 'March 26'. After excision, exposed posterior wall of fissure was stimulated without effect. The ensuing pyramidal degeneration is described in Chapter 4, and the effect of the excision on behaviour in Chapter 8.

The inter-areal frontiers (e.g. arm-face) under minimal faradic stimulation were sharp. They could, however, be blurred when minimal stimuli
were applied rapidly and successively to a row of points which crossed the
frontier ('deviation of response'). Thus, when jumping along such a row
from hand to face area, the lower border of hand area 'trespassed' into
face area. 'The responses of hand given by the hand area points thus
trespassing were always similar to the last hand responses obtained from
the portion of the hand area above them; and they were accompanied by
"angle of mouth" movement, either simultaneous with them or almost so.'
By jumping in the opposite direction along the row, the face area was
made to trespass into the hand area. 'As to how far such deviations . . . are
traceable to shuntings of route in the cortical structure itself, or how far
they are referable to shuntings in subcortical paths and centres, that is a
question towards whose solution our observations contribute little or
nothing.' The reader will probably conclude, as we have done, that
T. Graham Brown's attempts to settle this question (1915a, b, c, d; 1916a,
b) were inconclusive. Such 'shuntings' could be due to a combination of
physical diffusion of stimulus in the cortex with lowering of threshold by
physiological facilitation in cortex and in the related subcortical apparatus.
Two hypotheses can be proposed, neither of which can be rejected on the
evidence available.

1. Localization is abrupt. Minimal stimulation of the face area excites
movements of the face, and also lowers the thresholds of the face area
and of the related subcortical apparatus. When minimal stimulation is
applied to the adjacent arm area, current spreads into the face area;
although the intensity of the spreading current is normally too low to
excite the face, this low intensity becomes supraliminal during the
period of lowering of the face threshold.

2. Localization is minute and overlapping. The 'face area' contains
'subordinate' 'arm' elements and vice versa. Prior stimulation of the face
area excites the more numerous 'leading' face elements and facilitates the
subcortical face apparatus, so that this apparatus now discharges in
response to stimulation of the less numerous, subordinate face elements
within the arm area.

Modern experiments in which the pia-covered cortex has been stimulated with trains of repetitive pulses from electronic stimulators, or with
60 Hz alternating current, are all subject to the same essential uncertainty
about diffusion of the stimulus, but, as far as they go, they do not support
abrupt localization. Thus, Woolsey *et al.* (1952), who stimulated macaques
and Java monkeys unifocally with 60 Hz a.c., concluded that 'foci for
different muscles' are not 'discrete entities', as in a mosaic. 'Rather there
is very extensive overlap in the cortical motor patterns. . . . Nevertheless,

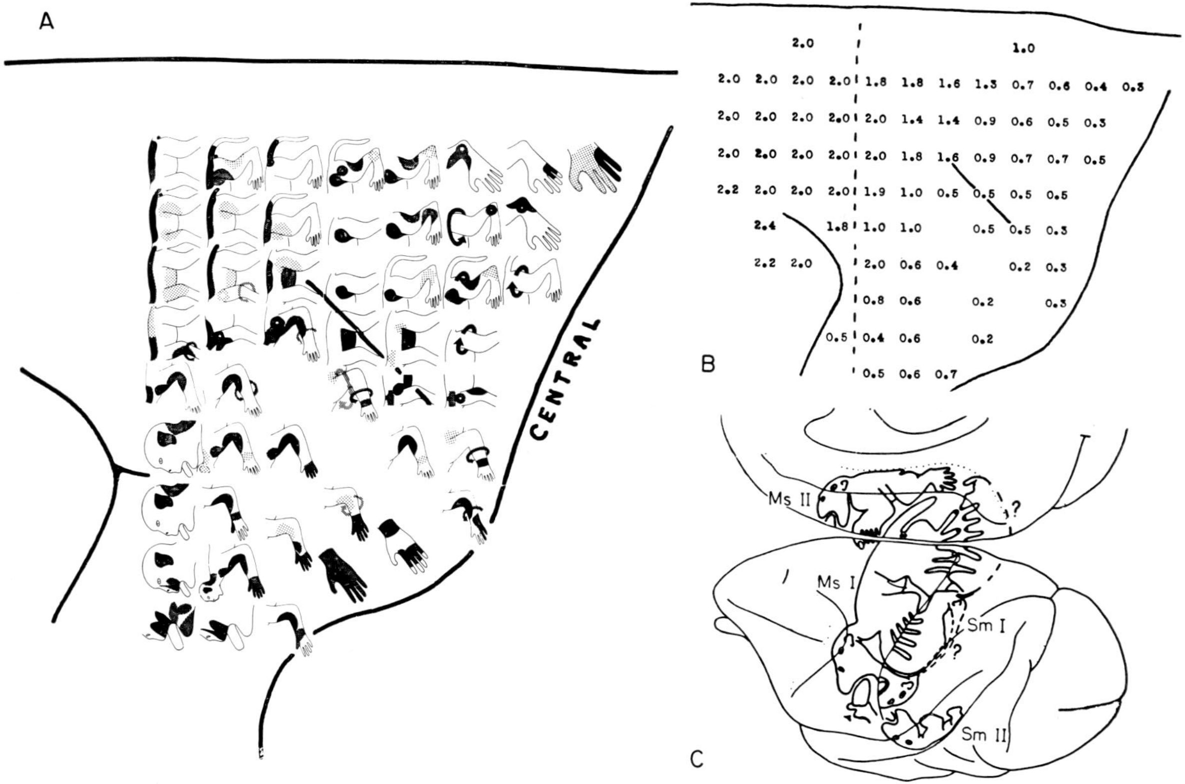

FIG. 2.6. A. 'Motor figurine chart' showing responses evoked by near-threshold stimulation of a monkey's cortex with 60 Hz sinusoidal alternating current in trains of 2 s duration delivered at 2 min intervals. Explanation in text (Woolsey *et al.*, 1952). We are grateful to Dr. Clinton N. Woolsey for giving us a copy of the original of this Figure.

B. Strength of near-threshold currents used in A, in mA RMS.

C. 'Simiusculi' drawn on dorsolateral and medial outlines of monkey's brain, showing precentral (MsI) and supplementary (MsII) motor areas. Somatosensory receiving areas (SmI; SmII) also marked. (Woolsey, 1964.)

the centres of the foci form a pattern which reflects in general the arrangement in the periphery' (Fig. 2.6A).

2.5 Investigation by 'faradic stimulation' of projection from 'middle level' to 'lowest level'

With the exception of François-Franck (1887—cf. Chapter 1.3), none of the pioneers of electrical stimulation was content to ask questions simply about the structure of the output: about the 'horizontal' map of the projection area (sections 2.4 and 2.6) and the 'vertical' structure of the descending projections to brainstem and spinal cord. Matters became confused by failure to disentangle experiments on localization from experiments on function, and *facts* of localization from *concepts* of function (Phillips, 1966, 1973, 1975). Ferrier (1886) wrote of areas being 'truly motor' in the structural sense of being 'in direct connexion with the motor strands of the crus cerebri and spinal cord', but he was much more interested in his motor 'centres' in a functional sense, as 'not merely the centres of impulse, but also the centres of registration and reproduction of volitional movements' (1886, p. 443). He evidently regarded faradic stimulation as a tool that was capable of mapping these specific functions, insisting on 'the definite purposive combination of muscular contractions, which is the very essence of the reaction, and key to its interpretation'. So he rejected galvanic stimulation as a tool, on the grounds that it 'causes only a sudden contraction in certain groups of muscles'. Presumably he regarded it as capable only of mapping 'centres of impulse'. We shall show in sections 2.6 and 2.7 that the modern counterpart of 'galvanic stimulation' is a valuable method of differentiating between groups of muscles which receive more direct and less direct connexions from the cortex.

Jackson agreed that the responses evoked by faradic stimulation had 'evidently a purposive or volitional character' (Ferrier, 1876). 'The artificial movements I have seen Ferrier produce by locally applied faradic currents to limited spots on the surface of the cerebral hemisphere of a monkey simulate the movements of health, whereas a convulsion is but a "clotted mass" of innumerable movements, produced by an excessive, sudden, and abrupt cerebral discharge.' (1875; 1931, p. 39.) And Schäfer (1900) commented: 'Undoubtedly the most striking character of many of the movements which are provoked by cerebral excitation is their co-ordinated and purposeful nature.' It was left to Sherrington (1900a) to discover that this character was due to the fact that the responses in question were coordinated within the segmental motor apparatus of the 'lowest level'. Thus, in monkeys with chronically isolated spinal cord, he could evoke coordinated flexion and adduction of thumb, retraction then protraction of shoulder, extension of wrist and flexion of elbow and fingers by electrical stimulation of the palm of the hand, or the dorsal branch of the ulnar nerve. 'Movements regularly and widely elicitable as local reflexes are liberally represented in the motor cortex . . . the local reflex movements obtainable from the bulbo-spinal animal and the reactions elicitable from the motor cortex of the narcotized animal fall into line as similar series.' (Sherrington, 1906.) Nineteenth century critics had said that 'there is no more significance in the statement that movements are represented in the cortex than there is in the statement that movements are represented in the skin' (Bates, 1957). The 'movements' in question are 'represented' in the spinal cord, and the segmental motor apparatus (Fig. 1.4) can be addressed from cortex or from skin. Whether we stimulate cortex, skin or nerve, the 'faradic' stimuli send impulses in unnatural combinations of axons, and in abnormally synchronized volleys, into the spinal cord. The segmental apparatus elaborates simple coordinated movements in response to an unpatterned jangle of excitation and inhibition—as when reflex stepping is elicited by faradization of afferent nerves (Sherrington, 1906).

We should not, *a priori*, expect that such stimulation, when applied to the cortical surface, should be able to evoke, in the cortex itself, the natural neural patterns of 'voluntary movements'. The discharges of the cortical neurones would be unnaturally synchronized. Questions about voluntary movements can be answered only by conscious man, and here the answer is decisive. The artificial synchronization of neuronal discharges disrupts the natural patterns of voluntary activity (Penfield, 1958). 'The effect of the electrode is to interfere with the patient's ability to make voluntary employment of the cortex near the electrode. He may be able to move the foot and the face at will, but he cannot direct the movement of the hand while hand cortex is being stimulated. Sometimes the electrode produces no movement and then this interference is the only effect of the stimulating current. When it does produce movement, it is by virtue of conduction of impulses from the cortex to ganglionic areas of the cerebrospinal axis.'

Thus faradic stimulation is disqualified, equally with 'galvanic', as a tool for evoking natural function in the projection area. This leaves us free to concentrate on its merits as a tool for mapping the outputs that are available for selection by the intracortical activities that it cannot itself evoke. It is true that glimpses of possible 'horizontal' transmissions, which would be important in the selection processes, were obtained by Leyton and Sherrington (1917) in their development of Brown and Sherrington's discovery (1912) of the 'instability of a cortical point': the response expected from one 'point' could be 'deviated' or even 'reversed' as the result of prior stimulation of another 'point' (section 2.4). But the faradic mode of stimulation was too crude to lead to more significant insights.

Section 2.4 has already raised doubts about the reliability of faradic stimulation for the accurate mapping of outputs, since the extent of its physical and physiological diffusion in the cortical tissue could not be measured. This section will look at its capacity to resolve the structure of descending connexions, excitatory and inhibitory to the segmental motor apparatus, and possibly also to the motoneurones of the 'final common path'.

All the responses we have so far considered have been excitatory. But the fact that cortical stimulation can inhibit spinal reflexes as well as exciting movements was discovered by Bubnoff and Heidenhain (1881). In Sherrington's experiments, inhibition always featured prominently. Thus: 'A. S. Grünbaum and myself have seen that in the chimpanzee and gorilla any single manual digit can be moved isolatedly by stimulation of the cortex. We must not forget, however, that with even a small *movement* the field of inhibition may yet be wide, for I have on occasion noted inhibition of muscles of the shoulder when the thumb was moved under cortical excitation, the shoulder previously being unrelaxed.' (Sherrington, 1906.)

In some patients with Jacksonian fits, there are also brief attacks which seem to be purely inhibitory (Holmes, 1927), though they may well be due to disruption of normal cortical activity by localized excitatory epileptic discharges which are too 'weak' to discharge the corticofugal neurones.

By giving faradic stimulation to a cortical point for several seconds on end, Leyton and Sherrington (1917) could evoke from the cortex of chimpanzee, orang-utan and gorilla 'combinational sequences' of movement which were, 'so to say, eloquent of purpose in most instances'. These were the movements we have already considered as being coordinated by the segmental motor apparatus. But their main purpose in these culminating experiments on anthropoids was '"localization" of the primary movement' by brief applications of faradic stimulation. Such movements, 'elicited by somewhat minutely localized stimulations, are, broadly speaking, fractional, in the sense that each, though coordinately executed, forms, so to say, but a unitary part of some more complex act, that would, to attain its purpose, involve combination of that unitary movement with others to make up a useful whole. . . . It is the isolated and restricted character of the primary movements elicited by punctate stimulation of the cortex, or, to repeat the term introduced above, their fractional character, which makes so equivocal any purpose that an observer, who would interpret their purpose, can assign to them.' 'This discrete "representation" of small local items of movement' is 'more evident in cat and dog than in rabbit, more evident in the macaque than in the cat or dog, in baboon than in macaque, in gibbon than in baboon, and in chimpanzee, orang, and gorilla than in gibbon.' Leyton and Sherrington's conception of the motor cortex was as a 'synthetic organ for motor acts', building up from the coordinately executed local items, 'larger combinations varied in character and serviceable for purposes of different and varied kind'. 'It would seem that in order to preserve the possibility of being interchangeably compounded in a variety of ways, successive or simultaneous, these movements must lie, as more or less discrete and separable elements, within the grasp of the organ which has the varied compounding of them.'

This evidence suggests that in the series of animals investigated, there is an increasing richness of descending excitatory connexions, by-passing the segmental motor patterns and addressing larger and larger numbers of smaller and smaller groupings of segmental output. There is an additional possibility, that an increasing richness of descending inhibitory connexions could be playing a part in the narrowing of the segmental output. Leyton and Sherrington probably had this in mind when they wrote of the motor cortex as an analytic organ, capable of breaking up 'compounds already constructed by lower centres'.

Such 'compounds' would be parts of built-in postural, defensive, and locomotor patterns ('segmental motor programmes', Fig. 1.4) involving fairly stereotyped reciprocal relationships between muscles working antagonistically at hinge joints. Hering and Sherrington's experiments on reciprocal inhibition from the monkey's cortex (Sherrington, 1906) were concerned with such muscles, which they called 'true' antagonists. In the suspended, lightly-etherized monkey, hip and elbow were held in flexed postures. Stimulation of an elbow-extensor point caused relaxation of biceps as well as contraction of triceps. 'The relaxation is usually so striking that merely to place a finger on it is enough to convince the observer that the muscle relaxes . . . the contracted mass becomes suddenly soft, melting under the observer's touch.' Conversely, stimulation of an elbow-flexor point caused relaxation of triceps, but only of that part of the muscle which extends the elbow: the part which retracts the humerus on the scapula remained tense.

'True' antagonists could never be made to contract together by stimulation of the internal capsule after removal of the cortex; their reciprocal responses are therefore organized at the 'lowest level' and are 'not chiefly or at all due to an interaction of cortical neurones one with another'. In the internal capsule, the area from which contraction of, for example, triceps, can be obtained is separate from the area from which it can be inhibited; and the inhibitory area 'corresponds with the area whence contraction of its antagonistic muscle can be evoked. Yet synchronous contraction of such pairs of muscles as *gastrocnemius* and *peroneus longus* is obtainable from the cortex.'

Sherrington excluded 'cases where one muscle fixes a joint enabling another muscle to thus act better on *another* joint—H. E. Hering's pseudo-antagonists'. Hering had found that cortical stimulation was able to evoke co-contraction of the wrist extensors and finger flexors. He called these 'pseudoantagonists'. Following Beevor (1904) we should call the wrist extensors 'synergists' and the finger-flexors 'prime movers'. This stereotyped pattern is familiar in the neurological clinic, in patients with cortical or capsular lesions who can grasp an object with their fingers, using the wrist extensors as synergists, but in whom the wrist extensors are found to be paralysed as prime movers when the patients try to dorsiflex their wrists. In the highly mobile forelimb of primates, in which the movements, and particularly those distal to the elbow, involve many muscles which act across several joints, we should not expect to find the more stereotyped antagonistic relationships that we find, for example, at the cat's knee. We shall see (Chapter 4, section 4.6) that the segmental reciprocal-inhibitory interneurones are subject to control by the cortex. One can imagine that the relationship between a muscle-pair could be switched from reciprocal action to co-contraction during the course of a complex sequence of movement, as fractional excitatory and inhibitory projections from the motor cortex are selected in appropriate combinations and sequences by a central programme.

About half a century separated Leyton and Sherrington's investigations of minimal 'local items of movement', made at a time when the only detector of corticofugal discharge was the contraction of muscle or the local relaxation of prevailing postures, from the modern era, in which the subliminal excitatory and inhibitory actions of circumscribed corticofugal volleys can be detected and measured by recording from interneurones and moto-neurones with microelectrodes (Chapter 4). During this period, attempts were made to discover the minimal detectable result of faradic stimulation of the cortex of primates. Was it 'an organized pattern of response involving reciprocal innervation of opposing muscle groups' or was it 'merely the reaction of a single muscle or part of a muscle' (Fulton, 1949)? Although this issue was essentially descriptive, the experiments were seen as an attempt to decide between alternative propositions: whether muscles or movements are 'represented' in the cortex. The antithesis was false, and was based on historic misunderstandings which are now best forgotten (Phillips, 1975).

Hines (1944), from her great experience of stimulating the cortex of monkeys and apes stated that weak stimulation with 60 Hz alternating current 'permits restriction of responses to single muscles', and that a particular muscle need not be the only one 'represented at a specific cortical point, but that it is the one predominantly represented there'. Her observations were by inspection and palpation of the intact parts. In their classical experiments, Chang *et al.* (1947) recorded simultaneous myograms from eight muscles acting across the monkey's ankle joint, and mapped the contralateral leg area with pulses at 60 Hz in trains lasting 4 s. 'Solitary responses' of single muscles were 'by no means the typical response to cortical stimulation; they appeared only under favorable conditions', usually in the distal muscles extensor digitorum longus and extensor hallucis longus (physiological flexors). When, as was usual, there was co-contraction of several muscles, some gave more tension than others, and some responded more promptly than others, when different points were stimulated. These criteria were used to map the cortical area for each muscle. The different muscles were 'not equally available to cortical stimulation', for peroneus longus never responded, and gastrocnemius, soleus, tibialis posterior, flexor digitorum longus and flexor hallucis longus (all physiological extensors) responded rarely. As the hamstring and femoral nerves had been cut, and the foot amputated, there was no evidence whether motoneurones of thigh muscles or intrinsic muscles of the foot were being activated from the same cortical areas.

Thus these fine experiments did not demonstrate that minimal responses are confined to single muscles. They were not of a nature to examine the alternative possibility of 'an organized pattern of response involving reciprocal innervation of opposing muscle groups' (Fulton, 1949). The crucial experiment would have required that some of the eight muscles should have exhibited background tonus, recorded by their myographs, so that if, for example, relaxation of a physiological extensor had been associated with minimal contraction of a physiological flexor this would have been recorded. Would solitary inhibition of a single muscle ever have occurred? Evidence of inhibition there was, but only with supraliminal stimuli; thus, a weak stimulus activated EHL and FDL equally, but a stronger stimulus to the same point gave a larger response of EHL and no response from FDL. Notice that the weak stimulus caused co-contraction, and not reciprocal response, of a physiological flexor (EHL) and a physiological extensor (FDL). To the stronger stimulus, the physiological flexor (EHL) responded alone. What was possibly an example of reciprocal inhibition was thus not obtained as a liminal response.

This classical paper, with its exemplary description of experiments, may be taken as the culminating attempt to use a faradic type of stimulation to map the minute localization in the motor area, and to discover whether there are circumscribed descending projections to the motoneurones of single muscles. Chang et al. (1947) interpreted their results in terms of overlapping fields of Betz cells for each muscle, each with a denser focus and a more diffuse fringe, and concluded that 'the representation of muscles stands midway between a strict mosaic pattern and diffuse representation'.

We have to remember that the motoneurone pools which are the ultimate targets of corticofugal motor projection are not, themselves, sharply marked off from one another in the spinal cord. Sherrington (1899) worked out this anatomy in the cervical enlargement of monkeys in meticulous experiments in which stimulation and degeneration were variously combined. The motoneurones of each muscle 'are scattered in a continuous series through the length of a series of spinal segments; and throughout this extent are commingled with the cells of a great number—in some cases as many as forty or more—of other muscles'. So the 'wiring' needed to connect a circumscribed area of cortex to a particular moto-neurone pool would have to be complex at the spinal end, even if it were simple at the cortical end.

2.6   Maps and thresholds of cortical stimulation. Preferential accessibility of distal parts

Different experimenters have devised different methods of recording the results of their somatotopic mapping of motor responses. The responses to be mapped are supposedly those determined by the structure of the output projection, and should therefore be repeatable at the same and at later explorations of the same individual (Bates, 1957; Craggs and Rushton, 1976). The problem of presenting the very voluminous results of the explorations within the limits imposed by publication is a formidable one.

Figure 2.5 (left) shows how Leyton and Sherrington's evidence (1917) was recorded in detail. It displays one part only of the map of an individual chimpanzee's cortex, namely, the arm area. The numbers refer to a list of 445 'primary movements' of arm, leg, face, trunk, head and eyes. The list was cumulative for the whole series of experiments; the individual maps did not contain all the numbers. 'Primary movements' were the first, and often the only responses from the various points; 'secondary' and 'tertiary' responses could develop from them, and were separately recorded in the list. Because of the differences between individuals, and the variation in cortical landmarks (sulci, arteries and veins), it was difficult to constrain the results into composite maps. Figure 2.4, therefore, is only an overall pictorial impression of all the chimpanzees of the series. The responses varied if the points were stimulated within a few seconds of one another (facilitation, deviation, reversal of response), but were repeatable if a longer period was allowed between stimulations and also if (as in the experiment of Fig. 2.5) the same brain was re-explored a few weeks later. Nevertheless, Leyton and Sherrington (1917) considered that 'the fixity of such localizations is as regards minutiae to some extent probably a temporary one'. In Fig. 2.5 (right) we have substituted explanatory letters for the numbers (see legend for key), in order to show the extent of the overlap between the responses from different points, and the relatively large area from which responses of thumb and index finger were obtained.

Woolsey *et al.* (1952) presented their results as 'motor figurine charts' (Fig. 2.6A), which are less tiresome for the reader than referring to numbers on a list. They used 60 Hz a.c., which probably elicits a larger range of minimal muscular responses than any other mode of electrical stimulation. Each point was stimulated three or more times, 2 min being allowed between stimulations, and the result entered on an enlarged tracing of the cortex as a diagram of the responding part. Shading, e.g. of the flexor or extensor aspects of the joints, was used to show the direction of movement, dense shading for prompt and strong responses, less dense for weaker responses. Such shading can be used to indicate flexion or extension of large joints, but cannot easily be used for the direction of responses of the digits. Thus, some of the fine detail that was actually observed may be missing from the charts. Such charts were published for individual experiments, and also a composite chart which needed but little 'tailoring' or 'editing', except in the face area, in order to give a fair picture of the series as a whole. The general pattern is also summarized in the 'simiusculus' of Fig. 2.6C with the caveat that this is 'an inadequate representation of the localization pattern, since in a line drawing one cannot indicate the successive overlap which is so characteristic a feature of cortical representation'.

In all such experiments it is important to specify the initial positions of the trunk and limbs, for the maps differ when these are varied (Gellhorn and Hyde, 1953). Relevant to this result is a clinical observation of Holmes (1927): if, during an attack of Jacksonian epilepsy, 'while there is vigorous clonic flexion of the forearm, the elbow be flexed as far as possible, the spasm may at once shift to its extensors. This may be due to the new position altering the relative excitability of the cortical flexor and extensor points.' It might also be due to reflex changes in the excitability of the spinal mechanisms.

Neurosurgical patients cannot be asked to submit to the many hours of stimulation and re-stimulation that the electroanatomist requires if he is to draw a complete and confident map of the projection areas of a monkey's brain. Penfield and Boldrey's (1937) map is therefore a composite one, assembling the fragments of evidence collected from a large number of cases, many of them stimulated under local anaesthesia (Fig. 2.7A). Figure 2.7B reproduces Penfield and Rasmussen's diagram showing the relative number of responses of each part evoked by stimulations of pre- and postcentral gyri with trains of pulses at 60 Hz. Figure 2.7C shows one of the well-known 'homunculi' which summarize the general pattern of localization, and to which Penfield and Jasper (1954) ascribe 'the defects,

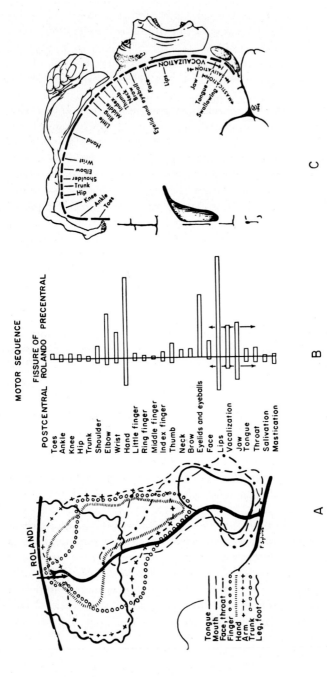

FIG. 2.7. A. Right peri-Rolandic cortex of human brain. Overlapping outlines show areas from which any motor responses of indicated parts were ever evoked in different individuals in a series of neurosurgical explorations (Penfield and Boldrey, 1937). Though symbols for 'trunk' appear in key; no trunk area appears on the map.

B. Proportion of motor responses elicited from precentral and postcentral gyri in series of neurosurgical explorations (Penfield and Rasmussen, 1950).

C. Vertico-transverse section of human right hemisphere (cf. Fig. 1). 'Motor homunculus' (see text). (Penfield and Rasmussen, 1950.)

and the virtues, of cartoons, in that they are inaccurate anatomically and yet they call attention to differences in the character of areas'. One must go to the individual protocols of Penfield and Boldrey (1937) to appreciate the details of the evidence that went into the maps and diagrams which summarize this uniquely valuable corpus of human observation.

A striking feature of all these maps is the unequal size of the cortical areas projecting towards the different peripheries. The largest areas are for fingers, toes, mouth and tongue. This is especially evident in Penfield and Boldrey's composite map (Fig. 2.7A). Further, the threshold current is lowest for toes, thumb and mouth (Boynton and Hines, 1933) and fingers (Woolsey et al., 1952; see Fig. 2.6A, B). Another indication of the *preferential accessibility* of these peripheries to cortical stimulation is that when the strength of stimulation at 50 Hz is adjusted to be above threshold for most parts of the baboon's precentral gyrus, the hand, face and foot respond most promptly, that is to say, the pathways leading to their motoneurones, require less *temporal summation* than those leading to the motoneurones of proximal muscle groups (Liddell and Phillips, 1950).

We recall Hughlings Jackson's finding (1931, p. 90) that focal convulsions 'mostly begin (1) in the hand, (2) in the face or tongue or both, (3) in the foot . . . when the fit begins in the hand, the index finger and thumb are usually the digits first seized: when in the face, the side of the cheek is first in spasm: when in the foot, almost invariably the great toe'. No explanation of such a selective impact of lesions which were usually 'ill-defined, coarse and widespread' was put forward until Walshe (1943) proposed that 'Jacksonian fits have their characteristic form of onset because the movements concerned are those that have the widest fields of low-threshold excitability' in the cortex.

These 'widest fields' can be demonstrated most clearly by stimulating unifocally with single rectangular pulses of long duration (5 ms); each pulse evokes only a brief flick of the responding parts. Figure 2.8 illustrates the results of such an experiment on a baboon (Liddell and Phillips, 1950). The threshold for the 'flick movements' of thumb and index was 1.2 mA, for foot 2.05 mA and for face 2.35 mA. With the strongest pulses (about 5 mA), most of the precentral gyrus and part of the postcentral gyrus were giving flick movements, yet these were confined to the distal parts of the opposite side of the body: 'clotted' contractions of all parts, which might have been expected *a priori*, were never seen. It is clear that the spinal and bulbar motoneurones concerned in these distal responses are *preferentially accessible* to cortical stimulation. They control the muscles that are used by the primates in their 'least automatic' activities.

It is interesting that Ferrier himself may have come very near to getting this result (1876, p. 132). When performing the experiments which led

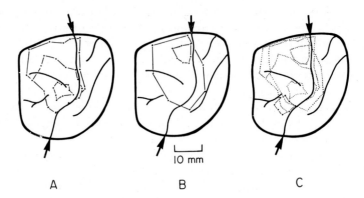

FIG. 2.8. Left Rolandic cortex of baboon. Arrows mark central fissure; precentral gyrus to left of fissure. Unifocal stimulation by single surface-cathodal rectangular current pulses, duration 4.5 ms.

A. Extent of areas for flick movement of thumb, index and minimus finger at strengths 1.2, 1.6 and 2.7 mA. At 1.2 mA, no other parts responded, and no responses were evoked from any part of the precentral or postcentral areas lying outside the innermost area on the map.

B and C show overlapping areas for other responses to stronger pulses.

B. Extent of areas for hallux and middle toe at strengths 2.05 and 4.7 mA.

C. Extent of area for angle of mouth, 2.35 mA. Dotted lines show overlapping areas of (A) and (B). *Scale*: 10 mm, below B.

him to prefer faradic to galvanic stimulation, he obtained, by galvanizing a particular part of the precentral gyrus, 'spasmodic and sudden jerks of the hand and forearm'. If he had weakened the stimulus to threshold, the response would surely have narrowed itself to thumb and index.

2.7   Dependence of maps, thresholds and preferential accessibility on the pyramidal tract

The question remains: are all the responses of the trunk and limbs that can be evoked by stimulation of the motor cortex (Woolsey's Ms1) mediated by the pyramidal tract which provides its most direct and conspicuous outflow? Although it was at first assumed that all responses to cortical stimulation were mediated by the PT, it was later discovered that some responses survived complete severance of both pyramids in the dog (Wertheimer and Lepage, 1896, cited by Sherrington, 1900b).

Comparative studies can contribute to the answer, in mammals in which the pyramidal decussation is small and the corticospinal fibres are few and short (Chapter 1, section 4). Figure 2.9 reproduces Woolsey's (1958) summaries of his group's maps for rabbit, rat and cat, which show that responses could be evoked in the same peripheries in all three species. In rat and cat, the corticospinal tract extends as far as the lumbar segments of the cord, but in the rabbit the tract is very poorly developed and ends at the third cervical segment. In the rabbit, therefore, the map of trunk and limbs is due to the cortico-rubro-spinal and cortico-reticulo-spinal outflow from the projection area.

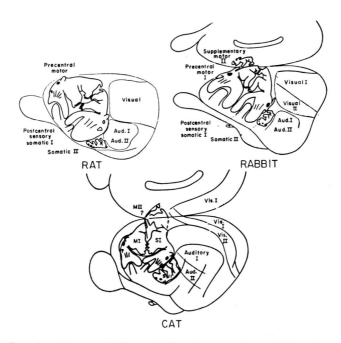

FIG. 2.9. Dorsolateral aspect of left cerebral hemispheres of rat, rabbit and cat. In rabbit and cat, medial aspect of hemisphere is also shown. *Precentral motor, MI and Supplementary motor, MII*: areas from which motor responses of opposite face, limbs and trunk can be evoked by electrical stimulation with 60 Hz sinusoidal alternating current. 'The orientations, proportions and relations of parts to one another are essentially correct. The diagrams are inadequate to the actual facts in that they do not indicate the successive overlap which is characteristic of the organization of the central nervous system.' (Woolsey, 1958.) The diagrams also show the cortical receiving areas for somatosensory inputs (somatic I and II, SI and SII), and for auditory and visual inputs (Aud. I and II, Vis. I and II) as mapped by the evoked potential technique. (Woolsey, 1958.)

In the brushtail possum or marsupial phalanger (*Trichosurus vulpecula*) the corticospinal tract is thicker, but extends only as far as the tenth thoracic segment. Hore and Porter (1971) have stimulated the possum's cortex with trains of 10 to 20 pulses (unifocal, surface-anodal) at 500 Hz. These evoke flick movements of contralateral parts, in the manner of single long pulses. Minimal stimulation of the forelimb area elicited flexion at elbow, forward flexion of the forelimb at shoulder, and flexion or extension of wrist and digits. These responses were abolished by pyramidotomy, but survived sectioning of the brainstem which spared only the paired pyramids. Near-threshold stimulation of the hindlimb area caused flick dorsiflexion of ankle and digits; stronger stimulation added flexion of knee and abduction of hip. All hindlimb responses survived pyramidotomy but were abolished by cutting the brainstem, sparing only the pyramids. Evidently the forelimb map depends on the integrity of the possum's short corticospinal tract; its hindlimb map depends on indirect pathways (cortico-reticulo-spinal etc.).

In primates, the extent to which the classical (faradic) motor map depends on the integrity of the PT, and is therefore an expression of the structure of the cortical origin of the tract, has also been studied by pyramidotomy. The surviving responses will give some measure of the relative contribution of the cortico-rubro-spinal and cortico-reticular projections to the results of electrical mapping of the precentral gyrus.

Lewis and Brindley (1965) mapped the baboon's cortex with 100 Hz a.c. in acute experiments, before and after cutting both medullary pyramids, and obtained a larger residuum of differentiated motor responses than the coarse synergies described by earlier workers (Tower, 1944). Although the thresholds of the responses of limbs and tail were raised, and the responses were more fatiguable, the pattern of localization in the precentral gyrus was similar to that seen before section. 'Though the number of kinds of response obtainable in any one animal was smaller after than before transecting the pyramids, most of the kinds of movement that could be obtained by near-threshold stimulation before the transection were obtained from at least one of our animals after it. . . . Conspicuous in their rarity or absence are movements of the thumb alone, extension of the elbow, flexion of the toes, and plantar flexion of the ankle.' Felix and Wiesendanger (1971) recorded electromyographically from distal muscles in monkeys. After pyramidotomy, some response was preserved, though the cortical threshold was raised, and longer temporal summation was needed.

Felix and Wiesendanger proved that the responses of the monkey's hand to single-pulse stimulation (Fig. 2.8) are mediated by the PT. They cut one PT and applied single pulses alternately to the motor areas of both hemispheres. The short-latency 'flick' response from the disconnected hand area was abolished, even when tested many weeks after the lesion, and even when the lesion involved only 30 per cent of the cross-section area of the PT; the control response of the other hand to stimulation of the opposite arm area remained normal.

The clearest demonstration of involvement of the pyramidal tract in producing some of the motor responses obtained by stimulation of the cerebral cortex in monkeys came from the studies of Woolsey *et al.* (1972). More than a year after complete section of pyramidal tract fibres on one side the thresholds for motor responses to stimulation of the apyramidal cortex was elevated at all points. But, more importantly, the responses to stimulation of this cortex never involved the distal joints of the forelimb and hindlimb—precisely those joints which were most readily moved by weakest stimuli from the normal control cortex on the other side (Fig. 2.10).

2.8 Summary

The contribution of this chapter to the model of Fig. 1.4 has been to trace the history of the discovery of the motor cortex ('middle level'); of the first attempts to discover the somatotopic arrangement of its clusters of corticofugal neurones; and of the first indications that these project partly to the segmental apparatus which coordinates simple patterns of movement, and increasingly, as one ascends the primate scale, to smaller and smaller groupings of output. The larger the repertory of smaller groupings, the greater the possibilities of combination and recombination by natural intracortical selector processes which cannot be evoked or imitated by repetitive (faradic) electrical stimulation.

The existence and approximate location of the area of densest motor outflow from the cerebral cortex of man towards the opposite half of the body was discovered by clinical and pathological study of cases of focal (Jacksonian) convulsion, and was later corroborated by electrical stimulation of the cortex in patients undergoing neurosurgical operations. Electrical stimulation of the brains of different mammals, and especially of primates, outlined their corresponding cortical areas with greater refinement and accuracy. This summary relates only to primates.

Within the general area are five sub-areas projecting towards arm, leg, trunk, face and head and eyes, and within each sub-area are projections towards the different muscle-groups; for example, in the case of the arm area, towards those which operate the joints of the arm, forearm and hand. Hughlings Jackson's clinical observations convinced him that the localization of the five sub-areas, and the localization within each sub-area, was overlapping; he supposed that the minutely patterned projections arising from *any* area or sub-area went towards muscle-groups of *all* parts of the body, but in different proportions from the different areas: thus, each area would have its *leading* projection towards a major target, for example towards a part of the hand, and *subordinate* projections, for example, towards more proximal parts of the arm and (more subordinate still) towards all other parts of the body. He distinguished such 'minute localization' from the 'abrupt localization' which he saw gaining ground in the writings of other workers, and which he rejected.

The results of 'faradic' mapping of the cortex of monkeys and apes gave no generally accepted evidence of overlap *between* the five sub-areas (inter-areal overlap) but we are aware of no critical experiment that

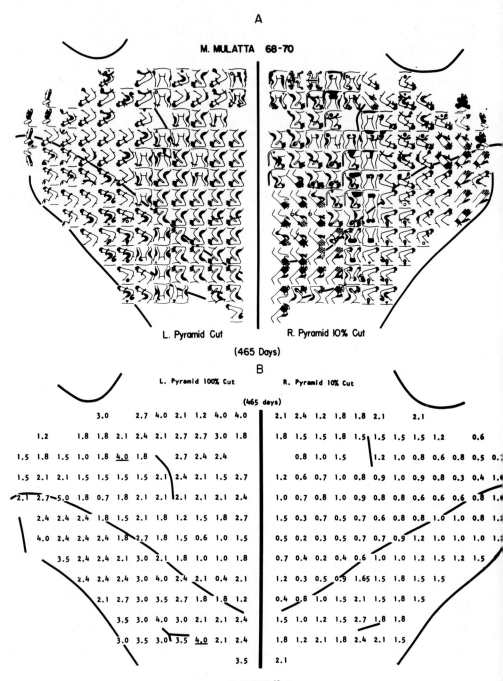

A

M. MULATTA 68-70

L. Pyramid Cut   R. Pyramid 10% Cut

(465 Days)

B

L. Pyramid 100% Cut   R. Pyramid 10% Cut

M. MULATTA 68-70
STIMULATION THRESHOLDS (mA, RMS, 60 cycles)

decisively ruled out any such overlap. Some degree of overlap *within* each of the five sub-areas (intra-areal overlap), however, is evident in every published map.

Though Ferrier believed that faradic stimulation was a tool which could evoke natural activity of the motor cortex, this belief has been untenable since the cortex has been stimulated in conscious man. The tool maps structure, not function. The responses taken by Ferrier as evidence of natural cortical activity were found by Sherrington to be the result of patterned activity in the segmental apparatus. Larger repertories of 'fractional' responses were found in the higher primates, their descending projections presumably by-passing the segmental apparatus and addressing the 'final common path' more directly. The restriction of such fractional responses to single muscles was not always demonstrable: it has certainly never been demonstrated that every muscle in the body can be activated in isolation by 'faradising' specific 'points' on the surface of the cortex.

We have to conclude that the method of minimal faradic stimulation of the pia-covered surface of the cortex, with response of muscles as indicator of excitation, has reached the limits of its resolving power. It cannot decide whether those minimal responses which involve more than one part of a limb depend on horizontal spread of current to adjacent 'abrupt' localizations, or whether the 'minute' intra-areal localization is actually overlapping. Thus, the minute structure of the fields of origin of the pyramidal projections cannot be reliably mapped by this method. The relative importance of direct electrical excitation of the corticofugal cells, and of synaptic actions brought to bear on them by direct excitation of afferent axons and cortical interneurones, is not revealed. Not only physical spread of stimulus, but also physiologically distributed excitation (Adrian, 1937), might blur the underlying corticofugal localization; on the other hand, that localization might be spuriously sharpened by coincidental stimulation of intracortical systems mediating 'lateral' and 'recurrent' inhibition. A further complication is that much of the projection arises from the walls of the deep central sulcus as well as from the surface of the precentral gyrus to which the electrodes are applied.

FIG. 2.10. A. Figurine map which illustrates the responses elicited by electrical stimulation of pre- and postcentral cortex of both hemispheres of a monkey 465 days after complete section of the left medullary pyramid at the level of the trapezoid body. There was some involvement in the lesion of the medial border of the right pyramid, probably less than 10 per cent of its fibres being interrupted. The consequence of pyramidal tract degeneration is a lack of indications of responses about distal joints of the fore- or hindlimb produced by stimulation of the left precentral cortex.

B. Threshold values for the stimulating current used to elicit the responses illustrated in (A). In each case the number refers to mA, RMS, of the 60-cycle sinusoidal current which produced the response.

(Woolsey et al., 1972.)

The projections towards different parts of the body are unequal in bulk. Those projecting towards hand, foot, mouth and tongue arise from wider areas, and these peripheries are *preferentially accessible* to cortical stimulation; they respond promptly to the weakest repetitive stimuli, and also to single 5 ms pulses. The responses of the hand to the single pulses are abolished by cutting the PT. Many of the responses which require a few seconds' temporal summation have been found to survive pyramidotomy, and are therefore mediated, at least in part, by indirect projections (cortico-rubro-spinal, cortico-reticulo-spinal). The PT thus emerges from these experiments as the 'hardest-wired' of the pathways leading from the cortex, and its corticospinal component as having its 'hardest wiring' to the segmental apparatus of the hand and foot.

Explanation of the facts of preferential accessibility, and resolution of the uncertainties about abrupt versus minute localization, need to be furthered by detailed studies of the cortical origin and subcortical connexions of the PT, by methods more discriminating than crude stimulation of the pia-covered convexity of the cortex and detection of the responses by inspection and palpation or by myography.

The last thirty years have seen the development of refined microanatomical and microphysiological methods, far surpassing, in their resolving power, any that were available to the pioneers. We shall illustrate the possibilities of these new methods by describing some of the advances that have been made so far by applying them to the PT, mainly in cats and primates: advances in knowledge of the properties of pyramidal tract neurones (PTN) and in explaining the actions of cortical stimulation upon them (Chapter 3); in the detailed description of the cortical origin and subcortical distribution of the PT (Chapters 4 and 5); and in identifying the excitatory and inhibitory inputs to the PT (Chapter 6). Such investigations, admittedly, do no more than specify the properties of a motor *apparatus*. Structure, however, offers possible clues to function (which we shall note along the way), and is an indispensable foundation for the investigations of function which we shall discuss in our final chapter.

3
Microphysiology of neurones of the pyramidal tract

3.1 Cells of origin of axons of the PT

These cells include the largest representatives of a type of neurone which is found in all areas of the neocortex and not only in the motor area. The large, pyramid-shaped perikarya of these motor cells were first stained and seen by Betz in 1874 and by Bevan Lewis in 1878; they were once commonly known as 'the giant cells of Betz', and they gave to the motor area its cytoarchitectonic name, 'area giganto-pyramidalis'. The name 'pyramidal' describes the shape of the perikaryon and owes nothing to the fact that pyramidal cells in this area contribute axons to the *pyramidal* tract; the PT, in turn, owes its name to the medullary *pyramid*, not to the fact that its axons come from pyramidal neurones. Since it is now known that the Betz cells form a small minority only of the pyramidal neurones of the motor area which contribute axons to the PT (Chapter 4), and that the majority is composed of smaller cells, it has become conventional to speak of 'pyramidal tract neurones' (PTN) and to divide the population into 'large' PTN and 'small' PTN; or 'fast' PTN and 'slow' PTN with respect to the different conduction velocities of their respective axons, the division (in the cat) being placed arbitrarily at 20 m s^{-1}.

The full ramification of the structure of cortical pyramidal neurones was not visualized before the development of the Golgi method from 1873–1886 (Fig. 3.1A, B, C). This method colours about 1 per cent only of the neurones in any preparation, but each of these is revealed in its entirety, against a clear background. The apex of the tapering perikaryon continues as the thick apical dendrite which runs at right-angles to the surface of the cortex, branches freely along its course and ends in profuse fine horizontal ramifications in the outermost lamina of the cortex. The dendrites are covered with spines, which were sometimes thought to be artefacts due to metallic precipitation, but whose reality was confirmed by

Ramón y Cajal by staining with methylene blue, 'a method which colours the cells and fibres while almost alive' (Ramón y Cajal, 1937). These spines have since been proved by electronmicroscopy to be areas of synaptic contact (Gray, 1959). The axon arises from the base of the pyramid (in the third or fifth layer in the case of small pyramidal neurones, in the fifth layer in the case of large) and runs vertically downwards into the sub-cortical white matter, sending several recurrent collateral branches back into the cortex (Fig. 3.1).

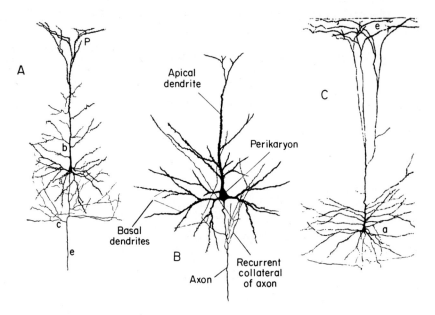

FIG. 3.1. A. Pyramidal neurone from neocortex of a rabbit, after Ramón y Cajal. The distance aP is about 1 mm. e, Axon; b,P, apical dendrite with branches covered with spines; a, soma and basal dendrites; c, recurrent collaterals of axon. The Golgi impregnation has picked out this cell and has not coloured the other neurones, axons, dendrites, neuroglial cells, and blood vessels with which the apparently empty spaces are in reality densely packed.
   B. Pyramidal neurone from sensorimotor cortex of cat (Sholl, 1956).
   C. Pyramidal neurone from human cortex (Ramón y Cajal).

3.2   Antidromic identification of PTN

In microphysiological experiments on cats, PTN have been identified by stimulating their axons in the ipsilateral medullary pyramid, and recording the antidromic impulse with a microelectrode located just outside the perikaryon (Fig. 3.2A). A corticospinal PTN can be identified by stimulating its axon in the contralateral corticospinal tract in the spinal cord.

In favourable conditions the microelectrode may penetrate the membrane without immediately killing the neurone, when the 'resting' membrane potential (about -70 mV) will be suddenly registered (Fig. 3.5), and the subsequent antidromic impulses recorded as positive-going action potentials up to 100 mV in amplitude (Fig. 3.5; Fig. 3.2B).

In extracellular records, antidromic impulses are recognizable by their constant latency, and by their ability to follow high frequencies of repetitive stimulation of the axon (> 500 Hz). When the latency is too short to include a synaptic delay (as in Fig. 3.2: conduction velocity of axon 44 m s^{-1}; latency 0.95 ms) the matter is not in doubt. When the latency is longer, another criterion needs to be added (Gordon and Miller, 1969). The period of unresponsiveness to antidromic stimulation, following the discharge of an orthodromic impulse by the PTN, must be equal to twice the conduction time plus the refractory period of the axon. This is because an earlier antidromic impulse would be blocked by collision with the orthodromic impulse, as explained in Fig. 3.3.

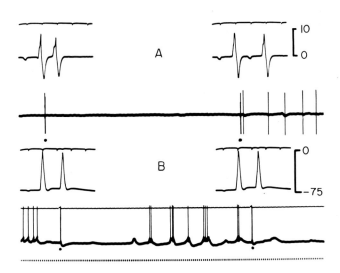

FIG. 3.2. Extracellular (A) and intracellular (B) recording from a fast PT neurone of a cat (conduction velocity 44 m s^{-1}).

A. Upper records show antidromic impulses evoked by stimulation of medullary pyramid. Time in ms; vertical scale 10 mV. Continuous record shows same pairs of antidromic impulses (marked by dots) and background discharge of impulses on slower time scale. Time, 10 ms (bottom of figure).

B. After penetration of the neurone. Paired antidromic impulses (above), and also on continuous record (below, marked by dots). Continuous record shows waves of excitatory synaptic depolarization of the neurone, some of which reach the firing level (-51 mV) and generate one or more impulses; also, waves of inhibitory synaptic hyperpolarization. Vertical scale 75 mV.

(Phillips, 1961.)

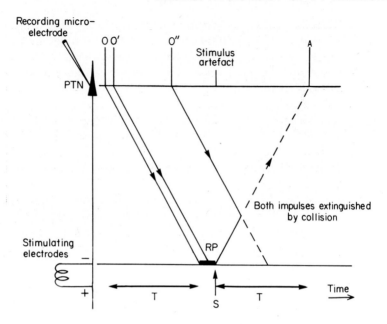

Fig. 3.3. Blocking by collision of an antidromic impulse by a preceding orthodromic impulse in a PTN.

Stimulation of axon at time S.

An orthodromic impulse arising in the PTN at time 0 (or at any earlier time) will not prevent the setting up of the antidromic impulse at time S and will not prevent the antidromic impulse from reaching the PTN at time A.

An orthodromic impulse arising at time 0' will make the axon refractory at the site of the stimulating cathode at time S; the stimulus will not therefore set up an antidromic impulse.

An orthodromic impulse arising at some later time, e.g. 0'', will collide with the antidromic impulse at the appropriate time and place. Both impulses will be extinguished, so no antidromic pulse will reach the PTN at time A.

T = Conduction time. RP = refractory period.

Minimum interval 0A = 2T+RP.

The top line shows the stimulus artefact and antidromic impulse as they would appear on the oscilloscope during an actual experiment: A would appear after 0, but not after 0', 0'', etc.

In intracellular records, the antidromic impulse can be recognized beyond doubt by a further criterion. As seen in the continuous record of Fig. 3.2B, the antidromic impulses (marked by dots) arise from a level of membrane potential below the normal 'firing level', without any prior synaptic depolarization; such depolarization precedes each one of the fifteen orthodromic impulses recorded during the same period (see also Fig. 3.5).

As it travels from the axon into the soma of the PTN, the antidromic impulse successively invades two distinct regions of excitable membrane, A and B, which can be tentatively identified with the initial segment of the axon (A) and the soma and proximal dendrites (B). Transmission from A to B may fail at high repetition rates. This is illustrated in Fig. 3.4, which is fully described in its legend.

3.3 The membrane properties of pyramidal tract neurones

Takahashi (1965) made intracellular recordings from identified PT neurones in cats. Although he obtained some intracellular records from slow PTN (axonal conduction velocity 11 to 18 $m s^{-1}$), he obtained a much larger sample of fast PTN (axonal conduction velocities above 21 $m s^{-1}$; mean velocity about 60 $m s^{-1}$). Although the cells with slower axonal conduction velocities tended to have lower membrane potentials after impalement than the cells with fast axons, their antidromic spikes were larger, i.e. they showed a greater overshoot of the spike potential. In addition, the antidromic spikes of these PTN with slow axons had a longer duration than the spikes produced in neurones with fast axons (1.52 ± 0.23 ms compared with 0.71 ± 0.20 ms). The after-potentials also differed. PTN with fast axons showed a depolarizing wave (delayed depolarization) after the spike, whereas the slow axon cells did not show this. The delayed depolarization was also produced when a spike was generated in the PTN by a brief pulse of current passed across the membrane through the intracellular recording electrode. It was then followed by a hyperpolarizing after-potential, the amplitude and duration of which varied with the axonal conduction velocity of the cell studied. The after-potential in fast PTN was usually larger in amplitude and shorter in duration than that of the slow PTN cells. Current pulses superimposed on the hyperpolarization revealed that an increase in membrane conductance accompanied the hyperpolarization in the fast PTN and that the amplitude of the hyperpolarization was increased during imposed depolarization of the cell membrane.

When the current steps were applied in a depolarizing or a hyperpolarizing direction to the membranes of PTN, voltage changes with an overshoot (and an undershoot at termination of the step) were induced. Over a range of about 20 mV in the hyperpolarizing direction, the relationship between the amplitude of the current step and the amplitude of the voltage change was approximately linear for both fast and slow PTN. But non-linearities usually developed when more hyperpolarization was produced. Hyperpolarizing pulses of current within the 20 mV range were used to estimate the effective membrane resistances of fast and slow PTN having resting membrane potentials of more than −58 mV. There was a wide scatter of membrane resistance measurements from 1.5 to 15 $M\Omega$, but the cells with longer antidromic response latencies had significantly higher resistances (10.1 ± 2.5 $M\Omega$ compared with 5.9 ± 2.8 $M\Omega$). For the fast PTN group there was a linear correlation between membrane resistance and antidromic latency. The membrane time constants could not be measured satisfactorily from these records because of the overshoot and undershoot phenomena which meant the time course of potential change was not exponential. Nevertheless, a rough estimate of the approximate time constants of these cells showed variation from 3 to 15 ms with average values for the fast and slow groups which were not significantly different (6.7 ± 2.2 compared with 7.6 ± 2.3 ms).

Taken together, all these observations tend to support the concept of two groups of PTN in cats (Bishop et al., 1953; Lance, 1954; Lance and Manning, 1954). On the one hand, large cells with a large surface area have a low total membrane resistance, a brief spike duration and a brief after-hyperpolarization. To the pyramidal tract these cells contribute axons with fast conduction velocity. The small cells, with a small surface area, have a high total membrane resistance, a longer spike duration and after-hyperpolarization. They send slowly conducting axons into the pyramidal tract.

Of the other studies on the membrane properties of PTN in the cat (Koike et al., 1968a; Koike et al., 1968b; Koike et al., 1972) one that may be related to the different functions of cells with different conduction velocities is the study of the repetitive firing produced by maintained current stimulation through an intracellular electrode (Koike et al., 1970: see also Creutzfeldt et al., 1964). Like motoneurones (Kernell, 1966a), PTN with high stable resting membrane potentials were shown to maintain repetitive firing during long depolarizing current pulses. The initially high firing rate declined during the first 100 ms of the pulse (adaptation) and thereafter maintained a more or less steady rate which depended on the strength of the applied current. In general, PTN with slowly conducting axons were more sensitive to the passage of weak, near threshold currents across their membranes but, when the stimulus was strong enough to excite the cell, those with fast axons responded sooner after the onset of the current. Once made to fire, the impulse intervals tended to be longer for the slow PTN; but at a similar rate of firing there was much more variability in the impulse intervals for the fast PTN. It is perhaps significant that, in response to transmembrane current, 'fast PT cells showed more clearly than slow cells the tendency of double discharge with short intervals of less than 10 ms ("doublet") which were often far below the mean interval of the series' (Koike et al., 1970). The rate and degree of adaptation of the discharge of fast PTN was considerably greater than that of the slow PTN.

When maintained rates of firing in response to prolonged current steps were analysed, it was found that slow PTN showed a smaller increase in rate than fast cells in response to increases in current above rheobase. Maximum firing rates produced in the secondary range of higher current intensities (Kernell, 1966b) were lower for slow PTN (of the order of 250 impulses per second) than for fast PTN (of the order of 400 to 450 impulses per second). All these properties led Koike *et al.* (1970) to postulate that the fast and slow PTN might behave in a phasic ('kinetic') and tonic

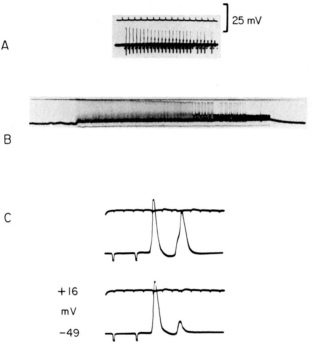

FIG. 3.4. A. Failure of antidromic impulses to travel from the A segment (? initial segment of axon) into the B segment (? soma and dendrites) of the membrane of a fast PTN (axonal conduction velocity 25 m s⁻¹). Extracellular recording. Medullary pyramid stimulated at 172 Hz. After the 7th impulse, A-B transmission becomes delayed, as shown by inflections on ascending (positive-going) phases of action potentials. The 20th, 24th and 26th impulses do not get beyond the A segment. Time 100 Hz. (Phillips, 1959.)

B. Intracellular recording from a fast PTN (conduction velocity 25 m s⁻¹). Antidromic stimulation of the medullary pyramid at 180 Hz for 1.2 s. After 0.7 s of stimulation, A-B transmission frequently fails. This A-B block is favoured by a concomitant synaptic depolarization of the membrane (see Fig. 3.6A) from −63 mV at the beginning of the stimulation to −54 mV at the end. After stimulation ceased, the membrane potential returned to its initial level. (Phillips, 1959.)

C. Intracellular recording from a slow PTN (conduction velocity 11 m s⁻¹). At critical interval of 2.4 ms between the two stimuli to the medullary pyramid, A-B transmission was sometimes partially blocked (upper record) and sometimes completely blocked (lower record). (Phillips, 1961.)

manner respectively in response to a particular, similar synaptic drive. But, in normal function of the cerebral cortex, the synaptic convergence on to these different cells may be quite different and the interaction of large PTN on small differs from that of small on large (Armstrong, 1965; Takahashi *et al.*, 1967). So the membrane properties of the cell need not be the principal determinants of firing patterns.

In intracellular recordings we may recognize rhythmic firing generated by the PTN's own pacemaker membrane, which is presumed to be located in the initial unmyelinated segment of its axon. In certain unmyelinated crab axons Hodgkin (1948) provided an explicit and beautiful model for the pacemaker membranes of central neurones and peripheral receptors. The model responded to a steady flow of depolarizing (outward) current across the membrane by a rhythmic discharge of impulses. As the current was increased smoothly, so the frequency of discharge rose smoothly, from 5 to 150 Hz. The frequency was proved to depend on the rate of growth of an active local depolarizing response of the membrane, and not on the brief refractory period.

In the regular discharge rhythms illustrated in the continuous records of Fig. 3.5A, A', and C, each impulse is preceded by such a sloping depolarization, which may be called a 'pacemaker potential' by analogy with cardiac pacemaker fibres (Phillips 1961). When this reaches the firing level (Eyzaguirre and Kuffler, 1955) the membrane discharges an impulse and repolarizes, and the cycle recurs. The steeper the rise of the pacemaker potential, the sooner the firing level is reached, and the higher the frequency of discharge. Theoretically, an interpolated antidromic impulse should 're-set' the rhythm and thereby prove that the pacemaker is intrinsic to the PTN. The experiment will succeed if the rhythm is regular, and the threshold of the PT axon is low enough (because of proximity to the stimulating cathode) to require only very weak stimuli to the medullary pyramid (Fig. 3.5C). Strong stimuli excite large numbers of PT axons, whose recurrent collaterals (Fig. 3.1) exert complicating synaptic actions on the impaled PTN, and confuse the picture. Thus, exact re-setting is not evident in Fig. 3.5A, A'. In the ideal experiment, the PTN would be stimulated in isolation by a pulse injected through the intracellular microelectrode.

In the experiment illustrated in Fig. 3.5A, A', the depolarizing current which determined the rhythmic firing of impulses was an artefact and was probably due to mechanical stimulation of the soma-dendritic membrane by pressure or traction by the microelectrode. In this record the maximum membrane potential was -57 mV, about 13 mV lower than in the later, less traumatic impalement of the same PTN (-70 mV in Fig. 3.5B'). The frequency of discharge (40 to 65 Hz), however, is by no means abnormal (e.g. in PTN of monkeys making conditioned movements for reward: Chapter 7), and may be regarded as the natural response to such a degree of depolarization, which would normally be generated by excitatory synaptic action and not by mechanical injury.

In the PTN, the frequency of firing would not depend solely on the rhythmic property of the pacemaker membrane. It would also be subject to the effects of after-hyperpolarization following each impulse and to the complicating effects of recurrent excitatory and inhibitory synaptic actions impinging on the membrane.

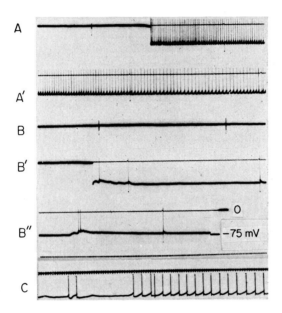

FIG. 3.5. Two penetrations of a fast PTN (conduction velocity 30 m s⁻¹) by a recording micropipette. Single pulses delivered to medullary pyramid at one-second intervals evoked antidromic impulses (marked by dots). First penetration during record A, shown by downward (negative) deflexion of baseline (maximum membrane potential -57 mV; see calibration at end of B″). At instant of puncture PTN began to discharge at 65 Hz.

An impulse was discharged each time the pacemaker potential reached the firing level (-52 mV). Record A′ is continuation of A, and ends 2.6 s after the penetration; after a further 16 s of repetitive firing at 40 Hz the micropipette was withdrawn from the neurone.

After an interval, it was advanced again during B and B′, re-crossing the membrane during B′. This second impalement was evidently less traumatic than the first: maximum membrane potential was -70 mV, and regular rhythmic firing was absent, as it had been throughout the periods of extracellular recording. Occasional synaptic potentials, some reaching the firing level (-52 mV) and generating orthodromic impulses (as in B″) occurred during several minutes' continuous recording. (Phillips, 1959.)

C. A fast PTN (conduction velocity 51 m s⁻¹) firing regularly at about 25 Hz. An interpolated antidromic impulse has re-set the rhythm. (Phillips, 1956a.)

There is, however, abundant evidence of rhythmic activity imposed on the PTN by structures lying upstream, e.g. by thalamocortical projections (Andersen and Andersson, 1968). Such a rhythmic input can be readily recognized in the continuous intracellular recording of Fig. 3.2B, and contrasted with the intrinsic pacemaker activity which is illustrated at the beginning of that record. The hump-like waves of depolarization represent surges of synaptic excitation, paced by some thalamocortical mechanism which is extrinsic to the PTN. Each wave brings the intrinsic pacemaker rapidly towards its firing level, and sometimes makes it fire repetitively. Possible sources of such afferent activity will be considered in Chapter 6.

3.4   Microphysiology and micropharmacology of synapses on PTN

The complex, branched dendritic surface of the PTN is richly endowed with synapses. There is great need for quantitative information of the connexions made with the PTN in the cat and other species (Chang, 1951) by the axons of other brain structures. Regional distribution of these synapses may be very important functionally and the potency of a particular input may depend very much on its connectivity with proximal or distal branches of the dendrites, with pedunculated or sessile spines or with a large or a small area of the dendritic surface. Details of the physiological actions exerted on PTN by synapses of different origins will be deferred to Chapter 6. Our immediate objective is to show that both excitatory and inhibitory synapses are applied to the membranes of PTN in the cat, and to consider some experiments that throw light on the identity of the chemical transmitters that are involved.

While recording intracellularly from a PTN, some of its synaptic inputs can be activated artificially in one of two convenient ways. One is to stimulate the medullary pyramid with pulses of different strengths, which implicate more or fewer PT axons. The pulses are at first strong enough to excite the axon of the impaled PTN for the purpose of antidromic identification and classification by conduction velocity. They can then be weakened, below threshold for this axon, so that the synaptic actions of the recurrent collaterals of neighbouring PTN can be studied without interference from the antidromic impulse and the after-potentials of the impaled cell (Phillips, 1959, 1961). The other plan is to stimulate the cortical surface, which was shown by Phillips (1956b, 1961) and by Sawa et al. (1963) to result in complex depolarizing and hyperpolarizing effects on the PTN.

An experiment of the first sort is illustrated by Fig. 3.6A, B. In A a 'fast' PTN (conduction velocity 25 ms^{-1}) responded to a single-volley activation of the recurrent axon collaterals of its neighbours by an excitatory postsynaptic potential (EPSP) which began 5.5 ms after the start of the volley in the medullary pyramid. In B, another fast PTN (conduction velocity 42 m s^{-1}) was exposed to 45 volleys in the recurrent collaterals of its neighbours, at a frequency of 420 Hz. The initial EPSP was cut short by a prolonged and profound inhibitory postsynaptic potential (IPSP) which lasted for about 0.5 s. The membrane potential was hyperpolarized from -60 to -74 mV.

Figure 3.6C shows synaptic potentials evoked by cortical stimulation with single long pulses, duration 10.5 ms, in a fast PTN (conduction velocity 38 m s^{-1}) which lay in the wall of the cruciate sulcus, 4.5 mm from the convexity of the overlying posterior sigmoid gyrus. Surface-anodal and surface-cathodal pulses excited this cell directly (at the 'make' and 'break' respectively of the long pulse), and both evoked an EPSP. The surface-cathodal pulse, however, evoked an IPSP following the pulse (Fig. 3.6C, b), presumably by selectively exciting an intracortical (or U-fibre) inhibitory pathway at some point between the deep-lying PTN and the convexity of the gyrus.

Excitatory and inhibitory synaptic actions can be detected indirectly in extracellular recordings from PTN. The excitatory synaptic actions may be powerful enough to initiate a discharge of impulses by an initially 'silent' neurone; weaker actions can be detected as an increase in frequency of discharge of a neurone that is already firing. The inhibitory synaptic actions cannot be detected by the extracellular method unless the PTN is already firing: they can then be measured in terms of the resulting reduction in its discharge frequency. In the case of polysynaptic inputs to the PTN, however, the method cannot distinguish effects due to post-synaptic changes in the PTN membrane (EPSP and IPSP) from changes in the prevailing patterns of excitatory and inhibitory input; thus, the discharge of a PTN could be slowed by reduction of a prevailing excitatory input (inhibition by disfacilitation), or accelerated by reduction of a prevailing inhibitory input (facilitation by disinhibition).

Much work has been done to try to specify the transmitter substances that are responsible for generating these EPSPs and IPSPs in the PTN. A major advance was D. R. Curtis' invention of multi-barrelled micro-pipettes for applying putative transmitters and their specific antagonists as closely as possible to the postsynaptic membrane (Curtis and Crawford, 1969). The method by-passes the blood-brain barrier, and produces steeply rising local concentrations of the substances, but it is not yet possible to deliver them entirely within the sub-synaptic cleft. One barrel records the discharge of impulses extracellularly: the others contain various candidates for the excitatory and inhibitory transmitterships. These are retained within their barrels by appropriate backing currents, and delivered iontophoretically by appropriate current pulses. Such experiments have found that 80 per cent of cats' PTN are excited by acetylcholine and some inputs to PTN are therefore from cholinergic neurones. The enzymes for acetylcholine synthesis have been found in synaptosomes isolated from the cerebral cortex (Whittaker, 1964).

The prolonged and profound inhibitions of cats' PTN are remarkable for their lack of sensitivity to strychnine, which is a potent antagonist for the shorter-lasting IPSPs of spinal motoneurones, at which site strychnine-

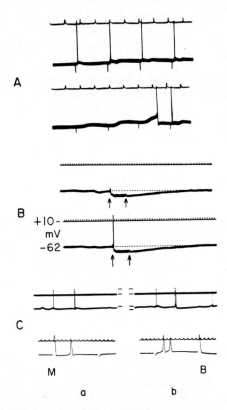

FIG. 3.6. Synaptic excitation and inhibition of PTN.

A. Intracellular records from a fast PTN, axonal conduction velocity 25 m s⁻¹, membrane potential −63 mV (same PTN as in Fig. 3.4B). Stimulation of medullary pyramid at 48 Hz. In upper record, stimuli were supraliminal for axon of this PTN. Following the 2nd, 3rd and 4th antidromic impulses are EPSPs, latency 5.5 ms. In lower record, pyramidal stimulus was reduced to about 60 per cent of its previous strength. The first three stimuli evoked incrementing EPSPs; the third generated an orthodromic impulse on reaching −49 mV. The next stimulus evoked an antidromic impulse and a smaller EPSP. Time 100 Hz. (Phillips, 1961.)

B. Fast PTN, conduction velocity 42 m s⁻¹. Repetitive stimulation of medullary pyramid, subliminal for this axon, with about 45 pulses at 420 Hz (between arrows). Intracellular recording with micropipette filled with 0.6 M K$_2$SO$_4$. Initial EPSP generated orthodromic impulse in lower record but not in upper record. In both records, EPSP cut short by sudden onset of IPSP which lasted for about 0.5 s. Time 100 Hz.

sensitive inhibition is probably transmitted by the amino acid glycine, since the inhibitory action of glycine is also blocked by strychnine (Curtis, 1969). But strychnine applied to the surface of the motor cortex causes abnormal synchronous discharge of PTN and 'epileptic' jerking movements can result. So some intracortical neuronal networks must be subject to strychnine-sensitive inhibition. The discharges of PTN are suppressed by γ-amino-butyric acid (Krnjević and Schwartz, 1967) and this pharmacological action, and also the action of the physiologically activated inhibitory synapses, are antagonized by bicuculline (Curtis and Felix, 1971). Possibly, therefore, a direct inhibitory transmitter for actions on the PTN surface is γ-amino-butyric acid.

3.5 The physiology of pyramidal synapses

Once caused to fire a nerve impulse, a PTN will influence the neurones with which it is synaptically linked. The most accessible of these synaptic influences for physiological study is the excitatory connection of corticomotoneuronal fibres with spinal motoneurones in primates. Examination of the synaptic potentials produced in cervical alpha motoneurones of the baboon by repetitive, weak, surface anodal stimulation of motor points in the cerebral cortex revealed increasing effectiveness of successive stimuli in the repetitive train (Landgren et al., 1962a). Not only did successive synaptic potentials summate because each depolarizing wave began before repolarization from the previous wave was complete, but the amplitude of the waves themselves increased (Fig. 3.7). It was reasoned that this effect could not have been produced by an increase in the number of corticomotoneuronal fibres activated by the successive stimuli because the amplitude of the pyramidal tract volleys set up by these repetitive stimuli showed no appreciable changes with repetitive stimuli (Fig. 3.8). Therefore, the increase in amplitude of the synaptic potentials was considered to be due to an increase in transmitting potency at the corticomotoneuronal synapses.

C. Intracellular recording from fast PTN (conduction velocity 38 m s^{-1}) located in posterior wall of cruciate sulcus, 4.5 mm deep from convexity of posterior sigmoid gyrus. Sweeps (below, time 1000 Hz) expand the central 18 ms of the continuous records (above, time 100 Hz). Rectangular current pulses of 10.5 ms duration were applied unifocally to surface of posterior sigmoid gyrus at point of entry of recording microelectrode: anodal (a) and cathodal (b). At threshold 0.2 mA (not shown) the pulses excited the PTN directly, at the make of the anodal pulse, at the break of the cathodal pulse. The responses illustrated are to pulses of 1.0 mA. These also show direct excitation at make (M) and break (B), but the anodal pulse (a) evoked in addition an EPSP which began about 3 ms after the start of the pulse, and generated an impulse. The cathodal pulse (b) evoked an earlier EPSP which generated two impulses, and was followed by an IPSP (compare upper records (a) and (b)). (Phillips, 1956b.)

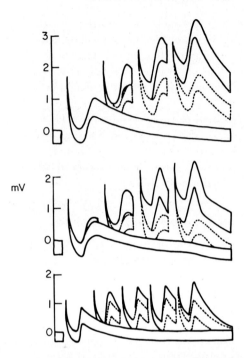

FIG. 3.7. Each set of tracings, from superimposed sweep records from single motoneurones shows, below (full line) monosynaptic potential evoked by single S +0.2 ms cortical pulse; above (full line), series of monosynaptic potentials evoked by the same pulses repeated at 200 Hz. Interrupted line shows the response expected from mere addition of the monosynaptic curves. Time: 5 ms separates shock artefacts. Above, median motoneurone, membrane potential −70 mV, shocks 1.3 mA. Centre, median motoneurone, membrane potential −72 mV, shocks 1.9 mA; note inhibitory action following crest of excitatory action in last response of repetitive series. Below, ulnar motoneurone, membrane potential −63 mV, shocks 1.3 mA. (Landgren *et al.* 1962a.)

When corticospinal neurones were made to fire repetitively by weak, single, long (5 to 10 ms) surface-anodal current pulses, EPSPs generated in cervical motoneurones sometimes showed clearly separate waves of depolarization. These waves each had a monosynaptic form and they, too, showed evidence of increasing synaptic potency of the successive volleys which must have been generated by the long current pulses. Strong, brief pulse stimulation has also been shown to cause repetitive discharge in populations of pyramidal tract axons (Fig. 3.15, Patton and Amassian, 1954) and sample records of the repetitive discharges of individual pyramidal tract neurones have been made by Kernell and Wu Chien-ping (1967a) (Fig. 3.19). With a strong cortical stimulus generating such repetitive firing, some of the later waves of the complex EPSP could be larger than the first monosynaptic wave (Kernell and Wu Chien-ping, 1967b).

In those experiments, the pyramidal tract volleys generated after the first tended to be smaller than the first. So recruitment of corticomotoneuronal axons was unlikely to be the explanation of the increasing size of successive EPSPs.

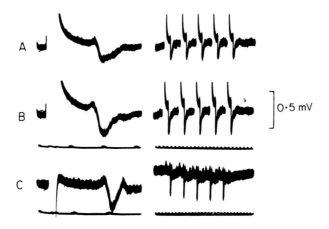

Fig. 3.8. Superimposed records of waves in lateral corticospinal tract, caused by single and repetitive surface-anodal shocks (duration 0.2 ms), to precentral gyrus near central fissure and about equidistant between superior and inferior precentral fissures; negative deflexion downwards. A. Stimulus 2.0 mA, single and repetitive, 250 Hz. B. Same experiment, stimulus 3.25 mA; time marker ms, for fast and slow sweeps for A and B. C. Another experiment, C7-8 level; singles 2.9 mA, tetani 2.8 mA; 250 Hz; time marker ms. (Landgren *et al.*, 1962a.)

It remained possible that some local interneurones in the spinal cord were caused to fire by the repetitive corticospinal volleys. A contribution of these local discharges could have caused the growth of the EPSPs either by contributing postsynaptic potentials or by influencing the corticomotoneuronal endings by a presynaptic mechanism. Addition of postsynaptic potentials caused by excitatory spinal interneurones was an unlikely mechanism because no separate waves of depolarization which could not be accounted for by repetitive corticomotoneuronal firing were seen. In addition, the maximum size of the complex synaptic potential achieved with repetitive corticomotoneuronal firing was related to the size of the initial wave of depolarization in a way that allowed the maximum size to be accounted for completely by repetitive firing in the same axons (Kernell and Wu Chien-ping, 1967b). Thus, although local interneurones may certainly be activated by repetitive discharge in corticospinal fibres and although, under some conditions, complex EPSPs produced over polysynaptic pathways may be recorded in spinal motoneurones after cortical stimulation (Phillips and Porter, 1964), these effects are unlikely to account for the growth of monosynaptic EPSPs seen with repetitive discharges in corticospinal axons.

In all the experiments on increasing effectiveness of corticomotoneuronal activity with repetitive firing, large numbers of pyramidal tract axons were activated by the stimulus and relatively large postsynaptic potentials were produced by the colonies of corticomotoneuronal fibres included. The sizes of subsequent postsynaptic potential waves were therefore influenced by changes in the membrane potential of the postsynaptic cell caused by preceding events. In general, the effect of this influence would have been expected to reduce the size of the potential change caused by the same quantity of transmitter producing the same change in post-synaptic conductance, because the subsequent ionic movement would be across a membrane already partly depolarized.

Shapovalov (1975) has drawn attention to the fact that the growth of successive monosynaptic EPSPs achieved by repetitive stimulation of the bulbar pyramids, while present, is less than the growth seen when the cortex is stimulated. With the limited number of observations available, it is not possible to evaluate the many factors which could affect the successive increases in EPSP size. Analysis of the contributions of cortical recruitment, interneuronal discharge or increased transmitter potency are further complicated by the fact that the degree of increase in cortico-motoneuronal EPSP size with repetitive stimulation varies in different motoneurones. Shapovalov (1975) reported that, when the EPSPs were large (in motoneurones supplying distally acting muscles) frequency potentiation was less evident than when the EPSPs were small (in the motoneurones of proximal muscles).

To study further the phenomenon of increasing effectiveness of suc-cessive volleys in a train of corticomotoneuronal impulses it would be desirable to examine the changes in synaptic potential produced by trains of impulses in single corticomotoneuronal fibres activated independently. It has not been possible to study the changes in size of unitary cortico-motoneuronal EPSPs (produced by a single impulse in a single cortico-motoneuronal fibre) in relation to preceding impulse traffic in that same fibre. But, with minimal stimuli applied to the cerebral cortex, the changes in very small corticomotoneuronal EPSPs which occur as a result of pre-ceding activity have been investigated. These small EPSPs, on occasion, may have been unitary because of the chance activation, within the population of corticospinal fibres, of only one corticomotoneuronal fibre making synapses with the test motoneurone. But, more often, the effects occurred by activation of a presumed small number of corticomotoneuronal fibres. In these experiments the possibility of cortical recruitment is reduced to a minimum. Thus, in Fig. 3.9, the paired small CST volleys, which had to be detected and recorded by computer-averaging technique, are identical in amplitude and waveform.

When two weak stimuli, each capable of causing a small D volley in corticospinal fibres (cf. section 3.6), were applied to the cerebral cortex, the corticomotoneuronal EPSP produced by the second stimulus was larger than the EPSP produced by the first if the interval between the two stimuli was short (Porter and Hore, 1969; Porter, 1970). The relationship between the size of the second EPSP and the duration of the interval between paired stimuli was investigated systematically. The relative increase in amplitude was termed facilitation, a name which had been used previously to describe the similar increase in size of end-plate potentials observed under some conditions at the neuromuscular junction. Facilitation of the synaptic response was defined as the difference in amplitude of the first and second depolarizing responses, expressed as a fraction of the amplitude of the first response (Fig. 3.9). Hence, for the pair of EPSPs,

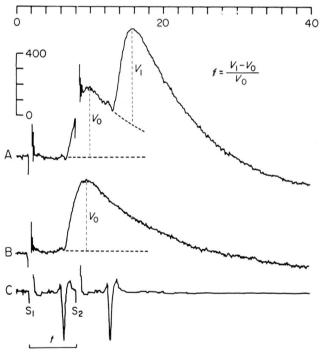

FIG. 3.9. Averaged EPSPs produced by single and paired cortical shocks. The Figure is redrawn from Fig. 6 of Porter and Hore (1969) to indicate the method of measuring facilitation (f) at an interval (t) between two cortical stimuli (S_1 and S_2). A indicates the average response of the cell to sixty-four applications of the paired stimuli at a rate of 1 s^{-1}. B indicates the average response of the cell to sixty-four applications of S_1 alone and C is the average corticospinal volley recorded simultaneously with the registration of A. Facilitation: $f = (V_1 - V_0)/v_0$. (Porter, 1970.)

V_0 and V^1, set up by each of two identical D waves in the corticospinal tract, the facilitation (f) would be calculated from the expression:

$$f = \frac{V_1 - V_0}{V_0}.$$

Since most of the EPSPs generated by weak stimuli were very small, computer averages of the responses were used to allow accurate measurements of amplitude and waveform to be made in the presence of physical and biological noise. Paired corticomotoneuronal EPSPs were generated with a series of different separations between the stimuli producing the train and, for each interval, the facilitation was calculated. These experiments were conducted in lumbar motoneurones of the anaesthetized monkey but similar results have been obtained for corticomotoneuronal influences on cervical motoneurones (Muir, 1975; Muir and Porter, 1976). Facilitation of the EPSPs varied in its magnitude from cell to cell. But the degree of this facilitation could not be related to the properties of the post-synaptic cell or the particular muscle innervated. All motoneurones which received a monosynaptic EPSP from the cerebral cortex exhibited facilitation of the amplitude of this EPSP with short intervals between the conditioning and the test stimulus.

In spite of the variation in the degree of facilitation from one set of corticomotoneuronal synapses to another, an average time-course of facilitation has been measured for a large number of motoneurones. This average facilitation time-course may be described approximately by a decaying exponential function with a time constant of 10 ms. (Porter, 1970; Muir and Porter, 1973). Figure 3.10A shows the corticomotoneuronal facilitation measured at a number of different intervals in 4 lumbar motoneurones and gives an indication of the range of variation encountered in a larger sample of different cells. Figure 3.10B plots the average facilitation measured in 24 lumbar motoneurones. The dashed line is the function $f = 0.85 \exp(-i_{\mathrm{T}}/10)$ where i_{T} is the interval in ms between the two stimuli. It shows that, on average, nerve impulses in corticomotoneuronal fibres not only produced a monosynaptic EPSP in motoneurones but also caused a change in efficacy at the synapses which was at first large and then declined at a rate which left no detectable facilitation after 50 ms. Impulses arriving in the same corticomotoneuronal fibres at intervals less than 50 ms from their predecessors would be more effective in depolarizing the postsynaptic cell than their predecessors. For roughly one third of the cells examined, the decay of facilitation did not show a smooth time-course but had a slight hump at an interval of about 5 ms. This elevated the observed average facilitation at the 5 ms interval above the theoretical line of smooth exponential decay.

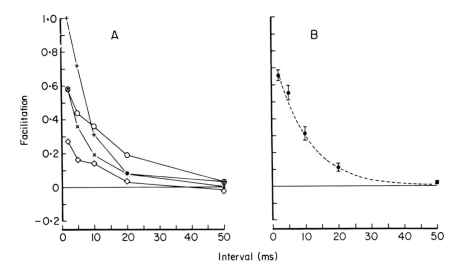

FIG. 3.10. Facilitation of the second EPSP of a pair with respect to the first, as a function of the time interval (i_T) between the two. A indicates the time-course of facilitation of corticomotoneuronal EPSPs in four different motoneurones. B shows facilitation values obtained by averaging over twenty-four cells, with vertical bars indicating ± 1 S.E. of mean. The dashed line is the function $f = 0.85 \exp (-i_T/10)$. (Muir and Porter, 1973.)

Under natural circumstances pyramidal tract neurones in monkeys have been shown to produce bursts of nerve impulses in relation to muscular contraction and movements of contralateral limbs (see Chapter 7). With some natural movements, the frequency of nerve impulse discharge during movement reached 100 Hz, and this could occur in pyramidal tract neurones with high conduction velocities. Conceivably some such pyramidal tract neurones could make corticomotoneuronal connections and their synapses would then be subjected to a number of sequential discharges with many intervals short enough to produce considerable facilitation. It was reasoned that the influence of this might be significant in rapidly promoting depolarization of motoneurones and efficiently bringing them to their firing level (Phillips and Porter, 1964). But it was not known precisely how the facilitation produced by one nerve impulse in a corticomotoneuronal fibre would be affected by the several impulses which could have occurred in that fibre in the preceding 50 ms. Accordingly, Muir and Porter (1973) tested the effect, on the amplitude of a minimal EPSP produced by a volley in a few corticomotoneuronal fibres, of two similar preceding volleys separated by a number of time intervals. They found that each of the first two volleys from a triplet of stimuli produced some facilitation of the amplitude of the EPSP generated by the third volley, provided that the intervals between the volleys were less than 50 ms. Figure 3.11 gives an example of the EPSP recordings from which measurements were made and Fig. 3.12 shows the average results obtained by expressing the facilitation of the third EPSP (V_2) with respect to the first (V_0) as a function of conditioning (first) interval and test (second) interval between the stimuli.

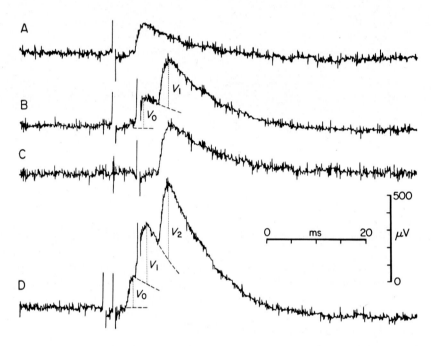

FIG. 3.11. Average corticomotoneuronal EPSPs produced in the one motoneurone by 256 repetitions of one, two or three identical cortical shocks. A indicates the average response to a single stimulus. B is the average response to a pair of stimuli spaced 5 ms apart. C is the result of subtracting trace A from trace B and indicates the time-course of the second of the EPSPs in B. A comparison of trace C with trace A allows an assessment of the increase in amplitude of the second response in B. D shows the average response to three cortical stimuli with intervals of 2 and 5 ms. Large amplitude deflexions of stimulus artefacts have been omitted for clarity. The time and amplitude calibrations apply to all four traces. Dotted lines indicate the method of measuring EPSP amplitudes. Facilitation is defined by $f = (V_n - V_m)/V_m$, where $n > m$. (Muir and Porter, 1973.)

It is clear that the third EPSP amplitude was affected by both preceding volleys and the magnitude of the combined facilitation was greatest when both the intervals were short (2 or 5 ms). Additionally, when the intervals were short, the amount of facilitation was affected by the order of these intervals and a larger effect on the EPSP resulted from an interval of 5 ms followed by one of 2 ms than by the reverse combination (Fig. 3.12).

Theoretically, then, the effect on the peak depolarization of a motoneurone could be dependent on subtle changes in the sequence of instantaneous frequencies and the precise temporal pattern of impulses in corticomotoneuronal fibres.

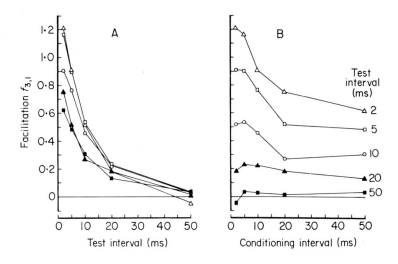

FIG. 3.12. In the graphs the average facilitation of the third EPSP of a triplet with respect to the first (unfacilitated) EPSP is plotted as a function of the test-interval (A) for various conditioning intervals and as a function of the conditioning interval (B) for various test intervals (indicated to the right of the graph). Consistent symbols have been used to identify the lines for particular conditioning intervals in A. Facilitation values used on the ordinate are defined by the expression: $f_{3,1} = (V_2 - V_0)/V_0$. (Muir and Porter, 1973.)

The observations summarized in Fig. 3.12B could be accounted for by considering that each corticomotoneuronal impulse generated an EPSP by release of transmitter from its terminals and additionally changed the state of the terminals so that release of transmitter by subsequent impulses would be facilitated. The effect on the amplitude of the third EPSP in the experimental results could be produced by the addition of facilitation from each of the preceding impulses and the magnitude of each contribution of facilitation could depend on the interval between the contributing impulse and the third (test) impulse. A reasonable approximation to the experimental results was obtained by considering such a model of additive facilitation components. The values from Fig. 3.12B have been replotted in Fig. 3.13 where they are compared with the theoretical curves obtained by the prediction that facilitation of the third EPSP will be given by the sum of that expected from the test (second) interval (i_T) and that from the conditioning plus test (first plus second) interval $(i_\mathrm{T}+i_\mathrm{c})$. Considerable correspondence was found between the experimental observations and the graphs of the expression:

$$f_{3,1} = 0.85 \exp{(-i_\mathrm{T}/10)} + 0.85 \exp{[-(i_\mathrm{T}+i_\mathrm{c})/10]}.$$

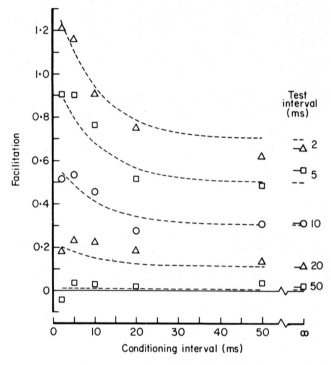

FIG. 3.13. The mean values of $f_{3,1}$ which were plotted as a function of conditioning interval (i_c) for each test interval (i_T) in Fig. 3.12 are plotted here in the same manner. Also included to the right are the average values of unconditional facilitation (symbols preceded by short continuous line). The dashed lines are graphs of the function $f = 0.85 \exp{(-i_\mathrm{T}/10)}$ $+0.85 \exp{(-(i_\mathrm{T}+i_\mathrm{c})/10)}$ for each of the test intervals used. The Figure illustrates the degree of correspondence between the experimental data and this mathematical model. (Muir and Porter, 1973.)

In some of the experiments it was possible to perform the subtraction illustrated in Fig. 3.11C and to compare the full-time course of the facilitated EPSP with that of the control EPSP. This comparison should give a sensitive indication of the effects of recruitment of additional corticomotoneuronal fibres or of the effects of interneurones in contributing to the facilitation. Although small changes in rise time of the facilitated EPSP were seen in some cells these were not consistent and roughly equal numbers of cells showed a slight increase and a slight decrease in rise time.

The half-widths, on the other hand, showed a tendency to increase with facilitation. The mean half-widths for facilitated EPSPs was 13 per cent greater than that for control responses. But there was no significant correlation between change in half-width and either interstimulus interval (and degree of facilitation) or the time-course of the control EPSP. The explanation of these results is not at present clear. The fact that some of the facilitated EPSPs had shape indices identical with those of the control responses suggests that the transmitter action had the same duration in both cases. The discrepancies in shape indices for the remaining EPSPs could have been caused by prolongation of transmitter action at the same boutons, by invasion of the test impulse into more boutons of the same fibres (perhaps distributed at different distances from the recording electrode along the dendrites of the motoneurone) or by impulses in other fibres (corticomotoneuronal or interneuronal). It is not possible to be certain about the contribution of other neurones, but, from all the evidence quoted above, these are unlikely to have played a major role in the facilitation process.

Although the precise mechanism of corticomotoneuronal facilitation is unknown, it is likely that a change in availability for the release of transmitter occurs in the presynaptic terminals and it is possible that the phenomenon may be important in the initiation of motoneuronal discharge by natural pyramidal tract activity (Porter, 1970). It is clear from Fig. 3.12B that the precise temporal order of intervals within a burst of corticomotoneuronal activity will determine the amount of facilitation and hence the peak amplitude of depolarization achieved by a given impulse in the burst. There is additional evidence indicating that the time of initiation of electromyographic responses in hindlimb muscles of the anaesthetized monkey depended on the temporal order of the unequal intervals between D waves set up in the corticospinal tract by weak repetitive stimuli delivered to a motor point on the cerebral cortex. Moreover, the peak amplitude of the complex EPSPs set up in motoneurones by a large number of corticomotoneuronal volleys, and the time of occurrence of the peak, were critically dependent on the temporal pattern of stimuli used to elicit the volleys (Porter and Muir, 1971). Muir (1973), using a generalization of the expression for facilitation which approximated the results for triplet stimuli described above, has been able to account for these observations on the basis of summation of similar facilitation effects from each volley of corticomotoneuronal impulses. So the process may be assumed to occur in a similar way when large numbers of nerve impulses follow one another in rapid succession along corticomotoneuronal fibres.

The measurements of the time-course and magnitude of facilitation have been made in anaesthetized animals. But predictions from these measurements, about the influence which temporal order of impulse activity in corticomotoneuronal fibres may have on the time of initiation of motor unit discharge, may be tested under natural circumstances in a free-to-move monkey (Porter, 1972). It has been found that the time of onset of electromyographic activity in a muscle is highly dependent on the time of occurrence of the peak instantaneous frequency of impulse discharge in pyramidal tract neurones whose activity was related to the contraction of those muscles (see Chapter 7). This correlation between neuronal activity and the time of onset of muscle contraction could arise as a direct result of the synaptic phenomena including facilitation at corticomotoneuronal terminals.

Facilitation of synaptic transmission with repetitive volleys in presynaptic elements has also been demonstrated at other terminations of cortical efferent fibres. Hence corticoreticular, corticorubral, corticopontine and corticointerneuronal synapses in the spinal cord have been shown to exhibit facilitation of the synaptic effects produced by repetitive stimuli (Magni and Willis, 1964b; Allen et al., 1971; Lundberg, 1964). Facilitation is also evident in the monosynaptic excitatory action of the recurrent collaterals of small on large PTN (Fig. 3.6A). Although the property of facilitation is poorly developed for the endings of group I afferent fibres on spinal motoneurones (Fig. 3.14), it has been demonstrated for rubrospinal connections with motoneurones in the monkey and for the influences of spinal interneurones on motoneurones in the cat (Shapovalov et al., 1971; Kuno and Weakly, 1972). How the phenomenon contributes to the functions of these connections in regulating motoneurone firing has not been examined at all.

If one assumes that the duration of transmitter action at corticomotoneuronal synapses is brief and of a similar duration to that at the synapses of group I afferent fibres on the same motoneurones, it is possible, from the records of minimal EPSPs, to make some deductions about the relative distributions of these synapses on the soma-dendritic surface of motoneurones. Porter and Hore (1969) found that, in a population of 57 motoneurones supplying *flexor digitorum longus* and *extensor digitorum longus* muscles of the monkey hindlimb, minimal corticomotoneuronal EPSPs were, on average, smaller and of slower rise-time and longer duration than minimal group I monosynaptic EPSPs in the same cells (see also Jankowska et al., 1975b). But the two groups overlapped extensively within a single population of shape indices. This could indicate a general tendency for the corticomotoneuronal synapses to be distributed on more peripheral dendrites of the motoneurone than group I synapses. In the majority of cases addition of the minimal EPSPs from corticomotoneuronal and group I synapses occurred linearly. This could indicate that, in these cells, the synaptic effects were exerted on spatially separate and non-interacting regions of the dendritic surface. But it is not clear how many contacts are made between a given corticomotoneuronal fibre and the surface of a motoneurone.

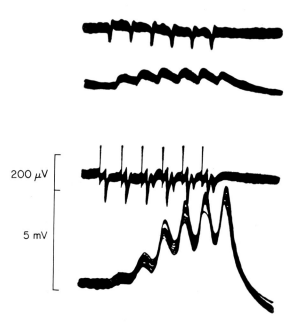

Fig. 3.14. Intracellular records from α motoneurone of median nerve of baboon.

Upper pair: group IA volleys repeated at 200 Hz (upper record); monosynaptic EPSPs evoked by them in motoneurone (lower record).

Lower pair: corticospinal volleys repeated at 200 Hz (upper record); monosynaptic EPSPs evoked in motoneurone (lower record). Strength of cortical pulses adjusted so that first CM EPSP was similar in size to first group IA EPSP.

(Phillips and Porter, 1964.)

3.6 Actions of cortical surface stimulation on PTN: thresholds for firing and thresholds for minimal motor response

Patton and Amassian (1954) were the first to distinguish experimentally between direct and indirect stimulation of PTN by single electrical pulses applied to the pia-covered motor cortex of cats and monkeys through conventional bifocal ('bipolar') electrodes. They recorded the resulting volleys in the medullary pyramid or in the contralateral CST. The first volley (the D wave) was the response of the PTN to direct electrical excitation by the electrical pulse. A sequence of later volleys (the I waves), which long outlasted the pulse, was explained as the PTN's response to repetitive synaptic bombardment, presumed to result from the activation of chains of cortical interneurones by the pulse. The D wave survived more than 2 min of asphyxia without attenuation, but the I waves were selectively abolished by asphyxia (Fig. 3.15), as well as by injury to the cortex, or removal of the cortex and stimulation of the underlying white matter, or by poor general state of the preparation (haemorrhage, too-deep barbiturate anaesthesia).

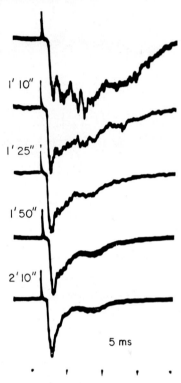

FIIG. 3.15. Records of D (direct) and I (indirect) volleys, evoked by stimulation of pericruv ate cortex, from contralateral CST of cat at C_{1-2} level, to show virtual abolition of I colleys by asphyxia, and survival of D volley. Times after onset of asphyxia shown at beginning of each sweep. At 2′10″ (bottom record) the amplitude of the D volley is scarcely smaller than that of the control (top record). Note that in CST of cat the D volley is recorded as a monophasic positive-going wave, from axons injured by the penetrating electrode. (Patton and Amassian, 1954.)

In following the experimental development of these discoveries, we shall deal with cats and primates separately. Our tasks will be, first, to sort out the direct and indirect actions of surface stimuli on the underlying PTN; second, to make quantitative comparisons between the electrical 'thresholds' (amplitude and duration of single rectangular current pulses of either polarity delivered unifocally to the pia-covered convexity of the cortex) for evoking discharges of PTN and for evoking minimal motor responses; and third, to describe the output of PTN at the threshold of motor response, that is, to specify the necessary conditions for motor response in terms of temporal and spatial summation of PTN impulses. For this analysis it is simplest if the current pulses flow between a single focal electrode on the cortical surface and a remote electrode of large area, so that current density is maximal at the point of contact of the focal electrode with the cortex. This is the 'unipolar' method preferred by Leyton and Sherrington (1917) because it 'gives minuter localization'.

3.6.1 EXPERIMENTS ON CATS

The lowest-threshold focus for motor response from the cat's cortex is near the lateral end of the cruciate sulcus; at this focus a large population of 'Betz' cells is usually to be found on the convexity of the lateral part of the anterior sigmoid gyrus where it is continuous with the coronal gyrus. Flick movements of the contralateral forelimb are evoked by single pulses of duration 10–20 ms, with the surface-anodal (S+) threshold usually, but not always, lower than the surface-cathodal (S−). Typical values are 0.75 mA anodal, 1.2 mA cathodal (Livingston and Phillips, 1957). That anodal thresholds are lower than cathodal was first discovered in the dog by Fritsch and Hitzig (1870).

An experiment in which intracellular records were made from a fast PTN (conduction velocity 53 m s^{-1}) located in this region is illustrated in Fig. 3.16 (Phillips, 1956b). The geography is shown in A. The PTN is as near as it can be to the convexity of the anterior sigmoid gyrus, and the long axis of soma and apical dendrite would be orientated at right angles to the surface at point A. Threshold for flick flexion of elbow was 740 µA, S+, 10 ms at point A. The threshold for a single impulse from the PTN was 48 µA, S+. At 100 µA, S+, four impulses were discharged during the pulse (Fig. 3.16B, 1) and at 245 µA, eight impulses, two of them confined to the initial segment (B, 2). This current was still only one-third of the threshold for minimal motor response. At motor threshold, a burst of eleven impulses was fired, but the amplitude of the last eight of these was much reduced by the depolarization during the pulse (impulses confined to distal part of initial segment, or first node of myelinated axon?) and there could be no proof that they had travelled along the axon. Assuming that they did so, this trebling of the amplitude of the stimulating pulse had only increased the number of impulses from 8 to 11. Therefore, it begins to look as if spatial summation of the impulses of many PTN, as well as temporal summation of their high-frequency discharges, is a necessary condition of minimal motor output from the spinal cord.

S-pulses evoked fewer impulses from the PTN (Fig. 3.16B, 3, 4): in response to 740 µA, which, unlike S+, was still below motor threshold, it fired three impulses only (not illustrated).

To gain some measure of the area of cortex contributing spatially summating PTN, the cortex was stimulated at point C (Fig. 3.16, A), 4.6 mm caudal to point A, and also at two other points B and D, lying at about the same distances medially and laterally from A. It is reasonable to

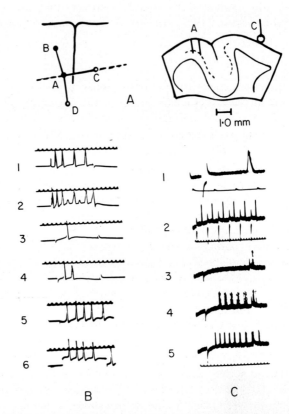

FIG. 3.16. A. Tracing of parasagittal section through lateral end of cruciate sulcus of cat is illustrated on the right. Intracellular microelectrode introduced into anterior sigmoid gyrus at A, between limits marked by lines, and recording from PTN at depth indicated by them. Stimulation of PTN at overlying point A, and also at C, 4.6 mm distant. Dotted line indicates layer of PTN somata but not sizes or positions of individual PTNs. Plane of section (dashed line through A-C), and other stimulated points B and D, are indicated on diagram of cortical surface on the left. Threshold for flick flexion of elbow with 10 ms, S+ pulse at point A was 740 μA.

B. Intracellular records from PTN at A. (Conduction velocity 53 m s⁻¹.) Stimulation with single pulses, duration about 10 ms, at points A and C.

1. Point A, 100 μA, S+. Four impulses, mean frequency about 500 Hz.
2. Point A, 245 μA, S+. Eight impulses (two in initial segment only), mean frequency about 800 Hz.
3. Point A, 100 μA, S—. One impulse.
4. Point A, 245 μA, S—. Two impulses.
5. Point C, 480 μA, S+. Five impulses, mean frequency about 500 Hz.

suppose that the current needed at points C, B and D to excite the PTN at point A would, if applied at A, excite PTN as far distant as C, B and D to a similar level of activity.

The results of stimulation at point C (Fig. 3.16B, 5, 6) were also representative of those at points B and D. The PTN at A discharged five impulses during an S+ pulse and four impulses during an S— pulse, strength 480 µA, delivered at point C. (The selective action of S+ pulses was not evident at these horizontal distances, with the larger currents that were necessary to reach the distant PTN.) Thus, even below motor threshold, PTN contained within a circle of radius 4 mm were firing a burst of impulses. It is of course unlikely that all these PTN projected to the relevant spinal segments, but it is highly probable that some at least of the outlying ones would have done so, for if not, the disparity between PTN thresholds and minimal motor threshold is unintelligible.

Figure 3.6C has already illustrated the direct and indirect excitation of a fast PTN lying 4.5 mm from the surface by pulses applied to the overlying posterior sigmoid gyrus.

A larger sample of PTN can be collected by extracellular recording from their axons in the contralateral CST. Although the PTN cannot be located as accurately as in the experiments with intracortical recording and histological reconstruction, their approximate position can be established by finding the lowest-threshold point (the 'best point') on the cortical surface. These experiments are important as a control of the values of PTN thresholds. Some degree of depolarization by injury might have been responsible for a spurious lowering of thresholds in impaled PTN, and so it proved: thresholds were 3–4 times higher in unimpaled cells. But it was confirmed that large populations of PTN were fired at high frequency by pulses which were subliminal for motor response (Hern *et al.*, 1962).

Figure 3.16C illustrates an experiment in which the lowest-threshold

6. Point C, 480 µA, S—. Four impulses during pulse, mean frequency about 500 Hz. (Phillips, 1956b.)

C. Records from single corticospinal axon taken with silver-filled micropipette inserted into contralateral CST of cat at C_{4-5} level. Stimulation at lowest threshold focus for flick flexion of forelimb with 14 ms S+ pulse; position corresponding to point A in Fig. 3.16A; threshold 650 µA.

1. Single short pulse, S+, 400 µA, evoked all-or-nothing impulse at constant latency, 2.1 ms.

2. Same pulses repeated at 250 Hz.

3. Single 14 ms pulses, S+, at PTN threshold 165 µA.

4. Single 14 ms pulses, S+, 220 µA.

5. Single 14 ms pulses, S+, 295 µA.

Each record composed of 20–30 superimposed sweeps. Note that burst of axonal impulses lags behind cortical pulse on account of conduction time to cervical cord. Time, 1000 Hz. Voltage scale 0.5 mV.

focus for minimal motor response coincided with the best point for the sampled CST axon, and corresponded approximately with the position of point A in Fig. 3.16A. Record 1 shows its all-or-nothing response to a short pulse, S+, 400 μA, at constant latency; in record 2, it followed a train of short pulses at 250 Hz. Record 3 shows the responses to 20–30 single S+ pulses, duration 14 ms, at the PTN's threshold, 165 μA. Strengthening the pulse to 220 μA elicited six impulses at a mean frequency of about 500 Hz, with some temporal variation in different trials (record 4). Strengthening it to 295 μA elicited nine impulses, with less temporal variation, frequency initially over 650 Hz, falling to 500 Hz (record 5). These impulses, of course, had all travelled down the CST axon (cf. the uncertainty in the intracellular experiment of Fig. 3.16B). The threshold for minimal movement was 650 μA, S+, 14 ms. This pulse caused repetitive firing of another CST axon whose best point lay 5 mm rostral to the best motor point. In the largest example of horizontal spread encountered in this series, the threshold for minimal motor response was 1.2 mA, and a PTN at a distance of 7 mm discharged one or two impulses in response to each long pulse.

The regular repetitive discharges of PTN during the passage of long pulses are readily interpreted as the rhythmic response of their pacemaker membranes to a steady flow of cathodal (depolarizing) current. The existence of such a cathodal 'stimulating fraction' of the total current would depend on appropriate orientation of the long axis of the PTN in relation to the lines of intracortical current flow. Thus, in the vertically orientated population of PTN at point A, Fig. 3.16, a fraction of the current from a surface-anodal pulse should enter by the dendrites and flow outward (cathodally) through the axons. This is analogous to the well-known rhythmic firing of single primary afferent axons in response to anodal polarization of a sensory surface containing cutaneous or lateral line receptors (cf. Hern et al., 1962). It is remarkable that the explanation of the efficacy of S+ stimulation of the cortex in terms of the 'virtual cathode established in the deeper and more excitable regions' was first proposed by Ferrier (1886) when discussing the results of Fritsch and Hitzig (1870).

3.6.2 EXPERIMENTS ON BABOONS

Sampling of single axons in the contralateral CST, combined with the use of weak, brief (0.2 ms) cortical pulses, has displayed the direct and indirect actions of surface stimulation on populations of PTN with special clarity. The axons thus sampled are those of fast PTN, from whose impulses the D volley is built up (Fig. 3.17A). The D volley is conducted at about 60 m s⁻¹ (Fig. 3.17B).

Figure 3.17C shows the brachio-facial genu of the Rolandic sulcus, and marks with a filled circle the lowest-threshold point (S+, 0.2 ms, 1.15 mA) for stimulation of a PTN underlying the convexity of the precentral gyrus. The latency of response of its axon in the contralateral CST was unvarying (2.2 ms), as shown by the exact superimposition of 59 responses (record D). Therefore, the utilization time at the cortex and the axonal conduction time were unvarying, and stimulation must always have taken effect at the same part of the neurone. These pulses were too weak to excite enough PTN to give a recordable multi-unit D volley in the CST.

The focal anode was then moved away from the best point along occipito-frontal (O-F) and mediolateral (M-L) axes (Fig. 3.17C), and the latency and S+ threshold were re-measured at several points on these axes. The latency remained constant at 2.2 ms. Evidently the same part of the neurone was still being stimulated, by physical diffusion of current. The threshold rose with distance in a roughly parabolic curve (Fig. 3.17G, full line); this illustrates that the current applied at the cortical surface needed to be increased as a function of the square of the horizontal distance in order to maintain the same current density through the responding PTN membrane. All this evidence points to direct stimulation of the PTN membrane by the S+ pulses.

The responses to S− pulses delivered near the best point differed in two respects. First, the threshold was higher (1.85 mA instead of 1.15 mA). Second, the latency was longer; in some responses it was increased by 0.65 ms, in the remainder by 1.55 ms (record F). The conduction time from cortex to C5 segment cannot have altered, so these alternative delays must have arisen within the cortex. The spike potentials were not exactly superimposed, showing that the latencies were slightly variable. The stronger stimulus has evoked a small D volley, latency 1.85 ms. We shall see that the PTN that are directly stimulated by S− pulses are those that lie in the rostral wall of the central fissure.

When the focal cathode was applied to points at increasing distances along the O-F and M-L axes, the latencies were longer than the 2.2 ms that was constantly measured in response to S+ pulses, and there were sometimes alternative latencies, as in record F. In 50 superimposed records taken from each point, the pattern remained constant at that point. The threshold rose with increasing distance, but the points (θ) did not lie along a simple curve (Fig. 3.17G). All these features are in contrast with those of the responses to S+ pulses, and compel the conclusion that the S− pulses excited this PTN indirectly, by stimulating intra-cortical or local U-fibre pathways which contributed excitatory synapses to it.

The results with unifocal S+ and S− stimuli suggest that the actions of conventional bifocal ('bipolar') stimulation would be complex, and experiment bears this out (Phillips and Porter, 1962). For record E, the dipole straddled the best point. The threshold was 2.1 mA, and the latency 1.4 ms longer than that of direct (S+) stimulation. The results of placing the dipole in different positions along the M-L axis are shown in

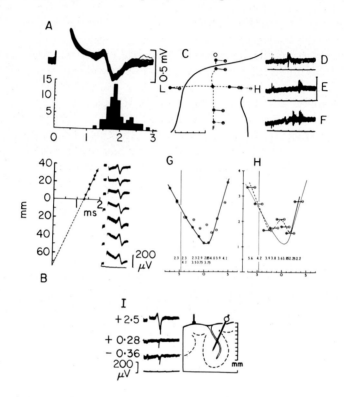

Fig. 3.17. Direct and indirect stimulation of fast PTN by unifocal S+ and S− electrodes, and by bifocal electrodes about 1.5 mm apart. Responses recorded from axons in contralateral CST at C₅ level.

The CST axons investigated in these experiments are those of fast PTN, whose impulses constitute the D volley.

A. *Above*: D volley evoked by S+, 0.2 ms, 2.8 mA pulse delivered to precentral arm area, recorded from contralateral CST at C₅₋₆ level. About 20 superimposed traces.

Below: times of arrival of impulses at C₅₋₆ level in 68 CST axons in six experiments (Landgren *et al.*, 1962a).

B. Conduction velocity of D volley along contralateral CST in cervical segments of spinal cord. Precentral arm area stimulated with S+, 0.2 ms, 4.5 mA pulses. Time of arrival at each locus was measured as point of reversal of D wave from positive-going to negative-going. Slope 59 m s⁻¹. Extrapolation (dotted line) suggests that D volley originated 75 mm from rostral recording locus. Shortest distance between this locus and the stimulated point in baboons of this size was 77–84 mm. (Phillips and Porter, 1964.)

Note that in the baboon the D volley can easily be recorded as a triphasic wave by a focal electrode resting on the dorsolateral surface of the cord, overlying the large CST. This is in contrast to the cat, in which the smaller CST yields nothing that can be recorded from the uninjured tract by ordinary amplification (Hern *et al.*, 1962).

Fig. 3.17H. When it was on the medial side of the 'best point', so that the anode was nearest to the PTN, the latency indicated direct excitation. As the dipole was placed in more lateral positions, and the cathode came nearer to the PTN, the threshold rose and the latency jumped to an 'indirect' value. As the cathode passed the 'best point' the threshold fell and then rose again, and the latency lengthened progressively as the dipole approached and straddled the central sulcus and finally crossed over to the postcentral gyrus.

The results with other PTN which were located on the convexity of the precentral gyrus were similar, and are interpreted as follows. Their long soma-dendritic axes are orientated at right-angles to the cortical surface. Threshold S+ stimuli would therefore hyperpolarize the dendrites and depolarize the axons. Stimulation by outward-flowing transmembrane current would thus take place in the deepest layer of cortex or outermost layer of white matter: at the axon hillock, the initial segment, or the first node of the myelinated axon (cf. Landau et al., 1965).

Threshold S— stimuli would have opposite effects. Hyperpolarization of the axon would discourage direct excitation, but the dendrites would be depolarized and the intracortical neurones and axons in the outer layers would be stimulated. Synaptic firing would occur after recovery of the axon from the depression induced by the brief pulse. The different latencies of response would be explained by the excitation of alternative converging pathways.

We now consider the PTN which are located in the anterior wall of the central sulcus, whose long axes are orientated at right angles to the sulcus and, therefore, roughly parallel to the surface of the brain. At threshold,

C. Filled circle marks lowest-threshold point for S+ stimulation of PTN, on convexity of precentral gyrus. Path followed by this anode during exploration of cortex is marked by dotted lines: OF, occipito-frontal; ML, mediolateral. Scale in mm.

D. Response to S+ pulses at filled circle: threshold 1.15 mA, latency 2.2 ms. No D volley.

E. Bifocal stimulation, dipole straddling filled circle. Threshold 2.1 mA, latency 3.6 ms.

F. S— stimulation, 0.5 mm medial to filled circle, threshold 1.85 mA. Alternative latencies 2.85 or 3.75 ms. Note D volley, latency 1.85 ms. Time 1000 Hz. Voltage 0.5 mV. All records formed from about 50 superimposed traces.

G. Full line and ⊕ : S+ thresholds for points along line LM in C. Vertical line corresponds to intersection of LM with Rolandic sulcus. Latency 2.1 to 2.2 ms. ⊖ : S— thresholds along line LM. Latencies noted at each locus.

H. Heavy broken line and ⊕—⊖ : bifocal thresholds along line LM. Latencies noted at each locus. Thin line: S+ thresholds from G. (Phillips and Porter, 1962.)

I. Recording from single PT axon in contralateral CST. Threshold for S+ pulses to convexity of precentral gyrus was 2.5 mA. These pulses elicited a large D volley but no I volleys. Thresholds for stimulation with focal electrode buried in anterior wall of Rolandic fissure were 280 μA anodal and 360 μA cathodal. The cathodal pulse elicited a small D volley. Time 1000 Hz. Broken line in tracing of brain-slice marks grey-white boundary. (Phillips and Porter, 1964.)

which is higher than for cells on the convexity, S+ and S— pulses both excite these PTN directly, but the best point for S+ is near to the edge of the fissure and the best point for S— is on the convexity of the pre-central gyrus. This is intelligible on the assumption that the outward current needed to excite the impulse-generating membrane at the axonal pole of the PTN would be provided by an anode located near to the Rolandic fissure, that is, nearest the dendritic pole, or by a cathode located more rostrally, nearest the axonal pole. Direct stimulation of deeply-situated PTN by S— pulses explains the small D volley seen in Fig. 3.17F.

Evidence that surface stimulation of moderate strength is capable of exciting PTN in the wall of the Rolandic fissure is shown in Fig. 3.17I. The buried electrode excited this PTN at lower threshold, with a minimal D volley. The surface anode did not 'reach' this PTN until it had been strengthened sufficiently to elicit a considerable D volley.

For surface stimulation, therefore, anodal pulses are to be preferred to cathodal or bifocal pulses. At threshold, a 0.2 ms S+ pulse selectively stimulates a population of vertically orientated PTN immediately under-lying the point of contact, and by-passes the interneuronal and synaptic complexities of the outer layers of cortex. As the pulse is strengthened, the directly excited population enlarges to include PTN lying a few mm distant horizontally, and also in the depth of the Rolandic sulcus. In spite of the wide spatial summation of single impulses, such pulses evoked no motor response, unless repeated at high frequencies, e.g. 6 pulses at 500 Hz. The brief synchronous train of D volleys evokes a 'flick movement' of the type mapped by Liddell and Phillips using 5 ms pulses (Chapter 2, Fig. 8).

The optimum duration of a single long pulse is shorter for the baboon (5 ms) than for the cat (10–20 ms). The shorter period of temporal sum-mation of PTN impulses that is needed for flick movement in the primate is the physiological corollary of the monosynaptic corticomotoneuronal (CM) connexion that will be described in Chapter 4. Section 5 has shown that repetitive activation of CM synapses increases their depolarizing action on spinal motoneurones, and brings them rapidly towards the firing level. In this section it remains only to demonstrate that the long pulses evoke repetitive firing of the PTN pacemaker membrane in the baboon, as they do in the cat.

Figure 3.18A shows the repetitive responses of a fast PTN, whose best point is shown at o on the map, to long S+ pulses of 150 and 220 μA applied at point o. Point m was the best point for flick movement of thumb and index. When point m was stimulated at 1.8 mA, the threshold for flick movement, the PTN near point o responded repetitively (record at bottom left). Although there was no evidence that this PTN made any connexions with thumb-index motoneurones in the spinal cord, the experiment emphasizes the limitations of surface stimulation in trying to decide between overlapping and abrupt localization, if PTN as far as 9 mm from the focal electrode may be made to fire repetitively during a minimal motor response.

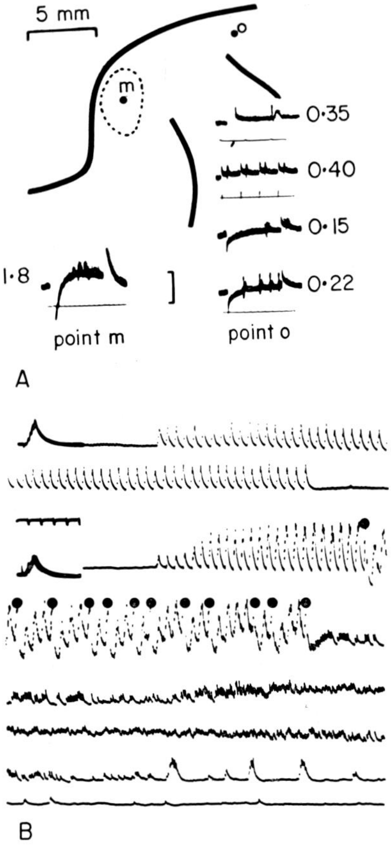

FIG. 3.18. Explanation of efficacy of single pulses of long duration in causing flick movements of the baboon's hand.

A. *Above*: map of right precentral gyrus of baboon, showing central, superior precentral, and inferior precentral sulci. o, Best point for PTN whose axonal impulses were recorded in contralateral CST at C_{5-6} level. m, Best point for flick movement of contralateral thumb and index.

Below, right: responses of PTN to single 0.2 ms S+ pulses, 350 µA; to 0.2 ms pulses, 400 µA at 200 Hz; and to single long S+ pulses, 150 µA and 220 µA.

Below, left: response of PTN at point o to long pulse at point m, at threshold for flick movement of thumb and index, 1.8 mA. Calibration 0.5 mV.

B. Selective action of long S + pulses on corticomotoneuronal colony of PTNs, recorded intracellularly as monosynaptic EPSPs in their target ulnar motoneurone (membrane potential −69 to −74 mV).

Top two lines: superimposed traces of EPSP (peak depolarization 7.5 mV) evoked by single 5.0 ms, 700 µA S+ pulses applied to contralateral precentral gyrus, followed by continuous record of responses to repetition of same pulses at 44 Hz for 1.4 s.

Third line begins with superimposed traces of EPSP (peak depolarization 6.0 mV) evoked by single 5.0 ms, 1.0 mA S− pulses, followed by continuous record of responses to repetition of same pulses at 44 Hz for 1.4 s. Note growth of EPSPs to about 15 mV. The ulnar motoneurone discharged an impulse (marked by dot) whenever one of these reached the firing level (−58 mV). Last of the twelve dots coincides with end of train of stimuli. Note epileptiform after-discharges by cells of the corticomotoneuronal colony, persisting for about 4 s.

(Hern *et al.*, 1962.)

The existence of the CM connexion has an important practical consequence: that by intracellular recording of EPSPs from motoneurones of a hand muscle, one can detect and measure the output of a part or of the whole of the *colony* of PTN that project monosynaptically to a target motoneurone (Landgren *et al.*, 1962b). Figure 3.18B illustrates the analytical power of the method in discriminating between the direct action of long S+ pulses on the PTN membrane and the indirect actions of S— pulses, mediated by cortical interneurones.

The top left record is of superimposed responses to single S+ pulses, duration 5 ms, below the threshold for minimal movement. The steep rise of the motoneuronal EPSP is marked by four ripples, showing that some members of the PTN colony were discharging four-impulse bursts in synchrony. The exact superimposition is striking. The pulses were then delivered at 44 Hz for 1.4 s. The discharges of the PTN colony varied little from one response to the next, and no after-discharge followed the train. The by-passing of the outer cortical layers was effectively complete. By contrast, the responses to single S— pulses (beginning of third line) were less exactly superimposed. Repetition of these pulses at 44 Hz for 1.4 s led to a large increase in amplitude and complexity of configuration of the EPSPs, and to the firing of twelve impulses (marked by dots where the action potentials went off the screen). For about 4 s after the end of the train of stimuli the membrane of the target motoneurone was bombarded by the epileptiform after-discharges of the PTN colony. Hern *et al.* (1962) argued that these complex and prolonged actions of S— pulses were due to intracortical bombardment of PTN and not to bombardment of the target motoneurone by spinal interneurones. If spinal interneurone pools had been stirred up by repetitive PT impulses, the complex actions should have been seen in response to S+ as well as to S— pulses.

It remains to illustrate the effects of very strong brief pulses on the PTN in the baboon. Their responses can be detected as D and I volleys from the dorsolateral surface of the cord, as single-axon records from the CST, and as monosynaptic EPSPs in target motoneurones. At such high intensities, the polarity of the pulse is immaterial. The intensities we have illustrated thus far were below the threshold for setting up I volleys.

In the series of Fig. 3.19A, the strength of 0.2 ms, S+ pulses was increased from 3.8 to 12.1 mA, and simultaneous records were taken from the dorsolateral surface of the cervical cord (lower traces) and from a sampled CST axon (upper traces). At 3.8 mA, the D volley was followed by a minimal I volley. The PTN fired during the D volley in most trials, at a fixed latency, and again during the I volley, though with a good deal of 'latency jitter'. At 12.1 mA the D volley was followed by three I volleys, to each of which the PTN contributed an impulse. In the records of series B, the counterpart of these events is shown in the EPSPs recorded in a target motoneurone, simultaneously with the D and I volleys recorded from the cord dorsum. These experiments (Kernell and Wu Chien-ping, 1967a, b) proved that the I waves are due to repetitive firing of the same fast PTN that contributed to the D wave. Since the I volleys are discharged after the end of the stimulating pulse, they cannot be generated by a flow of stimulating current through the pacemaker membrane. Patton and Amassian (1960) have proposed that the I waves are due to a 'periodic bombardment of Betz cells through chains of neurons with fixed temporal characteristics'. We have no knowledge of how widely these strong pulses spread horizontally within the cortex, or in depth, into the corona radiata or even into the basal ganglia and thalamus.

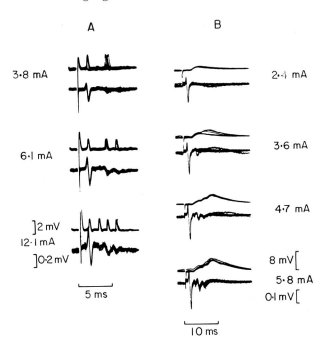

FIG. 3.19. Direct and indirect stimulation of baboon's PTN by very strong pulses applied to precentral gyrus.

A. Responses of single axon recorded from contralateral CST by a microelectrode (upper traces), and records of D and I volleys taken simultaneously from the dorsolateral surface of the cervical spinal cord overlying the point of penetration of the microelectrode. Strengths of S + cortical pulses, duration 0.2 ms, noted beside each pair of records. (Kernell and Wu Chien-ping, 1967a.)

B. Responses of corticomotoneuronal colony of PTNs, recorded intracellularly as monosynaptic EPSPs in their target ulnar motoneurone. Lower records show D and I volleys recorded simultaneously from surface of lateral corticospinal tract at same segmental level. Strengths of S + pulses to contralateral precentral gyrus noted beside each pair of records. (Kernell and Wu Chien-ping, 1967b.)

It is worth stressing that all the work of this section has been concerned with the 'large' and 'fast' axons which, in the primate, form the CM component of the CST, and that we remain ignorant of the properties and responses to stimulation of the very much larger number of small PT axons (cf. Towe, 1973).

3.7 Summary

This chapter has described the structure and properties of the PTN, the output cells of the cortical projection areas in the model of Fig. 1.4. Most investigations have been made on 'large', 'fast' PTN. Individual PTN have been identified by antidromic stimulation of their axons in the PT. The responses of their membranes to intracellularly applied currents and to the actions of excitatory and inhibitory synapses have been studied with intracellular microelectrodes. Multi-barrelled extracellular microelectrodes have been used to record their responses to microiontophoretic application of the excitatory and inhibitory transmitters, acetylcholine and γ-amino-butyric acid. Intracellular recordings from PTN, and extracellular recordings of their discharges from their axons in the lateral corticospinal tract, have been used to study the rhythmic discharges of their impulse-generating ('pacemaker') membranes in response to short pulses of polarizing current applied to the cortical surface. The direct response of this membrane to externally applied outward (cathodal) current has been distinguished from discharges evoked by the action of excitatory synapses. The distinction is best made in PTN which are orientated at right-angles to the surface of the brain: surface-anodal pulses excite the impulse-generating membrane directly because a fraction of the current penetrates the dendrites and flows outward (cathodally) through the axon, whereas surface cathodal pulses excite neurones and axons in the outer layers of cortex which supply excitatory and inhibitory synapses to the PTN. Repetitive cathodal stimulation differs from repetitive anodal stimulation in that it stirs up prolonged intracortical interneuronal activity. Single, very strong 0.2 ms pulses of either polarity cause repetitive bombardment of PTN by interneuronal networks, which force them to fire repetitively. These investigations have established the basic modes of response of PTN to stimulation of the cortical surface.

The synapses formed by PT axons on target neurones have a special property: their action on the postsynaptic membranes is markedly facilitated when the presynaptic impulses are repeated at short intervals. A detailed experimental analysis is given of this important effect, which enables the PT to adjust, by alterations in frequency, the power of its excitatory action on its targets. Certain intervals between two or three closely spaced impulses, discharged during a train of lower average frequency, are shown to be critically effective in depolarizing target cells. Such intervals are found to occur during natural activity (Chapter 7).

Current pulses applied at a 'point' on the cortical surface spread physically, as well as physiologically, to excite PTN several mm distant in all directions horizontally, as well as in the depth of the central fissure, even though these pulses evoke no muscular response. This creates difficulties for the use of surface stimulation in attempts to map the somatotopic arrangement of cortical projection areas. For any current strength, it will be necessary to calibrate the spread, and to specify the dimensions of the population of PTN centred on the stimulated 'point' (Chapter 5). Stimulation of closely adjacent points at motor threshold for the more 'excitable' point cannot discharge small, 'abruptly' segregated populations of PTN centred on those points, but must discharge larger and overlapping populations. Thus, stimulation near the edge of the face area (Chapter 2, section 4) would certainly spread to discharge PTN in the arm area and vice versa. Further attempts to solve the problem of 'abrupt' or overlapping 'minute' localization will be described in Chapter 5.

4
Origin, course and distribution of pyramidal axons in cats and primates

4.1 The PT as a paradigm of the charting of a central nervous pathway

As one of the most conspicuous pathways in the mammalian central nervous system, the PT has always been investigated by every new method as soon as it has become available, so that most of the methods of experimental neurology could be illustrated from the story of the PT, without much need to refer to other pathways. The general description given in Chapter 1 has now to be set firmly on its experimental foundations: first, by outlining the methods; second, by illustrating their detailed application in experiments on cats and monkeys.

Gross dissection of the human PT had led to error about its origin, and Reil had held that the grey matter of the brain was only laid on to the white without any real continuity (Jefferson, 1953). Until the discovery of neurones with the microscope, and the discovery that every axon arises from a cell-body with a nucleus and withers when disconnected from it (Wallerian degeneration), no understanding was possible (Liddell, 1960). Thereafter, it became possible to chart the origin and course of the PT by destroying the cortex containing its cells of origin and detecting the resulting degeneration in the white matter in sections at successively lower levels of brain and cord. Selective destruction of different cortical areas would distinguish those which gave origin to pyramidal axons from those which did not.

Until the mid-1880s, this anterograde degeneration was detected by allowing the animal to survive the cortical lesion for several months and then soaking the medulla and cord for a few weeks in ammonium bichromate, or staining them with carmine. Ferrier's monkeys (1884) and Sherrington's dogs (1885) were examined in this way. In one monkey which had survived for 19 months, 'the nerve fibres had almost entirely disappeared, their place being taken by connective tissue staining deeply with carmine'. In dogs, after 7 months, the affected pyramid was 'much shrunken, even although the cortical injury be not so large as a shilling piece'. It presented a 'smooth surface quite other than the sculptured face of a normal pyramid when hardened in Muller's fluid'. The shrunken pyramid was a mass of fine fibrous tissue, staining deeply with carmine, and containing scarcely a healthy nerve fibre.

The Marchi method, introduced in 1885, was a major advance. It detected the disintegrating myelin sheaths of the larger degenerating axons by blackening their fatty debris with osmium tetroxide. The black dots were seen against a clear background. The animal, or patient, had to die within a few weeks of the cortical injury, before the debris were removed by neuroglial reaction. Writing in 1909, Ramón y Cajal commented: 'La méthode de Marchi est lente à se repandre. Elle finit pourtant par s'imposer, et, grâce à son application par Marchi et Alghieri, Mott, Sherrington, Dejerine . . . elle a collaboré, ces dernières années, avec succes, à déterminer la voie pyramidal le long de la moelle épinière.' The method is ideal for charting the course of a compact tract such as the PT, which contains a small proportion of large myelinated axons scattered across its whole cross-section area; but it gives no information about the fine axons, and it cannot follow any of the axons to their fine unmyelinated endings.

Another method of following the course of the PT along the spinal cord depended on the fact, discovered by Flechsig in 1878, that different tracts become myelinated at different periods during postnatal development.The large axons of the PT are the last to acquire their myelin sheaths. Although the propriospinal axons in the dorsolateral funiculus are myelinated earlier, the large admixture of as yet unmyelinated PT axons results in visible pallor of this cross-section area in puppy and human infant. Flechsig at first visualized this by treatment with osmic acid. The Weigert method for staining normal myelin sheaths was introduced in 1884, and all subsequent investigators of the sequence of myelination have adopted it (Ramóny Cajal, 1909).

Microscopically visible pallor, and microscopically visible loss of the beautiful blue-blackened rings of myelin, enabled the course of the PT through internal capsule, cerebral peduncle, pyramid and spinal cord to be charted by the Weigert method in patients or animals who had survived appropriate cortical lesions for months or years, when the removal of the products of disintegrating myelin had long been completed, and the thick myelinated axons, and also the very much more numerous but still (in the 1880s) unseen thin axons, had been replaced by neurological scar tissue.

The staining of *intact* axons, as distinct from staining their myelin sheaths, became possible from 1873 onwards, when the Golgi method was introduced (Fig. 3.1); and Cajal, who made much use of it, introduced his own silver axon stain in 1901 and also mastered the formidable technical problem of colouring axons within the CNS with methylene blue. His discovery that thicker PT axons gave off thinner collaterals which descended from pyramid to spinal cord has already been noted in Chapter 1, section 1.4. Full awareness of the enormous preponderance of very thin axons in the PT came only in the 1940s, when Lassek (1948) used a silver method to stain the axons of the intact medullary pyramids in several species, counted the axons, measured their diameters, and compared the counts with the numbers of 'giant' pyramidal neurones in the motor cortex. The large disparities in every species disposed of the classical notion that all pyramidal axons arise from the 'giant cells of Betz'. Less than 3 per cent do so.

The tracing of *degenerating* axons (as distinct from their degenerating myelin sheaths) was not possible until the introduction, in the 1950s, of the Nauta method, a silver method which selectively stains dying axons as far as their terminal arborizations, revealing their characteristic varicosities, vacuolation and longitudinal fragmentation; the staining of intact axons is suppressed. It is important to verify these pathological appearances in disintegrating axons running for some distance in the plane of section. There remains, however, the problem of distinguishing the fine debris of axons passing through an area of grey matter from that of axons which actually terminate there—a problem which can be resolved only by visualizing degenerating synapses with the electron microscope. Silver staining of degenerating *boutons terminaux* in the spinal grey matter of primates within 72 hours of injury to the motor cortex was attempted by Hoff and Hoff (1934) with what seems, in retrospect, to have been a fair degree of success: electron microscopy has shown that degeneration involves initial swelling of the terminal argentophil neurofibrillar rings within the presynaptic bags of synapses of this type (Gray and Guillery, 1966).

The time factor creates a problem in the quantitative assessment of connectivity by staining degenerating axons. Some terminals and axons are undergoing degeneration, some degenerated elements are being removed and some have already disappeared entirely on any particular day soon after the injury is made. The staining method affects only those fibres in an appropriate stage of degeneration on that day and the continuously changing neural scene is viewed at only this one point in time.

Since the PTs are approximately symmetrical bilaterally, the loss of axons following cortical lesions can be estimated quantitatively by waiting until all degenerated axons have disappeared and then comparing the numbers of normal axons in the medullary pyramids on the two sides (van Crevel and Verhaart, 1963a, b). Until the 1950s, it was not appreciated that axolysis of the thinnest axons may not be completed in less than six months. Erroneous claims were therefore made that as many as 50 per cent of PT axons could survive destruction of the motor area, and that they must therefore have originated in outlying areas, e.g. in parietal, temporal or occipital lobes, or even in subcortical structures. Silver methods could be especially misleading in the period preceding complete axolysis, because the thinnest axons become swollen, and may, in transverse sections, be mistaken for, and included in the count of, intact axons of larger calibre. The Alzheimer–Mann–Häggquist methyl blue eosin method is good for axon counts of normal and depleted medullary pyramids: it colours the axons blue, their myelin sheaths red (even the sheaths of the thinnest axons), and glial cells and fibres blue (Van Crevel and Verhaart, 1963a). Results in the cat will be cited in section 4.2.

In addition to the *anterograde* changes in axons, myelin sheaths and synapses when the parent neurones are destroyed in the cortex, there are *retrograde* changes in the neurones when the axons are cut. This fact was exploited by Holmes and Page May (1909), who hemisected the spinal cord in dog, cat, lemur, monkey and chimpanzee, and searched the brains, and also the brains of human patients with injuries of the cervical spinal cord, for evidence of retrograde injury to cortical neurones. They found that the Betz cells showed characteristic swelling with loss of Nissl granules (chromatolysis) and eccentric displacement of the nucleus. These changes were already well known in other neurones after cutting their axons, and Holmes and Page May concluded that the contralateral CST originated from the Betz cells. In the cat, chromatolysed cells were found in the anterior and posterior sigmoid gyri, and in monkey and man, in the precentral gyrus. The positive result was reliable, but the absence of chromatolysed neurones from any area of cortex could not certify the absence of any projection from that area into the contralateral CST.

The use of two very recently introduced methods for tracing connexions, which depend on cellulifugal and cellulipetal axoplasmic transport, will be illustrated in Chapter 6. Injection of tritiated amino acids amongst a population of neurones results in the appearance of radioactivity in their axon terminals, which can be visualized by autoradiography (e.g. Jones, 1975). This is an anterograde method. A retrograde method is that of injecting horseradish peroxidase into a population of axon terminals, which results, after incubation with an appropriate substrate, in the appearance of granules in the perikarya of the cells of origin (e.g. Strick, 1975). Berrewoets and Kuypers (1975) used injections of horseradish peroxidase into the brain stem recticular formation, dorsal column nuclei and spinal cord of the cat, and Coulter *et al.* (1976) into the spinal cord of cats and monkeys, to identify the particular neurones in the pericruciate cortex which contributed axons to these regions. Although many labelled pyramidal neurones in layer V of areas 2, 3 and 4 contributed axons to the dorsal column nuclei, the giant Betz cells of area 4 were labelled only following injections into the spinal cord. Hence cortical fibres descending to the spinal cord and those descending to subcortical structures may, in part, derive from different sets of pyramidal neurones, and the corticospinal tract may have its origin in only a particular set localized in a particular region.

Since the 1940s, classical microanatomy has been increasingly complemented by microphysiological studies which, from our present standpoint, can properly be described as *electroanatomical*. Like classical microanatomy, electroanatomy can be retrograde or anterograde. The electroanatomical correlates of Holmes and Page May's experiments is the mapping of the area of origin of the PT by antidromic stimulation of the medullary pyramid, by recording the resulting evoked potentials at the cortical surface (Woolsey and Chang, 1948) or by recording the resulting antidromic impulses in single PTN (Lance and Manning, 1954). Like the chromatolytic observations, the recordings will be biased in favour of the large PTN. In 'anterograde electroanatomy', the unravelling of connectivity by making small lesions and tracing the course of the resulting degeneration is complemented by artificial excitation of small areas, by mapping with microelectrodes the small circumscribed areas of electrical response, and by precise timing of the response. This approach may sometimes disclose connections which have been missed by the microscopist, but its chief value lies in its ability to specify the *sense* of the synaptic connexions: inhibitory as well as excitatory, and in its ability to measure the relative quantity and timing of the antagonistic synaptic effects.

4.2 Cortical origin and calibre of PT axons in the cat

Using the Alzheimer–Mann–Häggquist method, van Crevel and Verhaart (1963a) found that the intact medullary pyramids of the cat each contain about 80 000 axons. Of these, 73 per cent are less than 2 μm in diameter; 20 per cent are > 2 to 4 μm in diameter; 5 per cent are > 4 to 6 μm in diameter, only 2 per cent thicker than 6 μm. Even the thinnest axons were surrounded by a ring of reddened myelin. Hemidecortication confirmed that all but a negligible fraction of the PT axons originate in the neocortex and that there is therefore no significant contribution from subcortical structures. The number of axons that had degenerated at any time was determined indirectly, as the difference between the counts of intact axons in the normal and in the depleted pyramid. The rates of degeneration of axons of different calibres were plotted in a series of cats. From the curves, the percentage of the total axons of one PT that had been severed by a particular subtotal ablation of neocortex could be estimated at any convenient time after the onset of degeneration—even before expiry of the six months that were needed for all the severed axons to disappear completely (van Crevel and Verhaart, 1963b). The results are shown in Fig. 4.1. The heaviest loss of PT axons followed abalations of pericruciate cortex (A); most of the remaining PT axons arise from the immediately adjacent pre- and postcruciate areas (B and C). Ablations of parietal, temporal or occipital cortex caused no significant degeneration of PT axons.

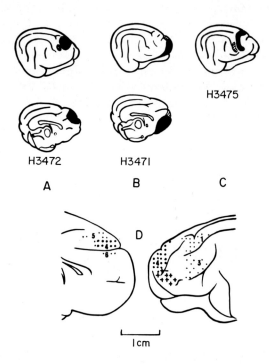

FIG. 4.1. Lesions of the left hemispheres of three cats.

The left-sided lesions in A, B and C are drawn on the lateral aspect of a *right* hemisphere; those in A and B are also drawn on the medial aspect of a left hemisphere.

Ablated cortex black, undermined cortex stippled (van Crevel and Verhaart, 1963b).

A. This lesion is estimated to have severed the following percentages (approximately) of PT axons of different diameters:

Calibre	% Axons severed
>0–2 µm	60
>2–4 µm	65
>4–6 µm	80
>6 µm	90

B. This more rostral legion is estimated to have severed the following percentages of PT axons:

>0–2 µm	15
>2–4 µm	10
>4–6 µm	10
>6 µm	5

Antidromic electrical mapping (Fig. 4.1D) gave results which agree remarkably well with those of van Crevel and Verhaart (Lance and Manning, 1954). The spectrum of conduction velocities ranged from 7 to 70 m s^{-1}. If we apply the working rule that conduction velocity is related to axon diameter by a factor of roughly 6 ('Hursh factor'), we can relate these velocities to the calibre spectrum of the PT axons, which extends from 1 to 12 μm. Van Crevel and Verhaart (1963a) found 2 per cent of axons thicker than 6 μm; Lance and Manning found 3 per cent of axons conducting faster than 60 m s^{-1}. The two peaks in the range of conduction velocities, at about 14 m s^{-1} and 42 m s^{-1}, led to the differentiation of slow and fast PTN (Chapter 3, section 3.1). The maps of Fig. 4.1 also agree with the map of the cat's 'area gigantopyramidalis' published by Holmes and Page May (1909). The cortical territory which contained their sample of giant cells is evidently roughly coextensive with the area of origin of the enormously greater number of fine PT axons as charted by van Crevel and Verhaart (1963a, b).

Intracellular injection of Procion Yellow dye into an antidromically identified PTN enabled its perikaryon to be visualized, after death, in lamina V of area 4 (Batuev and Lenkov, 1973).

4.3 Distribution of collateral and terminal branches of PT axons within the cat's brain

In transverse sections of the brain stem the PT looks as compact as a nerve. Classical human anatomy regarded the pyramids as composed only of unbranched corticospinal axons, destined for the motor nuclei of the contralateral spinal cord; corticobulbar axons (sometimes called 'geniculate fibres'), supposedly destined for the motor nuclei of the cranial nerves, left the internal capsule and cerebral peduncle and crossed the midline near to the nuclei.

C. This more caudal lesion, confined to lateral aspect of hemisphere, is estimated to have severed the following percentages of PT axons:

>0–2 μm	30
>2–4 μm	35
>4–6 μm	35
>6 μm	5

D. Summarizing diagrams of medial and lateral aspects of left hemisphere, showing distribution of antidromic spike potentials in multi-unit recordings with steel microelectrodes, following single stimuli to medullary pyramid in a series of cats. *Large dots*: consistent responses composed of many spikes. *Small dots and crosses*: variable and occasional responses (from Lance and Manning, 1954). Corticospinal neurones have been identified antidromically in somatosensory area SII, near to 3 in this Figure, by Atkinson *et al.* (1974).

But in longitudinal sections of the brain stem and internal capsule, staining of axons (e.g. by the Golgi method) in regions known to be occupied by the PT revealed abundant branching to Ramón y Cajal. Other workers do not seem to have taken much interest in the profuse branching shown in his beautiful drawings. We have already seen that he described how thick T-branches from axons in the medullary pyramid formed elaborate arborizations on neurones of the reticular formation. In this situation the destination of the branch is close enough to the PT for the connexion to be traced in one or a few adjacent serial sections. Other branches disappear from sight, heading for unknown destinations. In mixed populations of axons, for example, the internal capsule, there could be no proof that a branching axon was a pyramidal axon. Thus, in

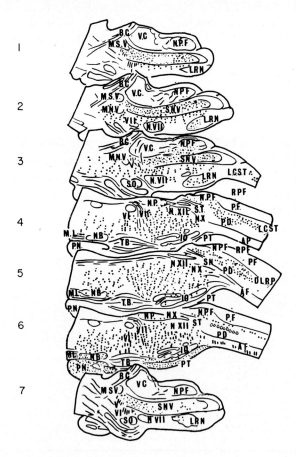

Fig. 4.2. Semidiagrammatic representation of the distribution of degenerating fibres within the medulla oblongata and cervical spinal cord, following destruction confined to the sensorimotor cortex (Kuypers, 1958).

Golgi preparations, Kemp and Powell (1971) was branches arising at right angles from axons in the cat's internal capsule and entering the adjacent caudate nucleus. Although Ramón y Cajal had accepted these as collaterals of corticofugal axons, Kemp and Powell rightly point out that one cannot know whether the parent axon is an ascending or a descending one. Not until the advent of the Nauta method did the great profusion of axons leaving the PT along its course become clear. But the extent to which these are terminal corticofugal axons which leave the tract completely at the level of their emission, or are *collateral* branches emitted by PT axons which descend further down the brain stem and even into the LCST cannot unfortunately be settled by examination of the fragmented axonal debris (Wallerian degeneration) resulting from a lesion of the sensorimotor cortex.

Kuypers (1958) made such lesions in cats, and was the first to reveal, with the then newly invented Nauta method, the surprising wealth of emission of axons from the PT in its course through the brain stem. Figure 4.2 gives a good impression of the host of axons streaming dorsally from the PT and reaching virtually every part of the pons and medulla. Figure 4.3 illustrates the distribution of some of the major connexions. In the cat there is no direct connexion to the motor nuclei of the cranial nerves. Corticofugal axons end in relation to groups of neurones which seem to represent the rostral extension of the intermediate zone of the spinal grey matter, and are presumably interneurones of the corticobulbar motor pathway. The projections to the 'sensory' trigeminal nuclei, to the dorsal column nuclei and to the lateral reticular nucleus are prominent. A remarkable feature is the rostral streaming of the bundles of recurrent pyramidal fibres (Figs 4.2 and 4.3, RPF) which, having crossed the midline in the pyramidal decussation, ascend again in the dorsolateral aspect of the medulla. It seems likely that we do not even yet possess the complete catalogue of the subcortical structures to which PT axons and their collaterals are distributed.

To distinguish critically, in any subcortical nucleus N, between collaterals of PT axons on the one hand (Fig. 4.4, C), and terminals of PT axons on the other (Fig. 4.4, T), a combined microanatomical and electroanatomical approach is necessary. Suppose that in a series of cats, a small lesion in a specific area of cortex is followed by fine axonal and synaptic degeneration in N. Suppose further that a weak stimulus (Fig. 4.4, SC) to the same area of cortex in a series of intact cats evokes postsynaptic activity that can be detected by a microelectrode in N. Then if this activity is due to impulses travelling in PT collaterals (Fig. 4.4, C), an antidromic volley evoked by a stimulus to the medullary pyramid (Fig. 4.4, PT) will invade these collaterals orthodromically (Fig. 4.4, arrows), and should therefore evoke the same postsynaptic response in N. For

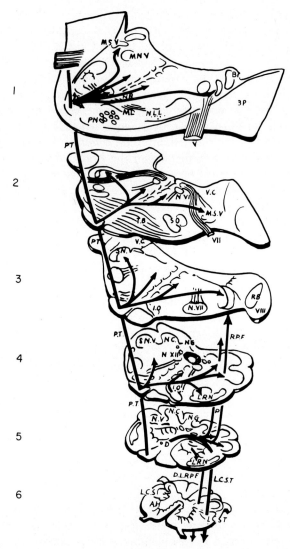

Fig. 4.3. Diagrammatic slices of pons (1), medulla (2–5) and cervical spinal cord (6) of cat, showing course of axons, degenerating as the result of lesion of sensorimotor cortex, streaming dorsally from the left pyramidal tract (P.T.) into the brain stem before crossing the midline at the pyramidal decussation (5, P.D.) to descend the cord as the lateral corticospinal tract (6, L.C.–S.T.). Amongst other destinations, pyramidal axons are distributed bilaterally to the main sensory nucleus of the trigeminal nerve (2, MSV) and its spinal nucleus (3, 4, 5, S.N.V.); to the lateral reticular nucleus of the opposite side (4, 5, L.R.N.); and to the dorsal column nuclei and spinal trigeminal nucleus of the opposite side (4, 5, N.C., N.G.), largely by recurrent pyramidal axons (5, RPF) which spring from the decussated pyramidal bundles and ascend the brain stem, giving off, in addition, descending branches (6, D.L.R.P.F.) to dorsal horn and intermediate region of the spinal grey matter. (Kuypers, 1958.)

example, PT collaterals have been proved, by this method, to enter the red nucleus (Tsukahara *et al.*, 1968).

Another method has been used by Endo *et al.* (1973). They recorded intracellularly from PTNs in the motor cortex; these were identified antidromically by stimulating the PT, and in some cases also the LCST (Fig. 4.4). They then stimulated several subcortical nuclei (e.g. Fig. 4.4, SN). If any of these received a collateral branch from the axon of the impaled PTN, that neurone would register an antidromic impulse. The latency was longer than when the PT was stimulated, because of slowed conduction in the thin collateral terminals; but if the stimulus SN was strengthened, the latency would suddenly shorten to the same value as the PT latency, SN having spread to stimulate the PT directly, at, or near to, the point of origin of the collateral. With intracellular recording, antidromic impulses can be distinguished from orthodromic impulses with absolute certainty (Chapter 3, section 3.2).

We do not yet know whether the axon of an individual PTN gives a collateral branch to every subcortical nucleus which lies along its path, or

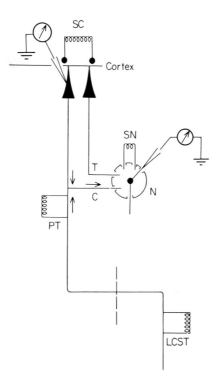

Fig. 4.4. Proof that pyramidal axon collaterals are distributed to a subcortical nucleus. Explanation in text.

whether an LCST axon, having emitted one or more intracranial collaterals, then proceeds to contribute collateral branches to interneurones,
cells of origin of ascending pathways, etc. in several segments of the spinal
cord. Endo *et al.* (1973) traced axon collaterals of fast (>20 m s^{-1}) and
slow (<20 m s^{-1}) PTN into subcortical sites which were presumed to
correspond to caudate nucleus, putamen, red nucleus, thalamic nuclei
VA, VL, VPL and CM, pontine nuclei, mesencephalic reticular formation,
and dorsal column nuclei. The antidromic stimulating electrodes were
aimed at these sites with the help of sterotaxic coordinates, but their
positions were not, unfortunately, verified histologically. These sites were
not all stimulated in every preparation. Of the sample of 187 PTN collected by Endo *et al.*, 119 (92/138 'fast', 27/49 'slow') were proved to emit
axon collaterals. Thirty-eight were shown to branch at two subcortical
loci and eight to branch at three.

A priori one would assume that the function of the PT collaterals would
not be merely to connect parts of the sensorimotor cortex to particular
subcortical nuclei. Such connexions could be provided by unbranched
pyramidal or parapyramidal axons travelling solely to those specific
destinations. The essential function of the collaterals would rather be to
send 'corollary discharges' to synaptic stations along 'parallel' pathways
whenever the parent PT axon is transmitting impulses to its ultimate
terminations. Such parallel pathways are both descending and ascending.
The descending pathways include the corticostriatal, cortico-rubro-spinal
and cortico-reticulo-spinal projections as well as the extrapyramidal
projections, e.g. corticostriatal and corticopontine originating outside the
sensorimotor cortex (Kemp and Powell, 1971). The ascending pathways
include all afferent projections to fore-brain and cerebellum. PT collaterals could provide, at points of synaptic convergence along their course,
'copies' of motor 'commands' for comparison with the afferent input
resulting from the movement (see Chapter 8).

Much combined microscopical and electroanatomical work will be
needed before we have the complete catalogue of the PT collaterals.
Until this has been done, we must restrict attention to the relatively few
cases of antidromically validated collaterals. It is more interesting to
consider them in putative functional categories rather than in the mere
order of their emission from the tract.

The first category (Fig. 4.5, 1, 2, 3) includes the Golgi recurrent collaterals which arise from the PTN within the cortex itself and are connected, directly and by cortical interneurones, to neighbouring PTN and
to corticorubral neurones. It includes also PT collaterals which enter the
striatum (Fig. 4.5, 4), red nucleus (Fig. 4.5, 5, 6) and bulbar reticular
formation (Fig. 4.5, 7). All these are representative of collaterals which
would transmit corollary discharges to parallel descending pathways. Such

pathways would include not only the major parapyramidal and extra-pyramidal projections, but also the subdivisions within the PT itself, mutually interconnected by 'lateral' synaptic interactions brought about by the Golgi recurrent collaterals at the cortical level.

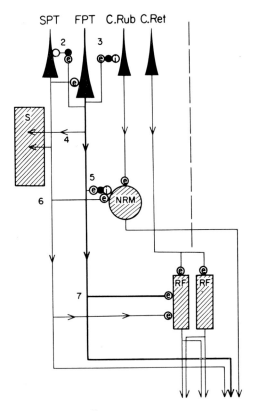

FIG. 4.5. Pyramidal axon collaterals within the cortex (1, 2, 3); to striatum (4, S); to large-celled part of red nucleus (5, 6, NRM); and to midline reticular formation of hind-brain (7, RF). SPT and FPT, slow and fast pyramidal tract neurones; C. Rub, cortico-rubral neurones; C. Ret, corticoreticular neurones. e, Excitation; i, inhibition.

The second functional category (Fig. 4.6) includes collaterals to the dorsal column nuclei, trigeminal nuclei and thalamus, which could adjust the gain and discrimination of the somaesthetic pathways which ascend to the cerebral cortex, and provide for comparison of afferent inputs with outgoing motor commands.

The third functional category (Fig. 4.8) includes collaterals which form part of the cerebro-cerebello-cerebral networks (Fig. 1.2) and control the inputs which ascend to the cerebellar cortex from the muscles, tendons, joints and skin.

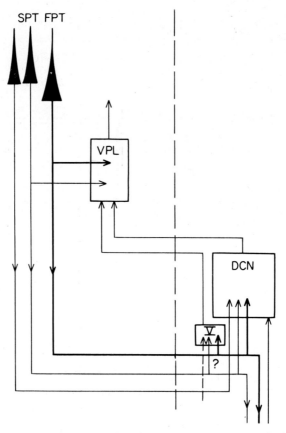

FIG. 4.6. Pyramidal axon collaterals and corticonuclear axons to somaesthetic relay nuclei.

4.3.1 GLOSSARY OF CORTICOFUGAL NEURONES AND AXONS

Before going further, it will help to avoid confusion if we can agree to adopt certain anatomical definitions. These are possibly not in general use; if they meet with approval it will be because they may be found helpful in planning the strategy and tactics of experimental work and in the interpretation of clinicopathological observations. The functional categories of neurones and axons will often cut across the anatomical groupings.

The pyramidal tract (PT) should retain its classical definition: axons composing the medullary pyramid (Marshall, 1936). This structure can readily be divided or stimulated.

Pyramidal tract neurones (PTN) are cortical neurones whose axons travel in the medullary pyramid, regardless of their terminal destination. They may give off axon collaterals in centrum semiovale, internal capsule, cerebral peduncle, and pontine 'pyramidal' bundles as well as in the medullary pyramid.

Parapyramidal neurones are cortical neurones located within the area of cortex which gives origin to the PT, but whose axons (and axon collaterals) leave the internal capsule, cerebral peduncle or pontine pyramidal bundles without ever reaching the medullary pyramid. Thus they would not be interrupted by pyramid section or excited antidromically by stimulation of the pyramid. They might terminate in mid-brain or pons, or travel further caudally in the medulla, dorsal to the PT.

Extrapyramidal neurones are cortical neurones located in areas of cortex outside the area of origin of the PT. They give rise to massive cortico-pontine and corticostriate projections. These are *extrapyramidal projections*. We dislike, and shall not use, the unfortunate term 'extrapyramidal system' to lump together all the extrapyramidal cortical areas, basal ganglia, etc.—that is, all descending corticofugal projections other than the PT.

The axons of *corticobulbar neurones* terminate within the brain stem. They include parapyramidal and pyramidal axons distributed to the motor nuclei of the cranial nerves, to the trigeminal and dorsal column nuclei, etc. They include, also, extra pyramidal axons distributed to the pontine nuclei.

Corticospinal neurones are those PTN whose axons continue into the spinal cord.

Thus, the PT includes some corticobulbar and corticoreticular axons; corticoolivary axons; *corticonuclear axons* to the cuneate and gracile nuclei; and corticospinal axons. All these axons may have supplied collateral branches to striatum, thalamus, red nucleus and pontine nuclei before they enter the medullary pyramid. The corticospinal axons may also have supplied collaterals to the inferior olives, to the bulbar reticular formation, and to the dorsal column nuclei, before they enter the spinal cord.

The parapyramidal projection includes the corticostriate, cortico-thalamic, corticorubral and corticopontine axons, as well as the more rostral corticobulbar and corticoreticular axons. For all we know, any or all of these may emit collateral branches.

It is obvious that the major functional categories outlined at the end of the previous section do not respect these morphologically defined group-ings. Thus some corticobulbar and some corticospinal axons belong to functionally equivalent 'input-modulating' or 'motor' categories (cf. Fig. 1.2, p. 8). Conceptually, it may seem perverse to insist on the classical definition of the PT when by so doing one deliberately excludes so many axons belonging to the same functional groupings as those represented within the PT. The practical advantages, however, outweigh the con-ceptual disadvantages when it comes to such operational matters as the placing of lesions and the insertion of stimulating and recording electrodes.

4.3.2 COLLATERALS DISTRIBUTED TO PARALLEL DESCENDING PATHWAYS

4.3.2.1 *The Golgi recurrent collaterals*

These, to the number of four or more, are regularly present in neocortical pyramidal neurones, including those of the motor area (Fig. 3.1, p. 54); their endings ramify around other cells of the same type (Ramón y Cajal, 1911). To activate them selectively it is only necessary to send an antidromic volley along the PT, but it is also necessary to be sure that the pyramidal stimuli are too weak to penetrate into the medulla and initiate contaminating orthodromic volleys in the underlying medial lemniscus. This has been accomplished by applying four fine cathodes to the exposed pyramid so that they lie transversely across its thickest part, spanning 1.0 mm, and by stimulating them separately. By this means the ventralmost layer of axons in this thickest part could be dissected electrically, as it were, into four bundles, one of which would contain the axon of the PTN under investigation. Stimuli subliminal for this axon would excite fewer axons of other PTN, located ventrally to the 'index' axon and therefore still further from the medial lemniscus. Stimulation of the separate bundles at 400 Hz gave no motor response, showing that the stimuli were indeed well below maximal (Phillips, 1959). Such fractional pyramidal stimulation always evoked detectable changes in the membrane potential of the PTN. Since its own axon was not stimulated (except initially, for antidromic labelling) these changes were due to activity in the recurrent axon collaterals of its neighbours. They have already been illustrated in Fig. 3.6A, B (p. 64). The sequence of excitatory depolarization followed by inhibitory hyperpolarization was found invariably, but the proportions varied from one PTN to another, presumably because the excitatory and inhibitory connexions to the different PTN were different. In extracellular experiments, there were corresponding changes in excitability which could be detected by a testing cortical pulse, and when recurrent inhibitory action was sufficiently intense a testing antidromic impulse would fail to invade the PTN (Phillips, 1959, 1961).

Armstrong (1965) extended these studies, again using intracellular recording in identified PTN of the cat. He produced evidence for excitatory postsynaptic potentials in the pyramidal neurones with rapidly conducting axons which could have resulted monosynaptically from the activation of collaterals of PTN with more slowly conducting axons. A further study by Takahashi *et al.* (1967) strengthened this observation. EPSPs were produced in PTN with axonal conduction velocities greater than 20 m s^{-1} and these EPSPs were generated by activation of PT axons with conduction velocities less than 20 m s^{-1} (Fig. 4.5, 1). Armstrong's findings on inhibitory postsynaptic potentials can be explained by a disynaptic inhibitory pathway from the collaterals of fast PTN directed to the cells of origin of slow PT axons (Fig. 4.5, 2). Synaptic interactions between the fast and slow PTN in the cat are likely therefore to be complex. Any tonic discharge of slow PTN would facilitate the discharge of associated fast PTN. But bursts of impulses in the axons of fast PTN would be expected to inhibit the discharge of slow PTN over recurrent axon collateral pathways. Stefanis and Jasper (1964) suggested that the IPSPs produced by recurrent axon-collaterals must be generated at synapses close to the soma of the cell and the spike initiating regions, since they were of large amplitude, arrested spontaneous firing and could block the invasion into the soma of an antidromic impulse.

The recurrent collaterals of PTN also inhibit the cells of origin of the corticorubral (CR) tract (Tsukahara et al., 1968), one of the parallel parapyramidal projections whose cells of origin are intermingled with those of the PT. The inhibition is probably mediated by local interneurones (Fig. 4.5, 3). Of the possible functional meaning of the recurrent inhibition of PT and CR neurones we have little idea. The parallel CR projection (Rinvik and Walberg, 1963) excites the neurones of pars magnocellularis of the red nucleus (Fig. 4.5, NRM: Tsukahara and Kosaka, 1968). The rubrospinal axons project somatotopically along the length of the zona intermedia of the spinal grey matter (Nyberg-Hansen and Brodal, 1964), and their distribution overlaps with that of the somatotopically arranged PT projection from the forelimb and hindlimb area of the cortex. The physiological actions of the cortico-rubro-spinal projection have been worked out by Hongo and Jankowska (1967) and Hongo et al (1969a, b), and closely resemble those of the PT. The recurrent inhibition would thus be directed to the cells of origin of two parallel projections with similar effects on the spinal cord. 'Blunderbuss' firing of recurrent collaterals by antidromic pyramidal volleys can demonstrate the existence of recurrent facilitation and inhibition, but cannot reveal any patterned organization there might be. During naturally occurring movements, recurrent facilitation and inhibition could play a part in shaping the discharge patterns of populations of PT and CR neurones, improving the information content of their 'instructions' to lower levels (Tsukahara et al., 1968). It is also tempting to speculate that the powerful recurrent inhibition may have a general importance in tending to suppress the genesis of epileptic discharges, and that Jackson's 'discharging lesion' may be a biochemical lesion of the inhibitory transmitter apparatus.

4.3.2.2 Collaterals to the striatum

All areas of the cat's cortex (least, the visual cortex) give rise to cortico-striatal axons, but their richest profusion comes from the sensorimotor cortex (Kemp and Powell, 1971). That these include a proportion of PT collaterals has been established by Endo et al. (1973). Of 104 fast PTN that were tested by stimulation aimed at the caudate nucleus, only 7 supplied collaterals, and of 33 slow PTN thus tested, only 2. For the putamen the corresponding numbers were 5/91 and 2/24; and for the globus pallidus, 2/91 and 0/24. We are not aware of any experiments in which postsynaptic responses in the striatum have been investigated by antidromic pyramidal activation of PT collaterals.

The PT neurones receive a powerful inhibitory input when the caudate nucleus is stimulated (Klee and Lux, 1962).

4.3.2.3 *Collaterals to rubrospinal neurones*

The axons of fast and slow PTN have been shown, by antidromic pyramidal stimulation, to send collaterals into the red nucleus (Tsukahara *et al.*, 1968; Endo *et al.*, 1973). The large neurones which give origin to the rubrospinal tract were impaled with intracellular microelectrodes (Tsukahara *et al.*, 1968) and identified by antidromic stimulation of the tract in the spinal cord. Their responses to volleys in the PT collaterals were then investigated. To the collaterals of fast PT they responded with IPSPs, mediated by interneurones (Fig. 4.5, 5). The slow PT collaterals excited the rubrospinal neurones monosynaptically (Fig. 4.5, 6). Thus the parallel cortico-rubro-spinal projection is inhibited by collaterals of PTN at the level of the red nucleus as well as by the Golgi recurrent collaterals at the cortical level. In the sample of PTN collected by Endo *et al.* (1973), 23/120 fast and 4/28 slow neurones contributed axon collaterals to the stereotaxic locus of the red nucleus. This nucleus, of course, receives corticorubral axons (Fig. 4.5, C.Rub) as well as PT collaterals (Tsukahara and Kosaka, 1968). Intracellular injection of Procion Yellow dye into an antidromically identified CR neurone enabled its perikaryon to be visualized, after death, in the inner part of lamina III or outer part of lamina V of the cat's motor cortex (Batuev and Lenkov, 1973).

4.3.2.4 *PT collaterals to reticulospinal neurones*

The large cells in the pontine and bulbar reticular formation, which give rise to the reticulospinal tracts, have been impaled with microelectrodes, identified by antidromic stimulation of the tracts, and tested by cortical stimulation in anaesthetized and pyramidal cats (Magni and Willis, 1964a). The largest effects were from stimulation of sensorimotor cortex, and were bilateral. Monosynaptic EPSPs were recorded in 87 per cent of a sample of 359 reticulospinal neurones. IPSPs were rare. In the anaesthetized cats, corticoreticular axons travelling in tegmental pathways other than the PT (Fig. 4.5, C.Ret) could have been responsible; the recorded actions need not have been due to PT collaterals. In the pyramidal preparations the brain stem was injured electrolytically at the rostral end of the mid-brain, sparing only the pyramidal tracts and substantia nigra. There must remain therefore some uncertainty about the possible sparing of parapyramidal and other tegmental pathways, especially since some responses were obtained from stimulation of occipital and temporal lobes which, as we have seen, are not significant contributors of axons to the PT. Nevertheless, the collaterals described by Ramón y Cajal would probably have contributed corollary monosynaptic excitation to the fast parallel cortico-reticulo-spinal pathway (Fig. 4.5, 7). Antidromic pyramidal volleys will be needed to resolve this question.

4.3.3 DISTRIBUTION OF TERMINAL PYRAMIDAL AND PARAPYRAMIDAL AXONS
       AND PYRAMIDAL COLLATERALS TO ASCENDING SOMAESTHETIC PATHWAY

In Chapter 1 we distinguished a class of PT axons which interact with incoming peripheral inputs at the level of the dendrites and somata of second-order neurones (Fig. 1.2B, p. 8). The spinal representatives of this class will be considered below (section 4.4). The dorsal column nuclei and trigeminal nuclei will be considered now (Fig. 4.6).

4.3.3.1 *Dorsal column and trigeminal nuclei*

Collaterals of corticospinal axons, as well as terminal pyramidal ('cortico-nuclear') axons, enter the dorsal column nuclei and influence the primary afferent axons, the interneurones, and the second-order 'relay' neurones which project to the contralateral ventrobasal thalamus by way of the medial lemniscus.

Gordon and Miller (1969) recorded antidromic impulses extracellularly from 42 corticonuclear neurones whose axon-terminals were stimulated in the contralateral cuneate and gracile nuclei. These were all small PTN, with conduction velocities ranging from about 3 to 20 ms^{-1}. Accurate location of the stimulated sites was certified by plotting curves of threshold against depth and by histological reconstruction of the tracks. Stimulation of the contralateral corticospinal tract evoked antidromic impulses in plenty of pericruciate neurones, but since none of these was also invaded antidromically when the dorsal column nuclei were stimulated, there was no evidence of CST collaterals entering the nuclei. The cortical location of about half of the corticonuclear neurones was established by correlation of microelectrode positions with cytoarchitectonic boundaries in the individual brains. These neurones were all within, or near to the edges of, area 3a, which is 'a transitional zone between the typical "motor" cortex of area 4 and that of typical sensory cortex in area 3b'. Corticocuneate neurones, which are concerned with the forelimb, differ from cortico-gracile neurones (from the hindlimb) in their origin from areas 4 and 3b as well as from area 3a (Cole and Gordon, 1976b), and in their faster conduction velocity (Cole and Gordon, 1976a). There is no such dissimilarity in conduction time from the cuneate and gracile nuclei to the cortex, and Cole and Gordon (1976a) suggest that the function of the dissimilarity in corticofugal conduction time 'may be related to the differing time courses of sensory return from hind- and forelimb consequent upon their movement'.

Corticonuclear neurones were 'occasionally found' in the experiments of Endo *et al.* (1973) but were 'not further mentioned'. Of 73 fast PTN which responded antidromically to stimulation of the contralateral CST, 12 also responded antidromically to stimulation of the putative (stereotaxically determined) site of the contralateral dorsal column nuclei, and therefore, if this location was exact, contributed collaterals to them. Of 27 slow PTN whose axons continued into the contralateral CST, 4 also responded antidromically to stimulation of the dorsal locus.

Electroanatomical study of the actions exerted by the sensorimotor cortex on the dorsal column nuclei was begun by Magni *et al.* (1959). They stimulated sensorimotor cortex, internal capsule, and pes pendunculi in pyramidal cats in which the mid-brain tegmentum had been destroyed electrolytically, sparing the pes pedunculi. Trains of 5 pulses, duration 0.2 ms, amplitude 5 to 7 volts, frequency 300 to 500 Hz, which were adequate to evoke flexion of the contralateral limbs, elicited a characterstic negative-positive wave sequence which could be recorded from the surface of the dorsal column nuclei, and with which (and especially with the positive wave) all subsequent analysis has been concerned. The response was bilateral, but preponderantly contralateral. It was abolished by cutting the pyramid on the stimulated side, immediately rostral to the decussation. With the positive (P) wave, there was associated a depression of the amplitude of the wave elicited at the surface of the cuneate nucleus by a volley in the superficial radial nerve.

Analysis of the P wave was pursued by Andersen *et al.* (1964a, b, c). A single pulse to the sensorimotor cortex evoked no P wave in the contralateral cuneate nucleus, but 2 to 8 pulses at 220 Hz evoked P waves of increasing amplitude, up to about 0.7 mV. The same increase was found when the cerebral white matter was stimulated after removal of the cortex, and was therefore presumed to be due to repetitive facilitating events within the cuneate nucleus. The distribution in space of the P wave corresponded with the region in which the axons of the lateral division of the dorsal column (column of Burdach) ran along the surface of, and dipped down into, the cuneate nucleus. Electrode tracks which penetrated the nucleus showed that the P wave reversed its polarity at the level of the axon terminals (Fig. 4.7B, C). These details were established in histological reconstructions (sagittal sections). All this evidence pointed to the probability that the pyramidal axons can depolarize the membranes of the terminal arborizations of the primary afferent axons within the cuneate nucleus. Such 'primary afferent depolarization' (PAD) was already known as the basis of presynaptic inhibition in the spinal cord: the reduced transmitting potency of such depolarized presynaptic membranes had been revealed in the diminished amplitude of the excitatory postsynaptic potentials evoked by them in spinal motoneurones.

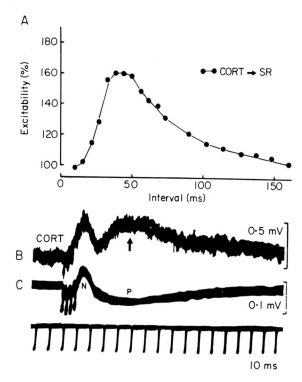

Fig. 4.7. Depolarization of primary afferent axons in the cuneate nucleus by cortical stimulation.

A. The time-course of the waxing and waning of electrical excitability of the terminals of primary afferent axons, following a brief train to stimuli to sensorimotor cortex at time 0, tested by microstimulation of the terminals at increasing intervals of time.

B. Electrical recording, from the site stimulated in A, by the same microelectrode, of the response of the terminals to the same cortical stimuli. The initial negative wave resembles that recorded from the surface of the nucleus in record C: the second negative wave is the mirror image of the surface P wave, recorded, at this depth (1.0 mm), from the active sinks of the depolarized terminals. Arrow marks its peak, which corresponds in time to the maximum of excitability in A.

C. The N–P wave sequence, recorded from the surface and evoked by the same cortical stimuli (modified from Fig. 2 of Andersen et al., 1964b).

The PAD evoked by repetitive pyramidal volleys was detected in the cuneate presynaptic terminals by testing their increased excitability by microstimulation within the nucleus. Figure 4.7A plots the time-course of the waxing and waning of excitability in terms of the size of the population of primary afferent axons firing an antidromic volley into the superficial radial nerve. The curve conforms with the time-course of the P wave recorded at the surface of the cuneate nucleus (Fig. 4.7C), and with its negative mirror image recorded amongst the terminals within the nucleus. The latter (Fig. 4.7B) was recorded at the same site, and with the same microelectrode, as that used for stimulating when determining the changes of excitability plotted in Fig. 4.7A.

In experiments on the 'lateral inhibition' exerted by one afferent nerve on the terminals of another, the PAD was recorded directly with an intracellular microelectrode inserted into the depolarized terminals, and possibly even into the very large synaptic boutons which are a feature of the cuneate nucleus (Andersen et al., 1964b). Unfortunately no intracellular records were taken from terminals depolarized by pyramidal volleys.

The reduction of transmitting potency of these synapses has not yet been demonstrated directly by intracellular recording from the postsynaptic (relay) neurones, but has been detected indirectly. A conditioning train of stimuli was given to the sensorimotor cortex, and followed by a testing afferent volley from a peripheral nerve, at increasing intervals of time. The size of the responding population of postsynaptic (relay) neurones was measured in terms of the amplitude of the volley recorded from the killed thalamic end of the medial lemniscus (Andersen et al., 1964d). The waning and waxing of population size, which is the statistical mirror of the unitary inhibitory events, again follows the time-course of PAD.

Interneurones in the cuneate nucleus were so classified because, unlike the relay neurones, they failed to respond antidromically to stimulation of the medial lemniscus. Extracellular recording from interneurones, many of which lay deeper in the nucleus than the 'relay' neurones, detected repetitive firing in response to stimulation of the somatosensory cortex. Some responded to single descending volleys; others needed two or more volleys. Latency was 3 to 42 ms (cf. conduction times of corticonuclear axons of 1.9 to 17.1 ms, measured by Gordon and Miller, 1969). It is assumed that these interneurones form axo-axonic synapses on the terminals of the primary afferent axons and that they are responsible for the PAD and, hence, for the presynaptic inhibition of the relay neurones.

Whether PT axons can impress postsynaptic inhibition on the relay neurones, presumably via hyperpolarizing interneurones in the cuneate nucleus, and, if so, what is the importance of postsynaptic inhibition in relation to the very prominent presynaptic inhibition, are questions which are still not settled. Intracellular records from the relay neurones were hard to come by, on account of their relatively small size and the pulsations of the medulla. Afferent volleys from forelimb nerves evoked IPSPs whose latency is systematically longer than that of the afferent-evoked EPSPs, suggesting an interneuronal link. Some IPSPs are of sufficiently long duration to account for inhibition almost as prolonged as that of the presynaptic variety (Andersen et al., 1964d). Unfortunately no intracellular records are available of inhibitory responses to cortical stimulation. There is, however, a fragment of evidence for postsynaptic pyramidal inhibition of cuneate relay neurones. Microstimulation among the presynaptic terminals and relay neurones evokes two orthodromic volleys which can be recorded from the killed end of the medial lemniscus: the first ('α spike') is due to direct stimulation of relay neurones, the second ('β spike') is due to monosynaptic excitation of relay neurones by electrically stimulated presynaptic terminals. In two cats out of four, prior cortical stimulation reduced the amplitude of the α spike, in the other two cats it had no such effect (Andersen et al., 1964d).

Of 78 antidromically identified cuneothalamic relay neurones collected by Andersen et al. (1964c), none was fired by cortical stimulation. Since it is difficult to be sure that an antidromic lemniscal volley is maximal, it is possible that some of Andersen et al.'s cortically fired interneurones were in fact relay neurones. Gordon and his colleagues (reviewed by Gordon, 1968) have recorded extracellularly from antidromically identified relay neurones in nucleus gracilis, and have found some that were fired by cortical stimulation. These workers have investigated systematic differences in the properties of the relay neurones in different regions of this nucleus, in electroanatomical experiments which offer important clues to the probable functional significance of the regional difference in architecture.

Nucleus gracilis contains relay cells of two types, spatially segregated into two groups which project to separate loci in the thalamus. The first group corresponds to clusters of neurones in the middle region of the nucleus (Kuypers and Tuerck, 1964). They receive signals from small receptive fields, and respond specifically to touching a claw, a footpad or a few hairs. These receptive fields are sharply circumscribed by lateral inhibition when adjacent fields are touched. This organization seems well adapted to extract one particular feature of the input, namely the shape of the outline of an object pressed against the skin. It has been shown theoretically by Gordon and Kay (Gordon, 1968; Kay, 1964) that a diffuse background of inhibition projected on to such a population of relay neurones will tend to sharpen the discrimination of outlines: increasing the background inhibition will restrict the response to the outlines alone before it suppresses all response. It is therefore interesting that the cortex supplies inhibition, and not excitation, to the cells of the clusters; the animal would thus be able to 'attend to' the contours of a stimulus in which it was 'interested'. A second group of relay neurones in the rostral pole of n. gracilis show excitatory convergence from large receptive fields of hindlimb and trunk. This apparatus would be insensitive to contour, but would extract from the total input another feature: the average intensity of stimulation. These neurones are excited, not inhibited from the cortex, which could therefore operate to adjust the sensitivity of 'attention' to the overall intensity of stimulation of a general region of the limb.

Tactile exploration of the environment entails active movement of the receptive fields of the body surface, and especially those of the face and of the distal parts of the limbs, over the surfaces of the objects being explored. The possible roles of interactions between motor output and afferent input in tactile and stereognostic exploration, in maintaining awareness of the positions of parts of the body and of the direction, range and velocity of movements, and in compensating for changes in the loading of the moving parts, will be considered in Chapter 8.

In the trigeminal nucleus, Darian-Smith and Yokota (1966a) found cortically evoked depolarization of primary afferent axons in experiments of the same type as those already described for the dorsal column nuclei. Of trigeminal neurones which projected to the contralateral posterior thalamus, 50 per cent could be excited from somatosensory cortex. There was also cortically evoked presynaptic inhibition of transmission through the nucleus (Darian-Smith and Yokota, 1966b).

4.3.3.2   *Collaterals to nucleus VPL of thalamus*

Shimazu *et al.* (1965) investigated the action of pyramidal collaterals on thalamocortical neurones of the ventrobasal part of the cat's thalamus. The tracks of the extracellular recording microelectrodes were not reconstructed histologically, but the VB neurones were characterized by their discharge of orthodromic impulses in response to stimulation of postcruciate cortex. Fifty-two neurones were tested by antidromic pyramidal volleys. It was obviously important to attempt to exclude unwanted orthodromic stimulation of the medial lemniscus, and this was done by restricting the strength of the stimuli to the pyramid so as to evoke, at the cortical surface, an initial antidromic potential of less than 60 per cent of maximal amplitude, and also by controls in which the pyramid was stimulated at sites both rostral and caudal to a complete transection. Fifteen VB neurones were excited, some repetitively, at latency 1.5 to 8.5 ms, and 'in about one-third of the neurons tested' there was also a subsequent period of depression: the latency of the cell's response to a testing volley in the medial lemniscus was lengthened during a period extending from 20 to 70 ms after the conditioning pyramidal volley. Tsumoto *et al.* (1975) have also backfired pyramidal volleys into collaterals entering the ventrobasal complex. Of 112 VB neurones, 31 were excited by single antidromic volleys in fast PT axons at monosynaptic latency, and 44 were inhibited by five volleys at 500 Hz; inhibition was disynaptic in the few cells in which intracellular recordings were possible. Strikingly, 22/31 of the monosynaptically excited cells were transmitters of responses to passive flexion of joints, but there was no report of experiments to discriminate between inputs from muscle and joint receptors; of the 44 cells that were inhibited, 34 were transmitters of responses to touching hairs, particularly in small peripheral receptive fields. We shall see that, at the level of primary afferent terminals, the PT characteristically suppresses inputs from the skin while not suppressing inputs from the muscles (section 4.1).

By antidromic stimulation at stereotaxic placements intended for nucleus VPL, Endo et al. (1973) detected the presence of collaterals of 25/134 fast PTN and 5/49 slow PTN.

4.3.4 COLLATERALS CONTRIBUTING TO CEREBRO-CEREBELLAR NETWORKS

The interconnexions between the fore-brain and the intermediate and lateral areas of the cerebellar cortex have already been outlined in a very general way in Chapter 1 (Fig. 1.2, p. 8). Figure 4.8, with its legend, fills in some of the details, for which some electroanatomical evidence will now be reviewed briefly. The pyramidal connexions are directed mainly towards the intermediate areas of the cerebellum, whose moderating influence on red nucleus, VL, and thence on motor cortex is exerted through nucleus interpositus (for reviews see Evarts and Thach, 1969; Allen and Tsukahara, 1974).

4.3.4.1 *Nucleus ventralis lateralis of thalamus* (Fig. 4.8, VL)

This is an important focus for convergence of impulses from the cerebellar nuclei and from the globus pallidus, and exerts a powerful excitatory action on PTN. Clare et al. (1964) stimulated VL, marking the positions of their electrodes by the Prussian Blue reaction. They concluded tentatively, from the times of arrival of an antidromic-evoked potential in the posterior sigmoid gyrus and of descending volleys in the PT or LCST, that they had stimulated collaterals of PT axons which ended in VL. Their conclusion was supported by Endo et al. (1973), who stimulated VL stereotaxically (but without histology) and recorded antidromic impulses from PTN. They found that 26/138 fast PTN and 7/30 slow PTN supplied collaterals to the nucleus.

The *pontine nuclei* (Fig. 4.8, PN) supply mossy fibres to the whole of the contralateral neocerebellar cortex. Some of their input comes from the PT. Allen et al. (1969) stimulated the white matter underlying the sensori-motor cortex, and also the cerebral peduncle, at sites whose distance apart was measured. Neurones of the pontine nuclei were identified by antidromic stimulation of the brachium pontis, their impulses being detected by an extracellular microelectrode. They were then excited orthodromically from the two sites. The difference in latency allowed the conduction velocity of the corticopenduncular segments of the axons to be calculated. Of 26 pontine neurones, 19 were excited by slow PTN only, 7 by both fast and slow. The total latency was short enough to indicate that the connexion was monosynaptic. Of the 26 neurones, 12 were also excited orthodromically by stimulating the PT. Thus, corticopontine pyramidal

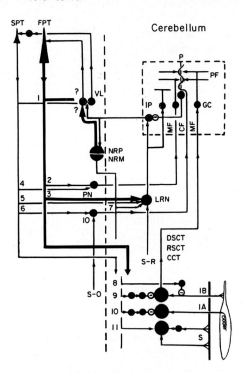

FIG. 4.8. Some of the connexions between the cat's PT and cerebellum, greatly simplified.
Key:
    Midline represented by broken line.
    Excitation:—→
    Inhibition:–⊖
    Action unknown: ?
FPT, fast PT neurones:
    1. Collaterals to ventrolateral nucleus of thalamus (VL).
    2. Collaterals to pontine nuclei (PN).
    3. Collaterals to lateral reticular nucleus (LRN) (tentative).
SPT, slow PT neurones:
    4. Collaterals to PN.
    5. Collaterals to LRN (tentative).
    6. Collaterals to inferior olive (IO) (tentative).
NRM, large-celled part of red nucleus:
    7. Possible rubrospinal collaterals to LRN.

axons certainly exist, but parapyramidal corticopontine axons, which could emerge from the peduncles rostral to the pyramid, are not excluded. The evidence does not show whether the PT endings are collaterals or terminals. For this discrimination, the experiment of Endo *et al.* (1973) would have been crucial if it had been controlled histologically. They collected 7/52 fast PTN and 4/28 slow PTN which responded antidromically to stimuli from electrodes which were presumed to have been successfully located within the pontine nuclei, as well as to stimuli to the PT.

The *lateral reticular nucleus* (Fig. 4.8, LRN) is another large station on the cortico-cerebello-cortical route. Microanatomical studies have shown that its inputs come to it from the spinal cord ipsilaterally (S-R), from the contralateral red nucleus (? as rubro-reticular axons or rubro-spinal collaterals: Fig. 4.8, 7), and from the contralateral sensorimotor cortex, though not from other cortical areas (Figs 4.2 and 4.3: Kuypers 1958; P. Brodal *et al.*, 1967). Künzle and Wiesendanger (1974) find that all axons travelling from sensorimotor cortex to LRN do so through the PT. P. Brodal *et al.* (1967) found a partial convergence between the descending and spinal inputs to the nucleus; but most of the spinal input is to the part of the nucleus which projects to the vermis (palaeocerebellum), whereas most of the rubral and cortical input is to the part which contributes mossy fibres to wide areas of the neocerebellar hemisphere.

The extent to which the LRN receives terminals of pyramidal axons, or collaterals of pyramidal and corticospinal axons, is not yet settled. Zangger and Wiesendanger (1973) stimulated subcortex and cerebral peduncle and found that LRN neurones were excited by fast and slow PT axons. These might have been PT axon terminals or PT or CST axon collaterals. In different experiments, LRN neurones were excited by stimulation of the

Spinobulbar tracts:
    S-0: Spino-olivary tract.
    S-R: Spinal inputs to LRN.
Spinocerebellar tracts:
    DCST: Dorsal spinocerebellar tract;
    RCST: Rostral spinocerebellar tract;
    CCT: Cuneocerebellar tract;
whose cells of origin are excited from skin (S), primary receptors of muscle spindles (IA) and tendon organs (IB), and send mossy fibres (MF) into cerebellar cortex.

From *corticospinal axons* these specific spinocerebellar inputs receive pre- and postsynaptic inhibition (8, 9, 10) and monosynaptic facilitation (11).

Cerebellum (mainly its intermediate region). Cortical Purkinje cells (P) are excited by granule cells (GC) via parallel fibres (PF), and by olivocerebellar climbing fibres (CF). P cells inhibit cells of cerebellar nuclei (e.g. nucleus interpositus, IP).

IP excites VL, both directly and via small-celled part of red nucleus (NRP).

VL excites FPT monosynaptically and SPT disynaptically.

(Modified from Phillips, 1977, by kind permission of Instituto della Enciclopedia Italiana, Rome.)

dissected lateral funiculus of the spinal cord, rostral to T3. This was done five days after hemisection at T3, at which time it was assumed that conduction in the ascending tracts would already be abrogated, and that the excitation could only be due to antidromic impulses in descending tracts. Both fast and slow latencies were measured. Since the rubrospinal tract travels with the LCST in the lateral funiculus, and the red nucleus is known to project to the LRN (Walberg, 1958), this experiment does not prove that collaterals of corticospinal axons enter the LRN, though it seems highly likely that they do so. The proof will require experiments of the Endo *et al.* type, with histological verification of the location of the antidromic stimulating electrodes in the LRN, and antidromic stimulation of the dorsolateral funiculus (which need not be dissected for this experiment).

The *inferior olive* sends climbing fibres to all parts of the cerebellar cortex. Its ventral lamella supplies the intermediate region (Fig. 4.8, 10, CF). Armstrong and Harvey (1966) placed micropipettes in the ventral lamella, and verified the recording sites histologically, and, in some experiments, by electrophoretic deposition of Fast Green dye. They stimulated the paramedian lobule and recorded antidromic field potentials and the antidromic action potentials of single neurones in the olive. The same neurones responded orthodromically to cortical stimulation, at a minimum latency of 8 ms. If this response depends on a direct cortico-olivary connexion, then it must be made by slow axons. The only evidence of monosynaptic connexion was the inability to shorten the latency by strengthening the stimulus. The crucial electroanatomical experiments to determine whether pyramidal or corticospinal collaterals (as distinct from cortico-olivary pyramidal axons) are responsible have not yet been reported, so the collateral that is drawn at 6 in Fig. 4.8 remains provisional.

4.3.5   CORTICOBULBAR AXONS TO NUCLEI OF CRANIAL MOTOR NERVES?

In the cat, no corticobulbar axons reach the motor nuclei of the cranial nerves (Walberg, 1957; Kuypers, 1958). The oculomotor, trochlear and abducens nuclei of rodents, carnivores, and primates appear to receive their corticofugal inputs indirectly, 'conveyed by a phylogenetically old indirect system in which relays occur in the reticular formation' (Carpenter, 1971). Of the cat's cranial motor nuclei in general, Kuypers (1958) concludes that the corticobulbar axons which control them terminate in relation to cell-groups which represent the rostral extension of the spinal cell groups which receive the terminations of the corticospinal tract. Porter (1967) made intracellular records from antidromically identified motoneurones of the hypoglossal nucleus, and measured their responses to surface-anodal stimulation of the face area. The latency of the EPSP was as long as 12 ms when the cortical stimulus was minimal; it shortened, e.g. to 6.3 ms, when the stimulus was increased. This is the expected result when a pathway includes interneurones. The latency of a monosynaptic EPSP would not have changed. The interneurones were found in the region of the spinal trigeminal nucleus, which was explored with an extracellular microelectrode. They were foci of excitatory convergence from the lingual nerve and from the cortex. They fired repetitively, and the EPSPs in the motoneurones showed steps on the rising phase which presumably represented repetitive bombardment by the interneurones. We know of no work on the cortical control of cat's trigeminal, facial or accessorius motoneurones.

4.4   The corticospinal projection in the cat

In classical studies the Marchi method clearly revealed the disintegrating myelin sheaths of degenerating corticofugal axons, streaming out of the LCST and into the dorsal horn and intermediate region of the grey matter as the result of lesions of the contralateral sensorimotor cortex; but it could not trace the distribution of their fragmenting unmyelinated arborizations amongst the neurones of different laminae. The nature of the nexus between CST axons and motoneurones remained in doubt. Uncertainties about the distribution of CST axons were not removed until the Nauta method had been invented. Kuypers' (1958) studies of the PT in the brain stem were paralleled by those of Chambers and Liu (1957) on the spinal cord and dorsal column nuclei.

The degenerating axons enter the base of the dorsal horn, and their fine terminals can be seen as disintegrating pericellular arborizations in the nucleus proprius of the dorsal horn and intermediate region. There is an important difference between the distribution of CST axons from the more caudal ('somatosensory') and more rostral (motor) area (Fig. 4.9), which must have functional implications. The projection from the more caudal area ends dorsomedially in the cord, in laminae IV to VI of Rexed (1964), where it would be in a position to control the transmission of incoming impulses from muscle, joints and skin, not only locally, to destinations within the spinal segments, but also remotely, to destinations in the fore-brain and cerebellum. The projection from the more rostral area is distributed preponderantly to the more ventrolateral parts of the dorsal horn and intermediate zone, in Rexed's laminae V to VII, adjacent to the interneurones which send their axons to the motoneurones of the ventral horn (Nyberg-Hansen and Brodal, 1963). Here it would be in a position to influence reflex transmission, both exteroceptive and proprioceptive, and motor output. The cat has no CST endings in relation to the somata and proximal dendrites of the motoneurones (Fig. 4.17), but another carnivore, the raccoon (*Procyon lotor*), a semi-arboreal animal whose digits have retained their primitive pentadactyl structure, does have sparse corticomotoneuronal connexions (Petras and Lehman, 1966; Buxton and Goodman, 1967; Wirth *et al.*, 1974).

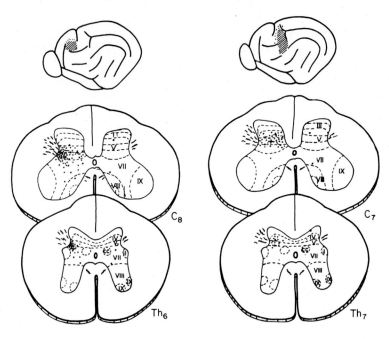

Fig. 4.9. Projections from cat's somatic motor forelimb area (left) and somatosensory forelimb area (right) to spinal cord. See text. (Nyberg-Hansen and Brodal, 1963.)

We have already given examples of the value of electroanatomical and electrophysiological studies as an adjunct to microscopy in answering questions about the origin and distribution of the PT, and of the special value of antidromic experiments in detecting the collateral branching of its axons. Using the antidromic method, Asanuma *et al.* (1976b) found that 70 per cent of 200 CST neurones sent axons only to the cervical enlargement, but that the remaining 30 per cent of the 200 supplied branches both to the lumbar region and to the cervical.

The methods of investigating the depolarization of primary afferent axons by volleys in the PT (presynaptic inhibition, PAD) have already been illustrated in some detail in the cuneate nucleus. These methods have been much employed in work on the actions of LCST volleys on primary afferent arborizations in the spinal cord, operating selectively on the inputs from particular classes of receptive fields (groups Ia, Ib and II from muscles; inputs from skin, etc.). Postsynaptic excitation and inhibition by the LCST of second-order neurones which give rise to ascending spinal tracts, and which can be 'labelled' antidromically by stimulating the appropriate tract, have been detected, timed and measured by intracellular recording. The actions on interneurones, and on motoneurones identified antidromically as belonging to different muscles or groups of muscles, have been investigated similarly. Actions of conditioning LCST volleys, mediated by interneurones to populations of motoneurones, have been detected, timed and measured by plotting the time-course of the enhancement or depression of a testing monosynaptic reflex, evoked by stimulating group Ia afferents in the appropriate muscle nerve and recording the response from the central end of the cut ventral root.

The results of some representative experiments will now be given.

4.4.1 ACTIONS ON AFFERENT INPUTS TO SPINAL SEGMENTS AND ASCENDING SYSTEMS

The LCST can depolarize the terminal arborizations of the thickest axons which come from the skin, of the group Ib axons from the Golgi tendon organs, and of the group II axons from the secondary endings of the muscle spindles. It cannot block the group Ia input from the spindle primaries (Carpenter et al., 1963; Andersen et al., 1964e; Andersen et al., 1964a, b). PAD is believed to be mediated by axo-axonic synapses, and to cause the terminals to release smaller quantities of excitatory synaptic transmitter. Intracellular investigation of motoneurones show that the amplitude of the EPSPs that are evoked by volleys in one of these presynaptically inhibited inputs is depressed; the time-course of the depression, and of the recovery of the control amplitude, parallels the time-course of PAD in the primary afferent arborizations. Absence of postsynaptic inhibition can be shown by the absence of postsynaptic membrane hyperpolarization or conductance change. Presynaptic inhibition can selectively cut down a particular input without depressing, to an equivalent degree, the responsiveness of second-order neurones to other inputs. Thus the LCST could reduce the responsiveness of the 'final common path' to a particular input or inputs without also blocking its responsiveness to commands from the brain.

Figure 4.8 summarizes some of the actions of the LCST on primary afferents and second-order neurones which signal to the cerebellar cortex along the dorsal spinocerebellar, rostral spinocerebellar and cuneocerebellar tracts (DSCT, RSCT and CCT). Transmission from the receptive fields of the skin can be enhanced by monosynaptic facilitation of second-order neurones (Fig. 4.8, 11). Transmission from the primary endings of the muscle spindles and from the Golgi tendon organs (Ia, Ib) can be depressed by disynaptic inhibition of second-order neurones (Fig. 4.8, 10, 9). The input from the tendon organs can also be reduced by pre-synaptic inhibition (Fig. 4.8, 8) (Oscarsson, 1965).

4.4.2 ACTIONS ON MOTOR OUTPUTS: INTERNEURONES, MOTONEURONES AND FUSIMOTOR NEURONES

For many experiments it is important to restrict to CST axons the volleys one sends down the spinal cord. This can be achieved by transecting the hind-brain from the dorsal aspect with a special tool which spares only the medullary pyramids, and ventilating the lungs with a pump (Lloyd, 1941) or by 'transecting' the rest of the brain stem by electrolysis ('pyramidal preparation' of Agnew et al., 1963). Stimuli can then be delivered to the motor cortex, or to the PT rostral to the lesion. In the experiments to be described, even maximal single PT volleys will evoke no motor output from the spinal segments. Adrian and Moruzzi (1939), who were the first to record from PT axons in the pyramidal decussation, were surprised to find them discharging 'spontaneously' in anaesthetized cats without causing any movement. For any motor output to occur in response to cortical or pyramidal stimulation (Brookhart, 1952), spatial and temporal summation are necessary: the first depends on the size of the PT volleys (number of axons discharged), the second on the number and frequency of the volleys. Such massive volleys probably have complex and conflicting actions and would be inappropriate if one wished to discover the effects of small PT volleys, discharged from circumscribed areas of cortex, on particular segments of the cord. For technical convenience, much work has been done on the lumbosacral segments of the cord although the CST makes its largest contribution to the cervical segments. Nevertheless, much knowledge of the interneuronal coupling between CST axons and moto-neurones has been gained from the actions of near-maximal volleys on the lumbosacral segments.

4.4.2.1 *Interneuronal coupling between CST axons and motoneurones*

Of such studies, Lloyd's (1941) was the first, and remains one of the finest. In pioneering research with extracellular microelectrodes, he built up a revealing picture of response beginning in the dorsal horn and then spreading ventrally to the motoneurones. He stimulated the PT rostral to the plane of section of the rest of the brain stem, and recorded the volley at successive segments as it travelled down the LCST, with a steel micro-electrode thrust into the dorsolateral funiculus. The expected triphasic spike potential was not found (cf. the LCST spike since found in primates: Fig. 3.17, p. 84); what was recorded was a positive-going wave, which was probably derived from axons injured by the penetrating microelectrode

(Fig. 3.15, p. 78). The fastest impulses travelled at about 60 m s^{-1} (cf. calibre spectrum of PT: section 4.2). No lower limit could be set to the conduction velocity of the finest axons, since the wave tailed off indefinitely. The temporal scatter of the volley increased as it travelled caudally: at the lumbar level the fastest impulses arrived 4.5 ms after the stimulus to the PT, and the slower continued to arrive for many ms. Thus there could be no certainty whether any delayed postsynaptic responses were monosynaptically generated by slower axons, or were polysynaptically generated by faster axons.

The grey matter was then explored with the microelectrode. To discharge interneurones in the dorsal horn, at least three LCST volleys were needed, frequency 400 Hz. These neurones were probably indirectly coupled to the CST axons, since they did not follow the frequency of the volleys. By contrast, some neurones in the intermediate region were 'driven' by volleys at 300 Hz. The background discharges of some neurones were suppressed by CST volleys.

The discharges of motoneurones were recorded from the ventral roots. In many of these pyramidal preparations, which were also decerebrated at intercollicular level and were under light Dial narcosis, the motoneurones were discharging tonically. Discharge attributable to a train of repetitive pyramidal stimulation lasting 245 ms, began about 15 ms after the arrival of the first volley at the lumbosacral level, and outlasted the stimulation by several hundred ms. This implied an indirect coupling between CST axons and motoneurones, and the interposition of interneurone pools that were capable of prolonged after-discharge and of bombarding the motoneurones repetitively. A more precise investigation of the coupling was achieved by plotting the facilitating action of conditioning pyramidal volleys on the excitability of motoneurones, as tested by a segmental monosynaptic reflex (Figs 4.10 and 4.11). This work was done before Lloyd had discovered that the afferent limb of the monosynaptic reflex is formed by group 1a axons of the muscle nerves. Renshaw had discovered that a stimulus to a dorsal root evokes a motor volley in the ventral root of the same segment at monosynaptic latency, and this was the stimulus used by Lloyd for testing the motoneurones. The reflex volley in the ventral root was not, of course, separable into the responses of motoneurones of different muscle-groups (e.g. flexors and extensors of a particular joint).

Figure 4.10 shows the changes in excitability of motoneurones caused by different numbers of pyramidal volleys at a frequency of 400 Hz. The relative amplitudes of the testing monosynaptic reflex are plotted as ordinates, the control value (amplitude of the test response in isolation) being 100 per cent. One to six conditioning pyramidal stimuli were given, the first at time 0, the second to the sixth at the times marked by arrows.

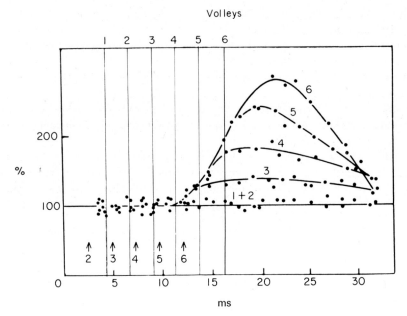

Fig. 4.10. Facilitation of spinal motoneurones by pyramidal volleys. Explanation in text. (Modified from Lloyd, 1941.)

We have added, to Lloyd's graph, six vertical lines to indicate the approximate times of arrival of the fastest impulses of the six volleys at the lumbar enlargement, at intervals of 4.5 ms after the corresponding arrows. The graph shows that one or two pyramidal volleys brought about no increase in motoneurone excitability. Thus, there can be no significant monosynaptic connexions between CST axons and motoneurones in the cat, whether from the fastest axons or from slower ones. The third volley, adding its effects to the subliminal facilitation of interneurones built up by the first two, must have discharged some interneurones which contributed excitatory synapses to the motoneurones. Figure 4.10 shows that the bombardment of the motoneurones began about 2 ms after the arrival of the third CST volley in the spinal segment, increased to a maximum in about 10 ms, and then died away. Four, five or six volleys generated effects with a similar time-course, but with shortening 'specific latency' for each specific volley. The crests of the curves correspond roughly with the time of onset of motoneuronal discharge in the experiments in which trains of stimuli lasting 245 ms were delivered.

To measure, with greater accuracy, the shortening of specific latency by temporal facilitation, Lloyd measured the specific latency of the responses to the third and sixth volleys in an experiment in which the

curves were defined by larger numbers of points (Fig. 4.11). Again we have
added vertical lines to indicate the arrival of the volleys in the spinal segment, 4.5 ms after the pyramidal stimuli. The specific latency of the
response to the third volley was about 2.8 ms, that to the sixth volley
about 0.8 to 1.8 ms. If the sixth specific latency had equalled the third,
the curves would not have diverged until time B. Such shortening of the
time between the 'specific' volley and the earliest excitatory synaptic
impact on the motoneurones would have been due to the discharge of
interneurones lying further downstream along the chains that link the
CST to the motoneurones. As Lloyd pointed out, the evidence of timing,
taken by itself, does not exclude a monosynaptic connexion between slower
CST axons and motoneurones: it is the absence of any detectable effect
of a single CST volley that excludes any *significant* monosynaptic connexion.

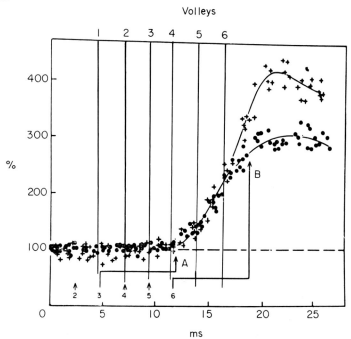

FIG. 4.11. Facilitation of motoneurones by 5 pyramidal shocks (circles) and 6 pyramidal
shocks (crosses). Arrow 3-A denotes the specific latency for the third pyramidal shock
(7.3 ms: specific latency for third volley = 7.3 − 4.5 = 2.8 ms). Arrow 6-B has the same
time span as arrow 3-A. Note that the curves diverge before B; hence there is progressive
shortening of latency in the spinal mechanism. (Modified from Lloyd, 1941.)

Much information about the interneurones that are interposed between
the CST axons and the different groups of motoneurones has come from
the experiments of Lundberg and his colleagues. Recording intracellularly

from 23 interneurones, some of which were proved to be genuine interneurones and not cells of origin of ascending spinal tracts, Lundberg
et al. (1962) found convergence of CST and segmental nerve volleys.
Some showed complex convergence from skin and muscle afferents.
Figure 4.12 shows records from a genuine interneurone which received
its only peripheral input from a cutaneous nerve—monosynaptic
excitation from the superficial peroneal (Fig. 4.12A). Very strong stimuli
to muscle afferents (biceps-semitendinosus, B, and anterior biceps-
semimembranosus, C) had no effect. One, two or three CST volleys
(D, E, F) evoked an EPSP with latency about 3 ms from the CST volley
(not shown). This need not have been monosynaptic. In other cells the
latency was shorter, and repeated volleys evoked an EPSP with steps on
the rising phase suggestive of presynaptic facilitation (Chapter 3). In
one neurone only was there postsynaptic inhibition from some nerves
and from the CST. Lundberg *et al.* concluded that these interneurones
were shared by reflex arcs and by the CST. Sherrington's early work
(1906) had found that similar motor responses could be elicited by
stimulation of the cortex or of the skin or peripheral nerves (Chapter 2).

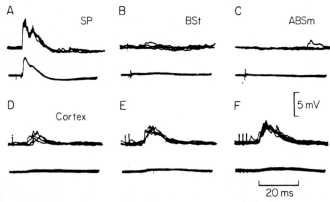

FIG. 4.12. Intracellular records from an interneurone of dorsal horn of lumbosacral spinal
cord (upper traces), showing convergence of excitatory synaptic actions from a cutaneous
nerve (A) and from the PT (D, E, F). Volleys in muscle afferents (high-threshold as well
as low-threshold) had no effect on this cell (B, C). Lower traces are of records from dorsal
root entry zone. (Lundberg *et al.*, 1962.)

Intracellular recording from the motoneurones detected the eventual
polysynaptic action of CST volleys, EPSPs predominating in flexor
motoneurones and IPSPs in extensor motoneurones. These effects are
illustrated in Fig. 4.13, which also shows the effects of convergence of
cutaneous and CST volleys on interneurones which are interposed
between these inputs and the motoneurones (Lundberg and Voorhoeve,
1962). A weak stimulus to a cutaneous nerve (A) had a minimal excitatory

action on a flexor motoneurone, and seven CST volleys had none (B). Together (C) they evoked an EPSP. The explanation is that the two inputs converged on common interneurones: when sent in together, with appropriate timing, they would have fired the interneurones, whose impulses would have evoked the EPSP in the motoneurone. Figure 4.13D, E, F shows a similar convergence of cutaneous and CST excitation on interneurones mediating inhibition to an extensor motoneurone. When spatial summation of the two inputs fires the interneurones the moto-neurone shows an IPSP.

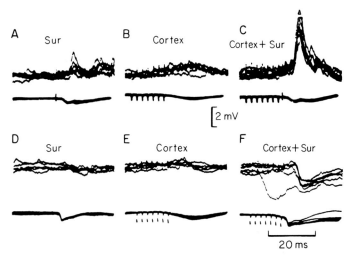

FIG. 4.13. A, B, C. Intracellular records (upper traces) from flexor motoneurone (posterior biceps-semitendinosus). Cutaneous (A) and corticospinal volleys (B) have no effect on motoneurone when delivered separately. Together (C) they evoke an EPSP.

D, E, F. Extensor motoneurone (triceps surae); no effect of cutaneous (D) and cortico-spinal volleys (E) separately; together (F) they evoke an IPSP. Lower traces are from dorsal root entry zone. Further explanation in text. (Lundberg and Voorhoeve, 1962.)

In addition to interneurones shared with reflex arcs, there are also propriospinal neurones which are monosynaptically excited by the CST and whose axons distribute monosynaptic excitation to motoneurones of several segments (Illert et al., 1974). These would by-pass the segmental reflex apparatus (Fig. 1.4, 3, p. 18). This appears to be their specific function, since none of them received inputs from peripheral nerves (cf. Kostyuk and Vasilenko, 1968).

4.4.2.2   Distribution of excitatory and inhibitory actions to interneurones and motoneurones of different muscle groups

Having given illustrative examples of the detailed working-out of some of the CST connexions by Lundberg and his colleagues, we can now summarize the main findings in a diagram (Fig. 4.14). Operating on the proprioceptive reflex networks, the CST reinforces the reciprocal inhibition of extensor motoneurones from the primary endings of the spindles of

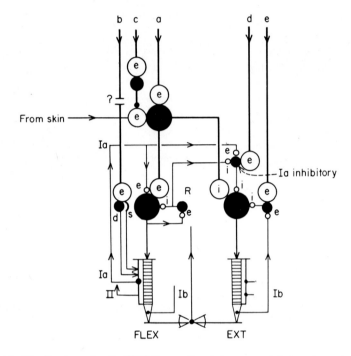

FIG. 4.14. Distribution of cat's CST (heavy lines) to segmental proprioceptive reflex networks (fine lines). Reproduced by courtesy of Istituto della Enciclopedia Italiana, Rome. Explanation in text. e, Excitation; i, inhibition.

Segmental Control ('proprioceptive') networks. A flexor muscle (FLEX) and an extensor muscle (EXT) are represented as acting antagonistically about a joint, depicted in the diagram as a hinged lever. Neither can shorten without lengthening its antagonist. The respective motoneurone pools are represented by large filled circles. The muscle spindles are represented in stylized form by a single unit in parallel with each muscle.

Ib. Disynaptic inhibition from Golgi tendon organs excited by active tension. (The circuit is drawn from the extensor only, to simplify diagram.)

1a. Monosynaptic excitation of flexor motoneurones and disynaptic inhibition of antagonist extensor motoneurones via Ia-inhibitory interneurones (Ia-inhibitory), by primary endings of muscle spindles (mixed signal of length and velocity) (circuit drawn from flexor only, to simplify diagram).

II. Secondary endings of muscle spindles (signalling length). Circuits not yet worked out.

d, s. Dynamic and static fusimotor neurones whose actions on the intrafusal muscle fibres adjust the velocity-measuring sensitivity of the primary endings and the length-measuring sensitivity of primaries and secondaries (Matthews, 1972), and can prevent unloading (and silencing) of the primaries and secondaries during contraction of the muscles.

R. Renshaw cells, mediating recurrent inhibition to some (but not all) motoneurones and also inhibiting the Ia-inhibitory interneurones of the antagonist pool.

flexor muscles by monosynaptically exciting the 'Ia-inhibitory inter-neurones' (d); it also reinforces the inhibitory feedback from the extensors' Golgi tendon organs (e). Operating at the exteroceptive level, the CST presynaptically inhibits the cutaneous input (c) and excites pools of inter-neurones which distribute excitation to flexor and inhibition to extensor motoneurones (a).

The predominance of excitation of flexor and inhibition of extensor motoneurones accounts for the facility with which flexion can be elicited by cortical stimulation, and the rarity of extensor responses noted by Sherrington (1906). 'This sparse occurrence of certain movements, e.g. extension of the knee . . . does not mean that this cortex is in touch with the flexors alone and not with the extensors. It means that the usual effect of the cortex on these latter is *inhibition*.'

Preston and his colleagues have worked out the detailed distribution of excitation and inhibition between the motoneurone pools of flexor and extensor muscles of the cat's fore- and hindlimb. The quantity and time-course of excitation and inhibition were plotted as the waxing and waning of facilitation of the monosynaptic reflexes from the group Ia fibres of the muscle's own nerves by conditioning trains of CST volleys (Preston *et al.*, 1967).

Figure 4.15 shows the long duration of the subliminal polysynaptic excitation of flexors, and of the polysynaptic inhibition of extensors, that follow a burst of 3 to 5 CST volleys (D and I waves: Chapter 3) in pyra-midal preparations in which the brain stem was destroyed electrolytically, sparing the pyramids. The reciprocal pattern of distribution is obvious. The flexor preponderance is the more striking when one remembers that this preparation resembles a decerebrate preparation, in which flexion reflexes are tonically inhibited and extensor reflexes are tonically facili-tated. The relationships between motoneurone pools are, however, more complex at the mobile wrist (not shown) than at the hinge-jointed ankle: the much greater range of wrist movements is less easily constrained into 'flexor' and 'extensor' categories, and the pattern of distribution of pro-prioceptive inputs is also complex (Willis *et al.*, 1966). The motoneurones of the intrinsic muscles of the forepaw received pure facilitation. Preston *et al.* (1967) and Corazza *et al.* (1963) propose that inhibition of extensor (anti-gravity) posture would be an important factor in the initiation of movements.

4.4.2.3   *Coupling between CST axons and fusimotor neurones and distribution of excitatory and inhibitory actions to those of different muscle groups*

Figure 4.14, b shows that CST axons are connected to static and dynamic fusimotor neurones. We shall see (Chapter 8) that such a connexion would be important for the 'servo-assistance' of movement (Matthews,

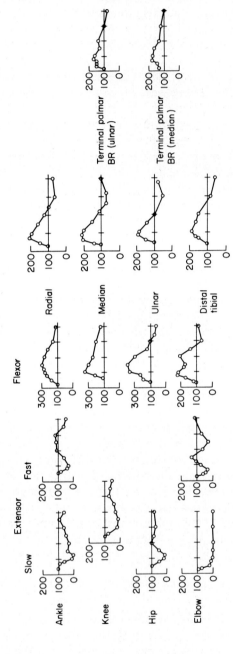

Fig. 4.15. Excitatory and inhibitory effects of PT volleys on motoneurone pools of different muscle groups of the hindlimb and forelimb of the cat.

In each graph, cortical stimulus was given at time 0; resulting changes in motoneurone excitability were tested by monosynaptic group Ia input at a succession of times thereafter (abscissae 10 ms intervals). The group Ia input, by itself, discharges a population of motoneurones whose size is measured by the voltage of the reflex volley in the motor axons. This size is represented as 100 per cent on the ordinates of each graph. If the effect of the 'conditioning' cortical stimulus is facilitatory, the 'testing' Ia volley will discharge a larger population of motoneurones (>100 per cent on ordinates); if inhibitory, a smaller population (<100 per cent). The curves therefore trace the time-course of the excitation and inhibition initiated by the cortical stimulus. Further explanation in text. (Preston et al., 1967.)

1972) and for the maintenance of a flow of information from the spindles of contracting muscles (which, without fusimotor activation, would be silenced by unloading) to cerebral and cerebellar cortex. The details of the synaptic linkage between CST axons and fusimotor neurones are not yet settled, and the uncertainty is marked by the query in Fig. 4.14, b. Different experimental methods are available and the choice between them depends on the information desired.

Excitation and inhibition of fusimotor neurones can be detected indirectly, by their effects on the discharges of single primary and secondary endings recorded from their axons in filaments of the dorsal roots. Simultaneous myography is essential. The method has many advantages: the muscle of the origin is known; the receptors can be classified by their responses to passive stretch and active contraction; and dynamic and static effects can be clearly distinguished. In a second type of experiment the fusimotor impulses can be recorded directly in filaments of the ventral roots, but the usual criterion of identity—small amplitude of the spike potentials by comparison with the amplitude of the spikes of the α motoneurones' axons—is not completely reliable; determination of conduction velocity is mandatory. Records from cut ventral roots are valueless if one wishes to study the functional relationships of different muscle groups, or if one needs to know whether the axons are of the static or dynamic type. If the records are taken from filaments split from different muscle nerves by microdissection (which requires very considerable skill), conduction velocity can be measured by stimulating the ventral root, and the destination of the axon is known, but not its static or dynamic function. In a third type of experiment, records from single fusimotor neurones are made with microelectrodes in the ventral horn. They can be referred to their muscle by antidromic stimulation of its motor nerve; the conduction velocity of their axons can be measured antidromically, but their static or dynamic properties cannot be established. In all these experiments we are limited to the sampling of single units, single fusimotor neurones or axons, or dorsal root axons which give the integrated effect of the several fusimotor axons supplying a single spindle. Although the synchronous discharge of a population of fusimotor axons could be detected in a muscle nerve, we know of no major, readily accessible monosynaptic input which could be used for testing the effect of CST volleys on the excitability of a fusimotor neurone pool, as the group 1a input can be used for testing the α motoneurone pools.

Fusimotor neurones are small and are very difficult to impale with intracellular microelectrodes for the recording of EPSPs and IPSPs. Corazza et al. (1963) collected a few, and found that stimulation of the PT evoked short-lasting EPSPs at polysynaptic latencies falling 'within the range of the shortest latencies measured in the α population'. Fidone and Preston (1969) investigated the mode of coupling by a new method. They recorded the modulation of the tonic impulse discharge of single fusimotor axons by single CST volleys, injected at a known point in time within an inter-impulse interval, and summed electronically the results of large numbers of trials. A single volley (D wave) had a detectable facilitatory or inhibitory effect. By contrast, α motoneurones required three to five CST volleys (D waves, or D and I waves). The central delay was measured by subtracting the conduction times of the fastest pyramidal axons and of the fusimotor axon from the total latency. The central delay was 3.6 to 4.3 ms, and varied so little from one preparation to another as to suggest a tighter synaptic coupling to fusimotor than to α motoneurones, either a dense interneuronal linkage between fastest CST axons and fusimotor neurones, or a monosynaptic connexion from slower CST axons. The modulation of tonic fusimotor activity by a single CST volley may last as long as 2 s, implying a long-sustained bombardment by interneurones.

Not much attention has yet been paid to the distribution of corticofusimotor action amongst different groups of muscles. Granit and Kaada (1952) were the pioneers of cortical and pyramidal stimulation combined with the recording of spindle afferents in dorsal root filaments and simultaneous myography. They were thus able to be sure, with the myograph at high sensitivity, that fusimotor actions could occur independently of contraction of the muscle. Their observations were limited to the gastrocnemius muscle, a 'physiological extensor' whose α motoneurones, as we have seen, are subject to inhibition from the cortex, but whose spindles would be stretched by active contraction of the dorsiflexors ('physiological flexors'). In principle therefore the gastrocnemius spindles could signal information of the movement of the ankle by their antagonists which can readily be activated from the cortex. In decerebrate or lightly anaesthetized preparations these spindles discharge tonically. They were accelerated by repetitive stimulation of motor cortex or PT, as also was the discharge of a fusimotor axon in the gastrocnemius nerve. The discharge of another gastrocnemius spindle was decelerated by stimulation of motor cortex and orbital gyrus. In a larger collection of records from ventral root filaments, Granit and Kaada found that stimulation of motor cortex or PT generally resulted in acceleration of fusimotor discharge before the axons of any α motoneurones began to fire. More rarely an α axon would fire before the onset of any fusimotor response. The prior activation of fusimotor neurones was part of the evidence for the original follow-up length servo theory of movement (Chapter 8).

In pyramidal preparations Fidone and Preston (1969), using their new method, collected 149 fusimotor axons to ankle extensors and 79 to ankle flexors. About 2/3 of the extensor fusimotors were decelerated, about 2/3 of the flexor fusimotors were accelerated by cortical stimulation. This distribution clearly corresponds with that of the cortical connexions to α motoneurones: inhibition of extensors, excitation of flexors. Co-activation of fusimotor and α motoneurones of flexor muscles (Granit's 'αγ linkage') would be appropriate if the cortex were involved in the initiation of servo-assisted movements (Matthews, 1964, 1972) (Chapter 8). The opposite type of distribution, found in the remaining 1/3 of flexor and extensor fusimotors, could be understood if the extensor spindles were used to signal information of movements of the joints, brought about by contraction of the flexors, to the cerebrum and cerebellum. Adjustment of the length- and velocity-sensitivity of these spindles by the brain could then be important. Static fusimotor axons are more common than dynamic fusimotor axons, and Fidone and Preston proposed the hypothesis that the facilitated extensor and inhibited flexor fusimotor neurones might be dynamic fusimotors. Vedel (1966) actually found that pyramidal stimulation enhanced the dynamic sensitivity of primary endings of soleus (ankle extensor) spindles. In some physiological extensors of the cat's wrist, Yokota and Voorhoeve (1969) saw acceleration of the discharge of secondary endings as well as increased dynamic sensitivity of primary endings in response to PT volleys which must, therefore, have excited both static and dynamic fusimotor neurones.

4.5   Cortical origin and distribution of PT axons in primates

In rhesus monkeys, Russell and DeMyer (1961) made selective lesions of the peri-Rolandic cortex and estimated the numbers of axons that survived in the PT. Adequate time was allowed for axolysis of the fine axons. Area 4 contributes 31 per cent and area 6, 29 per cent. The remaining 40 per cent of PT axons originate from the parietal lobe. The area agrees well with that mapped by recording antidromically evoked potential waves (Woolsey and Chang, 1948). The origin in man cannot be determined with the same degree of precision, since one cannot make well-circumscribed cortical lesions in previously healthy brains and verify their extent in serial sections after an appropriate survival period (cf. Fig. 4.18). It is believed that about 60 per cent of human PT axons arise from area 4 (Wiesendanger, 1969). In view of the remarkable accuracy of the maps of origin of the cat's and monkey's corticospinal tracts that were published by Holmes and Page May (1909), it seems probable that their map of the origin of the human CST is also accurate.

The fact that all these axons do not arise from large PTN has been mentioned in section 4.1. Lassek (1948) stained the axons of intact medullary pyramids by silver methods in man, monkey and chimpanzee, counted them, and compared their numbers with the numbers of giant pyramidal cells in the cortex. These cells were defined arbitrarily as having perikarya whose sectioned area, in the plane which included the nucleolus, was greater than 500 μm². The axons were up to 50 times as numerous as the giant cells. Branching of axons between cortex and pyramid can hardly be invoked to account for such a discrepancy. Thus, in man, there were about one million axons and only about 30 000 giant cells; in chimpanzee, about 800 000 axons and 28 000 cells; in monkeys, about 550 000 axons and 19 000 cells. The majority of the axons were thin, suggesting that they came from small PTN, and possibly from an area of cortex wider than the area gigantopyramidalis. Only in man were there many thicker axons: 2 per cent of the myelinated axons were 11–20 μm thick; 90 per cent were thinner than 4 μm, and more than 50 per cent were 1 μm thick. Lassek had estimated that 61 per cent of human PT axons were myelinated, but DeMeyer (1959), who used frozen and not paraffin sections, gives 93 per cent. In rhesus monkeys 62 per cent of PT axons are myelinated (DeMyer and Russell, 1958).

In rhesus monkeys, the PT and the corresponding corticobulbar projections contain contingents of axons with spatially differentiated (but overlapping) cortical origins, and different bulbar and spinal distributions (Kuypers, 1960); and these arrangements have functional implications. Figure 4.16, C charts the postcentral cortical origin of axons which end contralaterally in the nucleus proprius of the dorsal horn, and in the spinal trigeminal complex which is the headward extension of the nucleus proprius belonging to the face. These are marked, in the diagrammatic slices of the neuraxis, by hatchings which are parallel to those which mark the somaesthetic receiving area of cortex on chart C. From a wider area, extending also precentrally (chart D, open circles), arises the projection to the contralateral dorsal column nuclei (open circles) and to their cranial counterparts, the principal sensory trigeminal nuclei bilaterally (open circles). All these would be in a position to control the somaesthetic input from limbs, trunk and face.

On the motor side, a forward-spreading population of precentral axons passes to the medial bulbar reticular formation bilaterally (chart A and the two most rostral slices: parallel hatching); this, in turn, projects bilaterally by ventral reticulospinal tracts to the medial groups of motoneurones of the ventral horn, which innervate the muscles of the trunk and of the proximal limb segments. This indirect and bilateral pathway would allow cortical mobilization of the essential postural support on which the exploratory and manipulative performances of mouth and hands must always be securely based. Axons arising more caudally in the precentral gyrus (chart B, dots) end in the lateral bulbar reticular formation and the spinal intermediate zone, which probably contain the interneurones which control the bulbar and spinal motoneurones, as in the cat. The dots in the diagrammatic slices show their relationships with the motor nuclei of the trigeminal nerves bilaterally; with the nuclei of the facial nerves, mainly contralaterally; and their endings in the spinal cord, bilateral but preponderantly contralateral. Finally there are the corticomotoneuronal (CM) axons (chart B, solid squares) which go to the trigeminal motor nuclei bilaterally (rostral slice, solid squares), to the facial nucleus contralaterally (adjacent slice, solid squares) and to the contralateral motoneurone groups of the ventral horns (solid squares) which innervate the distal muscles of the limbs. Very few CM axons arise from the postcentral gyrus.

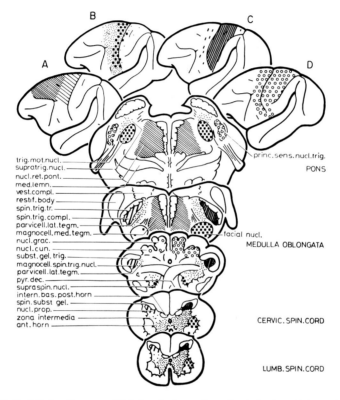

FIG. 4.16. Peri-Rolandic areas of left hemisphere of monkey's brain which send axons to specific destinations in the neuraxis, shown in diagrammatic slices of pons, medulla and spinal cord. Explanation in text. (Reproduced by kind permission of Professor H. G. J. M. Kuypers and Dr. J. Brinkman of the Medical Faculty of the Erasmus University, Rotterdam, and Istituto della Enciclopedia Italiana, Rome.)

There are virtually no CM endings in the newborn monkey (Fig. 4.17), although the CST is already present. These endings are present in adult profusion by 8 months, though the axons are still thinner than in the fully adult (Kuypers, 1964). CM endings are more numerous in chimpanzee than in rhesus, 'and seem to be almost as abundant as in man'. In gibbon and chimpanzee their numbers are comparable to those of CST endings in zona intermedia and dorsal horn (Petras, 1966).

Profuse endings in a human case, in which it should be noted that the precentral lesion involved only the most lateral part of the precentral gyrus (the face area), are illustrated in Fig. 4.18 (Schoen, 1964). The arrow indicates the contralateral terminations of the uncrossed ventral CST which partly decussates in the ventral commissure at segmental levels (C5, Th1, L3–4). It is probable that the axons which reached as far as L4 (Fig. 4.18D) had degenerated as a result of ischaemia and oedema of the leg area at the time of the stroke. The density of endings in the thoracic region may be related to voluntary control of the respiratory muscles in speech and song.

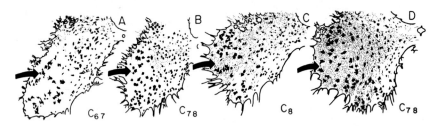

F$_{IG}$. 4.17. Ventral horn of spinal grey matter of cervical spinal cord. Adult cat (A) and newborn monkey (B) have no CST axon terminals in relation to cell bodies of laterally placed motoneurones. Such terminals are present in adult monkey (C); they are more profuse in chimpanzee (D). (Kuypers, 1964.)

The wealth of the endings in the chimpanzee explains how Leyton and Sherrington (1917) were able to see that some CST axons entered the chimpanzee's ventral horn, even with the relatively crude methods then available. Degeneration following excision of the 'area yielding primary movements of thumb, index finger, wrist and elbow' (in the experiment shown in Fig. 2.5, p. 33) was seen in the contralateral ventral horn of the 7th and 8th cervical segments. 'On the right side, the whole of the cross-area of ventral horn has scattered through it many degenerating fibres of very minute size; they give a "peppered" appearance to the grey matter there in contrast to the ordinary clean appearance of the corresponding grey matter of the left half of the cord. The peppering is perhaps most marked in the dorsolateral and ventrolateral cell-group regions, it is certainly least in the medio-ventral cell-group. Sections stained with Marchi show these degenerated fibres in the grey matter but slightly, although, when aware of them, one can detect the presence of a number of them by that method. The degeneration in the ventral horn is, however, much better revealed by the Schafer combination of the Marchi and

Kulschitzky methods; the minute blue-black ring surrounding the pale
axis cylinder . . . is altered to a minute blob containing no axis cylinder . . .
this kind of minute degeneration is scattered widely and liberally through
the ventral horn.' The Marchi degeneration in the contralateral CST,
which resulted from this lesion confined to the arm area, extended as far
as the last thoracic segment but was not detected in the lumbar enlargement.

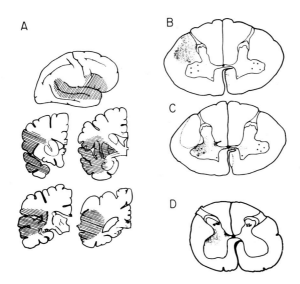

FIG. 4.18. A. Degeneration in human spinal cord, six weeks after cerebrovascular lesion
of lowermost part of right precentral gyrus, superior and middle temporal gyri and
lenticular nucleus (A).
    B. Degeneration of left crossed and right uncrossed corticospinal tracts at C5 level,
revealed by Häggqvist's method.
    C. Terminal degeneration of PT axons at same level, revealed by Nauta method.
    D. Degeneration of left crossed and right uncrossed CST continued at L3–4 level
(Nauta method). (Modified from Schoen, 1964.)

4.6   Electroanatomy of the Corticomotoneuronal projection of primates

Electroanatomical and microphysiological research on the projections and
collaterals of the PT in primates has lagged far behind that on the cat,
and the rest of this chapter will be concerned entirely with the actions of
CST axons within the ventral half of the spinal grey matter.

    Cooper and Denny-Brown (1928) noted Leyton and Sherrington's
finding of pyramidal 'collaterals' ramifying amongst the chimpanzee's
motoneurones, and pioneered the electroanatomical attack on the nexus
between them in monkeys. They stimulated the cortical arm area at

different frequencies and made beautiful electrical and mechanical records from mm. brachialis, triceps and flexor profundus digitorum of the contra-lateral forelimb. The fact that EMG waves could follow the cortical stimuli up to 180 Hz suggested that 'a direct synaptic relation seems most likely'.

At frequencies below 4 Hz there was no response, although stimulation was continued for >30 s. At slightly higher frequencies, after a 'summation period' measured in seconds (e.g. 7.6 to 14 s at 9 Hz), the motoneurones began to discharge in response to each volley. The first few responses would increase in size ('recruitment'). Figure 4.19 shows the relatively steady state attained by stimulation at 13 Hz. Each response appears as a discrete hump in the myogram and as a burst of motoneurone discharge in the EMG, consisting of a large 'primary wave' and smaller 'secondary waves'. The 'true latent period' (as distinct from the 'summation period') was measured from each cortical stimulus to the corresponding primary wave; it was about 14 ms, but could be reduced to about 9 ms by 'a light dose of strychnine'. Of this time, 2.5 ms was taken up in transmission from motor nerve to muscle. At that time there was no way of measuring the conduction time from cortex to spinal segment, and the value of the synaptic delay was unknown.

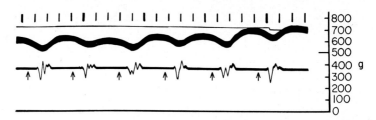

FIG. 4.19. Simultaneous isometric myogram (above: tension scale in g) and electromyo-gram (below) of m. flexor profundus digitorum of monkey. Cortical stimuli at 13 Hz. Arrows mark instants of stimulation. Each stimulus causes a primary wave in the EMG, followed by secondary waves. Time scale 1/50 s. (Cooper and Denny-Brown, 1928.)

The long summation period, and the period of recruitment, are evidently the manifestations of complex changes in background excitability which permit the motoneurones to discharge at a relatively fixed latency in response to the individual CST volleys. Cooper and Denny-Brown regarded these complex changes as the result of conflicts between excita-tory and inhibitory effects of the stimulation. In a muscle which was exhibiting background tonus under light anaesthesia, they noted the onset of inhibition 0.2 s after the start of stimulation at 50 Hz, which persisted for a further 3.0 s before the muscle started to contract. They regarded the 'summation period' of 3.2 s as 'the expression of the excitation breaking through a background of inhibition', and the occasional clonic after-discharges as examples of postinhibitory rebound (a familiar feature of Sherringtonian reflexology). Their results were not confused by reflexes from the contracting muscles, which, in some experiments, were excluded by cutting the dorsal roots (Sherrington, 1931).

The summation period showed 'remarkable constancy' for any stimulus frequency, provided that at least 30 s was allowed between stimulations. That the facilitatory process outlasted the stimulation period was proved by restimulating after shorter intervals. The summation period was then shortened, e.g. from 20.0 to 0.18 s. A subconvulsive dose of strychnine—which, as we now know, blocked inhibitory synapses in the spinal cord—also shortened the summation period.

Thus there was evidence of three effects: a probable monosynaptic action of CST volleys on motoneurones, and conflicting excitatory and inhibitory backgrounds of slow onset, prolonged duration and slow decay. In view of their slow time-courses, and of the intact neuraxis, there is no evidence to associate the two latter with the CST, or to dissociate them from it.

Bernhard *et al.* (1953) and Bernhard and Bohm (1954) performed experiments which were identical in principle with those of Cooper and Denny-Brown, but with the advantages that the delay at a central synapse (about 0.6 ms) had been discovered in the intervening years, and that technical advances in electronics and electrodes had made it possible to time the arrival of LCST volleys at any spinal segment, and to time the discharges of motoneurones into the ventral roots or motor nerves (Fig. 4.20).

Each cortical stimulus sent a fast volley down the LCST (velocity, 70 m s^{-1}) but this, by itself, failed to fire any motoneurones. Background facilitation was necessary, as in Cooper and Denny-Brown's experiments, and was readily generated by stimulation at 25 Hz. After 1 to 2 s, the motoneurones began to discharge irregularly, and each LCST volley caused a 'late' burst; after further prolonging the facilitation, there was also an 'early' burst (Fig. 4.20A). Subtraction of conduction time in LCST and motoneurone axons from the latency of the early burst left a central latency of only 0.7 ms. This proved that the linkage responsible for the early burst was monosynaptic. Late responses were more easily abolished than mono-synaptic responses by deepening the anaesthetic, as would be expected if they involved one or two extra synapses.

The nature of the build-up of facilitation was the subject of special study. It was evident in the irregular background firing of the motoneurones, unrelated in time to the LCST volleys, and outlasting the stimulation period. Tested by its facilitating effect on the monosynaptic reflex of the L7 segment, it was found to begin about 1.75 s after the onset of cortical stimulation at 25 Hz, to reach its maximum in 3 s, and to outlast the period of stimulation. With hindsight based on Kuypers' anatomical studies (Fig. 4.16), we can understand the significance of two further findings of Bernhard *et al.* (1953). The facilitation was evoked from a wider area of cortex than that from which a monosynaptic discharge could be fired into the L7 ventral root; and early and late responses were abolished by

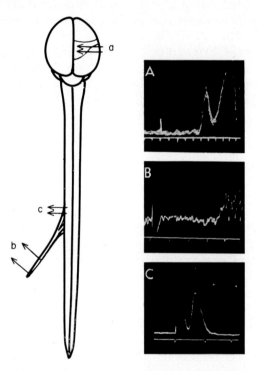

FIG. 4.20. Demonstration of monosynaptic corticomotoneuronal (CM) connexion in monkey. Hindlimb area stimulated repetitively at a; after a period of facilitation, early and late responses (A) recorded from L5 ventral root at b. Latency of early response was 4.7 ms (time scales in ms below each record).

B. CST volley recorded with microelectrode in dorsolateral funiculus (at c). Time from a to c, 3.6 ms. (Distance ac = 25 cm; conduction velocity, 68 m s⁻¹).

C. Time from root entry zone (stimulated near c) to recording electrodes at b, 0.4 ms. Result: 4.7−3.6−0.4 = 0.7 ms.

(Bernhard *et al.*, 1953.)

bilateral ventral cordotomy (but not by unilateral) although the LCSTs were conducting normally (Bernhard *et al.*, 1955). These findings implicate the bilateral cortico-reticulo-spinal projection in building up the background of facilitation on which the monosynaptic discharges of proximal muscle-groups must appear.

The background of concurrent inhibition seen by Cooper and Denny-Brown was also evident in Bernhard and Bohm's experiments. Thus, the monosynaptic response of triceps motoneurones would typically appear after 1 to 2 s of stimulation at 25 Hz, then disappear and reappear after after 8 to 10 s.

Bernhard and Bohm (1954) introduced the useful term *corticomotoneuronal (CM) system* to denote this special fast-conducting component of the monkey's LCST (70 m s^{-1}) which makes monosynaptic connexions with motoneurones. They discussed its probable importance in the refined cerebral control of the hands of primates, including man. The monosynaptic discharge was 'generally more pronounced' in the nerves of the forelimb, whereas the late response was dominant in those of the hindlimb. To compare the responses of proximal and distal groups in the forelimb, Bernhard and Bohm chose the nerves to biceps and triceps and the thenar and hypothenar nerves. No biceps or triceps responses ever occurred to a single LCST volley. Late responses were evoked from a wider cortical field than CM responses (cf. Kuypers' projections to interneurones and motoneurones, Fig. 4.16B). The CM projection from each precentral gyrus was distributed bilaterally to biceps and triceps; that to thenar and hypothenar muscles was exclusively contralateral, from cortical areas which were slightly larger than those for biceps and triceps. The distal nerves were characterized by a poverty of late discharges. They responded to a single LCST volley with a central latency of about 1.8 ms, which shortened to 0.8 ms when the volleys were repeated. The shorter value was accepted as monosynaptic, the longer was doubted: its explanation as a monosynaptic response had to await the appeal to intracellular recording, the discovery of presynaptic facilitation (Chapter 3, section 3.5), and the demonstration that the EPSP from one of the I waves, and not that of the D wave, would be the first to approach the firing level (Fig. 3.19B, p. 89).

Replicating Lloyd's experiments (cf. Figs 4.10 and 4.11), but without the brain stem lesion, Bernhard et al. (1953) sent down single volleys from the leg area and tested the effect on motoneurones of the L5 segment with the segmental monosynaptic reflex. They found that a single conditioning volley facilitated the test reflex, whereas at least three volleys had been needed in the cat. The facilitation began almost synchronously with the arrival of the LCST volley in the segment, reached its maximum in 12 ms and decayed in 40 ms. The start of the facilitation was undoubtedly monosynaptic, and its relation to the CST volley is in no way undermined by the intactness of the brain stem; but the continuing rise and prolonged time-course could have been due to a crescendo of impulses in tracts other than the CST (cortico-reticulo-spinal, etc.). In unanaesthetized pyramidal preparations (which are in deep coma, so general anaesthesia can be discontinued when the surgery is completed), Preston and Whitlock (1960) plotted similar facilitation curves. Their conditioning cortical pulses were strong enough to fire PTN repetitively (D and I waves) and also to discharge some motoneurones; such discharge was evident in records from motor axons as well as in twitches of thumb or hallux when appropriate areas were stimulated. The monosynaptic onset of the facilitation was confirmed; but in spite of the brain stem lesion, the remainder of the curve resembled that of Bernhard et al. (1953) (apart from an inhibitory erosion which we shall discuss presently). The pyramidal preparation, however, cannot altogether eliminate the possibility of excitation, by PT terminals or collaterals, of bulbospinal pathways which originate caudal to the brain stem lesion. Indeed, Preston and Whitlock (1960) could elicit the late facilitation separately, by stimulation of the bulb adjacent to the pyramids; so the crescendo of impulses that caused it could have been built up in bulbar as well as in spinal grey matter.

The absence of inhibitory erosion from the curves of Bernhard et al. (1953) was due to barbiturate anaesthesia, since Preston and Whitlock (1960) could remove the inhibition from their unanaesthetized pyramidal preparations by small doses of barbiturate. Examples of an inhibitory dip in a facilitation curve can be seen in Fig. 4.23, radial: the inhibition reached its trough 1.2 ms after the onset of facilitation; facilitation was then resumed and continued as long as in the curves of Bernhard et al. (1953). Such a latency of onset of inhibition suggested the interpolation of one or two sets of interneurones between the CST axons and the motoneurones. The experiment proves that the CST has an indirect inhibitory action on motoneurones. Preston and Whitlock (1960) were not able to separate the early excitatory and inhibitory effects by stimulating at different cortical loci, and could not, therefore, decide whether the CST can project inhibition independently of excitation. In the intact brain, however, parapyramidal pathways could have mediated some or all of the more prolonged inhibition seen in Cooper and Denny-Brown's experiments, and in the classical observations of cortical inhibition by Sherrington (1906).

Preston and Whitlock (1961) were the first to use intracellular recording from lumbar motoneurones for the detection and timing of the actions of CST volleys in monkeys. The EPSPs were prolonged and irregular in contour, showing that the initial monosynaptic impact was followed by delayed impacts due to bombardment by interneurones. The yield of IPSPs was disappointing, possibly because chloride-filled microelectrodes were used. The experiments with monosynaptic testing of motoneurone pools (1960) had shown the same stereotyped excitatory-inhibitory sequence in both ankle flexors and extensors, but 50 motoneurones showed pure EPSPs; 6 showed pure IPSPs; and only 3 showed the EPSP-IPSP sequence. In these 3, the EPSPs and IPSPs could not be separated by shifting the cortical electrode. Preston and Whitlock (1961) had therefore shown, in 6 motoneurones, that the CST can project inhibition independently of excitation. As evidence in favour of an interneuronal link in the inhibitory pathway from the CST, they reported a discharge of interneurones in the segment after the arrival of the CST volley and before the start of the IPSP in motoneurones.

Landgren *et al.* (1962a) recorded intracellularly from motoneurones of the ulnar, median and radial nerves of baboons. They chose these nerves in view of the special neurological interest attaching to the hand in primates, and of its preferential accessibility to cortical stimulation (Chapter 2, section 2.6). Since they were using minimal surface-anodal stimuli and recording only minimal synaptic actions which were strictly related in time to the small D volleys arriving in the C7–T1 segments, they felt justified in avoiding the extra surgical hazards of the pyramidal preparation. The pure CM-EPSPs revealed by minimal stimulation rose steeply to their crests and decayed exponentially in about 15 ms (Fig. 4.21A); in shape and time-course they were identical with the monosynaptic EPSPs evoked in the same motoneurones by group Ia afferent

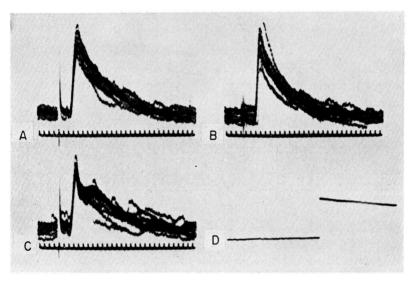

Fig. 4.21. Intracellular records from α motoneurone of deep radial nerve of baboon.
  A. EPSP evoked by unifocal surface-anodal pulses, strength 1.25 mA, applied to cortical area corresponding to that outlined in Fig. 4.7 (left). Time, 1000 Hz in A, B and C.
  B. Group IA monosynaptic EPSP.
  C. Same pulses applied to cortex at a point 3 mm distant from point stimulated in A. Note smaller EPSP and inhibitory erosion of its decaying phase.
  D. Calibrating 1.5 mV rectangular voltage step to amplifier input (Landgren *et al.*, 1962a).

volleys from the appropriate peripheral nerves (Fig. 4.21B). In some examples, however, the decay of the CM-EPSP was complicated by an IPSP which started 1.2 to 1.4 ms later than the start of the EPSP (Fig. 4.21C). Moving the focal anode to different cortical loci could alter the proportions of EPSP and IPSP in the same motoneurones, as in Fig. 4.21. These experiments with minimal stimuli proved that different populations of PTN could project different proportions of excitation and inhibition to a single motoneurone. In some cases almost pure IPSPs could be evoked.

Jankowska and Tanaka (1974) have shown that the inhibitory interneurones that are interposed between the LCST axons and the motoneurones are those that belong to the reciprocal inhibitory pathway from the group Ia input from the antagonistic muscles (cf. Fig. 4.14). Spatial facilitatory interaction of the two inputs could be demonstrated by an experiment based on the principle illustrated in Fig. 4.13D, E, F. The antagonistic group Ia volley and the LCST volley were timed to enter the lumbar segment synchronously. Each, by itself, was barely liminal; together they excited the interneurones and evoked an IPSP in the impaled motoneurone. The separate IPSPs evoked in the impaled motoneurone by supraliminal volleys from either source had identical waveforms. Identification of these inhibitory interneurones with the Ia-inhibitory interneurones was strengthened by another test. In the cat, the only known source of inhibition for these interneurones comes from the Renshaw cells (Fig. 4.14, R), the inhibitory neurones which are excited by the axon collaterals of the motoneurones and which mediate recurrent inibition to motoneurones and to Ia-inhibitory interneurones (Hultborn et al., 1971a, b). Not all of the motoneurones in a segment receive recurrent inhibition when the ventral root is stimulated antidromically; only those that do not do so are suitable for the test. From such motoneurones, identical IPSPs were recorded when either an antagonistic group Ia volley or an LCST volley was fired into the segment. Both IPSPs were suppressed by a suitably timed antidromic volley in the ventral root, in motoneurones in which a control ventral root volley evoked no IPSP.

Tanaka (1972) had previously performed an illuminating experiment on normal human subjects which suggested strongly that the excitability of the Ia-inhibitory interneurones is under cerebral control. The 'test preparation' was the monosynaptic H reflex of the triceps surae (extensor) muscle, elicited by a single volley in its low-threshold muscle afferents in the medial popliteal nerve. If the reciprocal Ia-inhibitory pathway had been in operation (Fig. 4.14), a burst of afferent volleys in the lowest-threshold axons of the antagonistic lateral popliteal (flexor) nerve should have reduced the amplitude of the H reflex. No such reduction occurred, however, when the limb was relaxed. This suggests that the Ia-inhibitory interneurones were, so to speak, turned off in the resting condition. Voluntary activation of the antagonist muscles by dorsiflexion of the foot caused a slight reduction in the amplitude of the H reflex, suggesting that the inhibitory interneurones had been somehow 'turned on'. This could have been due to corticospinal facilitation (Fig. 4.14, d), which would be expected to make these interneurones responsive to driving by the muscle spindles of the contracting antagonists in the process of 'αγ-linked reciprocal inhibition' (Hongo et al, 1969b) (The pathways can be followed in Fig. 4.14). In the 'turned-on' condition brought about by sustained voluntary dorsiflexion of the foot, a burst of three weak conditioning shocks at 300 Hz to the lateral popliteal (flexor) nerve depressed the testing (extensor) H reflex to about 70 per cent of its control amplitude; the inhibition reached its trough at 1.8 ms after the third shock, and recovery was complete after 6 ms.

Reciprocal innervation of antagonists has usually been regarded as a very hard-wired, deterministic affair, but this evidence suggests that the excitability of the inhibitory interneurones is under corticospinal control (and other control) and that it has to be actively sustained by the brain; co-contraction of antagonistic muscles (Chapter 8) could be procured by switching on their α and γ motoneurones while leaving the two sets of Ia-inhibitory interneurones switched off.

4.6.1 CORTICOMOTONEURONAL PROJECTION TO MOTONEURONES OF DIFFERENT MUSCLE GROUPS

The preferential accessibility to cortical stimulation of motoneurones innervating the intrinsic muscles of the hand (Chapter 2, section 2.6) finds a part at least of its explanation in the greater maxima of monosynaptic excitation that can be evoked in these motoneurones by LCST volleys. Figure 4.22 shows that the mean amplitudes of maximal CM-EPSPs are largest for motoneurones of the intrinsic hand muscles and extensor digitorum communis of baboons (Clough et al., 1968). These are the muscles normally employed by monkeys and men in the movements that are most severely impaired by lesion of the PT or of the arm area (Chapter 8). For elbow flexors (musculocutaneous nerve) and extensors (triceps nerves) the maximal CM-EPSPs are smaller. About half of the triceps motoneurones sampled by Phillips and Porter (1964) showed no CM-EPSPs, but showed early IPSPs and polysynaptic EPSPs and IPSPs. Early IPSPs were prominent in elbow flexor motoneurones (Fig. 4.23).

In motoneurones of hindlimb muscles, Jankowska et al. (1975b) found that the EPSPs are larger in the distal than in the proximal groups. The maximal EPSPs were not measured, but the amplitudes of EPSPs evoked by standard 0.2 ms surface-anodal pulses of strength 0.5 mA were compared. These weak stimuli are more effective in the leg area, where the

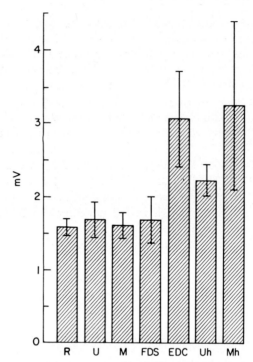

FIG. 4.22. Mean amplitudes of maximal CM EPSPs in motoneurones identified by antidromic stimulation of the following nerves: whole radial (R); whole ulnar (U); whole
median including 4 motoneurones from nerve to palmaris longus (M); flexor digitorum
sublimis (FDS); extensor digitorum communis (EDC); ulnar to intrinsic hand muscles
(Uh); median to intrinsic hand muscles (Mh). (Clough *et al.*, 1968.)

PTN are on the convexity, than in the arm area where many are buried
in the wall of the central sulcus (Chapter 5, section 5.2). The smallest
EPSPs were recorded by computer-averaging and could be measured
accurately. In motoneurones of distal muscle-groups supplied by the deep
peroneal nerve (including tibialis anterior, extensor digitorum longus, and
extensor digitorum brevis) the EPSPs ranged from 200 μV to 2 mV; in
triceps surae, from 100 μV to 1.2 mV; in motoneurones of hip and knee
muscles, from 100 to 300 μV. Not all motoneurones received monosynaptic
excitation from the cortex. This aspect of preferential accessibility is more
difficult to quantify: absence of response to submaximal stimulation of a
limited cortical area cannot prove absence of corticomotoneuronal connexion, but failures to evoke a monosynaptic EPSP occurred 'much more
often' in the case of motoneurones of hip and knee muscles than in the case
of distal motoneurones. This was so, even when the area of cortex that
was being explored systematically was giving 'a clear facilitation of the
respective monosynaptic reflexes'.

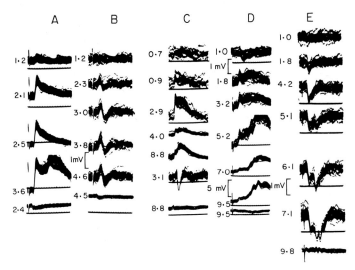

Fɪɢ. 4.23. A. Elbow flexor motoneurone (musculocutaneous nerve), showing monosynaptic EPSP evoked by increasing strengths of 0.2 ms pulses, surface anodal. Strengths noted in margin. Responses to I waves at 3.6 mA. Membrane potential − 75 mV.

B. Elbow flexor motoneurone showing monosynaptic EPSP followed by disynaptic IPSP. Increasing stimulus strengths noted in margin. Membrane potential − 63 mV. Calibration 1.0 mV for A and B.

C. Triceps motoneurone. Monosynaptic EPSPs followed by polysynaptic EPSP. Membrane potential − 68 mV. Disynaptic IPSP, just visible in response to 2.9 mA, unmasked in response to 3.1 mA; the motoneurone had been deliberately injured by stabbing, and membrane potential had fallen to − 43 mV. This illustrates that the full investigation of excitatory and inhibitory CST actions on a motoneurone requires that the resting membrane potential be shifted away from the equilibrium potential for inhibition, preferably by intracellular passage of depolarizing currents whose action is reversible.

D. Triceps motoneurone, m.p. − 62 mV. Threshold for IPSP (1.0 mA) is lower than that for EPSP (>1.0, <1.8 mA). Delayed polysynaptic excitation with strongest stimuli. Calibrations: 1 mV for C, 0.7–2.9 and 3.1 and D, 1.0–5.2; 5 mV for remaining records.

E. Triceps motoneurone. No EPSP, pure IPSP. Multiple responses to stronger stimuli, presumably due to I waves. Membrane potential − 63 mV. Calibration 1 mV. Bottom records in A-E are extracellular controls. Time 1 ms. (Phillips and Porter, 1964.)

The distribution of CST actions to the motoneurone pools of different muscle groups in the 'pyramidal' baboon is well seen in curves of facilitation and inhibition of the type already described for the cat (Preston et al., 1967). It is instructive to compare these curves (Fig. 4.24) with the corresponding curves for the cat (Fig. 4.15). The initial CM facilitation contrasts with its absence from the cat. For the pools of the proximal muscle groups, the general pattern of prolonged inhibition of extensors and facilitation of flexors is similar in cat and primate; but there is a striking difference at the elbow-joint, where inhibition predominates in the *flexors*. Preston et al. (1967) suggest that in the baboon 'we see the transition from quadruped to biped posture', and cite Woolsey et al.'s (1952) maps showing (in Macaca) extension of elbow in response to 60 Hz sinusoidal stimulation of the cortex (Fig. 2.6, p. 35), which contrasts with the virtual absence of extension of knee. In the pools of the distal muscle groups, the CM facilitation and the early (disynaptic) inhibition are followed by prolonged facilitation (Fig. 4.24); in the pools of the intrinsic muscles of the hand, the CM facilitation continues into the later phase of facilitation without interruption by an inhibitory dip.

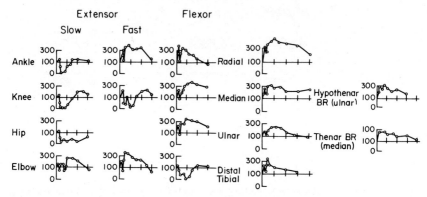

FIG. 4.24. Excitatory and inhibitory effects of PT volleys on motoneurone pools of different muscle groups of the hindlimb and forelimb of the baboon (cf. corresponding curves for cat, Fig. 4.19). Further explanation in text. (Preston *et al.*, 1967.)

4.7   Electroanatomy of corticofusimotor connexions in primates

Excitation and inhibition of baboon's fusimotor neurones by the CST has been investigated by recording from single axons in motor nerves (Clough and Sheridan, 1968; Grigg and Preston, 1971) and from fusimotor neurones in the ventral horn of the cervical spinal cord (Clough *et al.*, 1971).

Grigg and Preston used Fidone and Preston's (1969) modulation method (Fig. 4.4, 2, c) on the nerves to ankle flexors and extensors. They found that of 17 fusimotors that were facilitated, 9 responded at a central latency that was short enough (<1.0 ms) to indicate a monosynaptic CST-fusimotor linkage. Of 22 fusimotors that were not discharging spontaneously, none could be fired at monosynaptic latency by CST volleys. In distal nerves of the forelimb, Clough *et al.* (1971) saw EPSPs at monosynaptic latency in 6/19 fusimotor neurones investigated by intracellular recording, and disynaptic IPSPs in 4/19. But in a larger series of extra-cellular records, the latency of the earliest fusimotor impulse was always too long to be explained by monosynaptic excitation by the fastest CST axons (D volley). It was not possible to decide between monosynaptic excitation by an I volley or by slow CST axons, or polysynaptic excitation by fast CST axons. Many 'distal' forelimb fusimotor neurones could not be fired at all by CST volleys, and may represent a population over which the CST has less control.

Not surprisingly, these early fusimotor discharges had no detectable effect on the discharges of the primary endings of the muscle spindles (Koeze *et al.*, 1968), for single static or dynamic fusimotor impulses hardly disturb the rhythm of a primary ending (Bessou *et al.*, 1968). Prolonged repetitive stimulation of the cortex, and the clonic after-discharges that were seen occasionally, had excitatory and inhibitory effects on Koeze *et al.*'s spindle afferents; but these need not be ascribed to the CST, since the preparations were not pyramidal, so that other corticofugal pathways were open. It is, however, interesting that the sequence and balance of the effects on muscle contraction and spindle response could be altered by varying the level of anaesthesia, which shows that the cortex could control them independently.

Grigg and Preston (1971) found that 10/27 fusimotors were inhibited by CST volleys (central latency 1.0 to 7.3 ms, mean 4.5 ms), and Clough *et al.* (1971) saw IPSPs in 4/19 intracellularly recorded fusimotors (central latency 2.2 to 3.6 ms). An interneuronal link is probable, as in the case of α motoneurones. Koeze *et al.* (1968) reported that cortical stimulation caused slowing of the discharge of some spindle primaries of the finger extensors. Cortical inhibition of fusimotors would have obvious importance in the learning of manual skills, in which the relaxation of unnecessary muscles plays a well-recognized part.

The corticofusimotor apparatus could provide for the maintenance of signalling from the muscle spindles during shortening of the muscles. Functional implications for the servo-assistance of movement will be developed in Chapter 8.

4.8 Summary

The contribution of this chapter to the model of Fig. 1.4 (p. 18) has been to review the cortical origin, course and distribution of the PT in cats and monkeys, the animals on which most neurophysiological and behavioural research is being done. This has filled in many of the details concealed within the four arrows leading out of the cortical projection areas in Fig. 1.4, and has also filled in many details of the connexions outlined in Figs 1.1 (p. 6) and 1.2 (p. 8).

As important as the description of the known connexions, has been some explanation of the principles of the microscopical and electro-anatomical methods that have been used in tracing them, with illustrations of their detailed application in specific examples. These methods comple-ment one another at every point, each one often bringing up new problems for the others. A particularly productive example has been seen in the tracing of collateral branchings of PT axons, which has depended on methods of both classes. Since the information we now possess must be far from complete, the need to understand the power and limitations of the various methods will be evident to anyone who finds, in the course of his neurophysiological or behavioural research, that some essential piece of structural information is still lacking. Since microscopy cannot yet certainly distinguish between excitatory and inhibitory synapses, electro-anatomy is necessary to prove whether particular collateral or terminal distributions of the PT are mediating excitation or pre- or postsynaptic inhibition, and in what proportions, to the target organizations.

The cortical area of origin of the PT has been defined more accurately than was possible by classical electrical stimulation which used muscular responses as the detectors of corticofugal discharge, or by methods which could trace only the thickest myelinated axons. The discrepancy between the number of PT axons and the number of large PTN is so great that only about 3 per cent of the axons can arise from those cells. The actions of the very large number of fine axons are unknown; the majority of PT axons must be below the size of those of most of the 'small' PTN (conduction velocity less than 20 $m s^{-1}$) studied so far.

In its course in the cat, the PT emits collateral branches to the 'relay nuclei' of ascending pathways; to the pontine, olivary and lateral reticular nuclei which project to the cerebellum; to the striatum; and to neurones of parallel descending pathways (rubrospinal, reticulospinal). These would supply these structures with 'corollary' signals, some excitatory, some inhibitory, whenever the PTN discharged impulses to their ultimate terminations. Nothing is known in detail of PT collaterals in monkeys. Pyramidal and 'parapyramidal' corticorubral and corticoreticular terminals form parallel cortico-rubro-spinal and cortico-reticulo-spinal descending pathways.

In the spinal segments, connexions have been traced, in cat, to primary afferent fibres, tract cells and interneurones, and, in monkey, directly to motoneurones. These connexions are most profuse to the motoneurones of the distal muscles, and explain the preferential accessibility of the muscles of hand and foot to cortical stimulation. In both cat and baboon, there are connexions to fusimotor neurones, some of them monosynaptic in the baboon.

5
Structure of cortical projection areas.
Electrical stimulation II

5.1 Introduction

In this chapter we are working towards a description of the architecture and geography of the output channels that are available for selection by neural activities of the fore-brain and cerebellum which are nowadays called 'programmes' and which Hughlings Jackson called 'processes representing movements'. The description is in its infancy and may take many years to complete.

The experiments we have so far considered have not succeeded in resolving the fine grain of output structure of the motor area, that is to say, in determining whether localization is abrupt or whether it is minute and overlapping. Punctate, near-threshold faradic stimulation of the largest brains, those of apes, revealed the largest repertories of 'fractional' items of muscle-output, but the uncontrolled factors of spread of stimulus, and the confinement of electrode-positions to the convexity of the precentral gyrus when many of the projection areas were presumably located in the anterior wall of the central sulcus, make it impossible to draw conclusions about the size, shape and location of specific projection areas. The making of circumscribed cortical lesions and the tracing of degeneration by the Nauta method has not been pursued with very small lesions, or with lesions confined to cortex buried in the sulcus, so that the degree of somatotopy so far attained by this method is not much finer than 'arm' or 'leg' or 'face', and 'more rostral' or 'more caudal'.

Our full awareness of the wealth of collateral and terminal branching of PT axons is not yet twenty years old (Chapter 4). Rich as is the known branching in the cat, it may yet be found to be no less rich in the primates. The variety of destinations to which PT axons are now known to be distributed, compared with the classical assumption that all were travelling more or less directly to motoneurones, makes it necessary to ask questions about the arrangement of clusters of corticofugal neurones, collected within specific projection areas, which send axons to particular functional categories of destination related to the somatotopic subdivisions arm, leg and face.

The minimum possible output from the cortex is that of a single PTN. This sounds simple enough; but its axon may emit more than one collateral, and may, for all we know, make contacts with clusters of neurones in the brain stem and dorsal column nuclei before entering the LCST and giving off branches in several spinal segments, some to reflex interneurones, some to propriospinal neurones, some to Ia-inhibitory interneurones and some to fusimotor and α motoneurones, possibly belonging to more than one muscle. The quantitative distribution of its actions could well fluctuate from time to time, depending on background states of excitation and inhibition of its target cells at all these levels. It would be surprising, however, if clusters of PTN did not distribute their output preponderantly to some major target, even if that target were 'collateral', in the brain stem, with subsidiary targets in the spinal cord. The problem for the experimenter is to choose an identifiable target, and to map the cortical projection area or areas which contain the clusters of PTN which project to it. Of the many possible targets described in Chapter 4, the motoneurones of primates have the advantages that they receive monosynaptic connexions from the CST and that they can be labelled by antidromic stimulation of the nerves of particular muscles or muscle-groups. Thus to abstract them from the totality of Fig. 4.16 (p. 137) is not merely technically convenient, it is also physiologically significant, since the motor unit is the elemental basis of the organization of movement and posture (Sherrington, 1931). The localization of specific cortical areas projecting to single motoneurones is evidently the most elemental type of motor localization that can exist. It is, however, wise to remember that PTN which project to a particular motoneurone may well supply collaterals to other target areas. In the cat, some CST neurones supply collaterals to the cervical cord and then descend to the lumbar region (Asanuma et al. 1976b); Asanuma et al. (1976c) indicate that branching of 30 per cent of LCST axons occurs in primates.

5.2   Stimulation of cortical surface and intracellular recording from target motoneurones in baboons and monkeys

In the arm area of baboons, area 4 extends about 10 mm forward from the central sulcus along the convexity of the precentral gyrus, and almost to the bottom of the rostral wall of the sulcus, a depth of about 10 mm. We begin by considering what focal surface-anodal (S+) stimulation can discover about the location and architecture of the cortical projection areas which contain the *colonies* of CST neurones (Landgren *et al.*, 1962b) which project to target motoneurones. S+ stimulation selectively excites the PTN at their axonal poles (Chapter 3). Prompted by some of the more recent research that we shall consider in this chapter, we are allowing ourselves the liberty of developing some of the interpretations we placed on the results of these experiments at the time of their original publication.

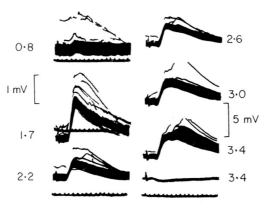

FIG. 5.1. Superimposed intracellular records of monosynaptic excitatory action of cortico-spinal volleys on a median nerve motoneurone at C7-8 level. Depolarization signalled by upward deflexion. Membrane potential −74 mV. Strengths of 0.2 ms S+ pulses noted in margin (in mA). Final record: extracellular control after microelectrode withdrawn from cell. Calibration of recording system: 1 mV for responses to 0.8 and 1.7 mA; 5 mV for remaining records. Time, ms. (Phillips and Porter, 1964.)

An exploring focal anode, delivering pulses of duration 0.2 ms at near-threshold strength, does not discover 'points' on the cortical surface from which minimal EPSPs are evoked in target motoneurones. It maps not points but areas. If, when such an area has been located, the anode is kept within it (at the 'best point': Landgren *et al.*, 1962b), and the current is progressively increased, the EPSP grows to a maximum (Figs 5.1 and 5.2). This proves that more than one PTN projects to the target moto-neurone. The strength which gives the maximal EPSP is that which excites every PTN of the colony. The thresholds are different for different target motoneurones, as would be expected if the rostral rims of their colonies lay at different depths below the point of contact of the surface anode with the cortex, that is, in the anterior wall of the central sulcus. The lowest thresholds are equal to the lowest thresholds measured for single CST neurones (Fig. 5.3B). These are the neurones that are located on the convexity of the precentral gyrus, with their apical dendrites and axons at right-angles to the surface. The rostral rims of the lowest-threshold colonies would therefore extend forward along the convexity. The rostral rims of those with higher thresholds would be at different distances below the surface of the brain, in the anterior wall of the central sulcus. The maximal stimuli for different colonies are also different (Fig. 5.2): smaller maxima suggesting more superficial location and greater compactness of the colony, larger maxima suggesting deeper location and possibly a less compact arrangement, but providing no critical evidence to distinguish between these possible architectural differences.

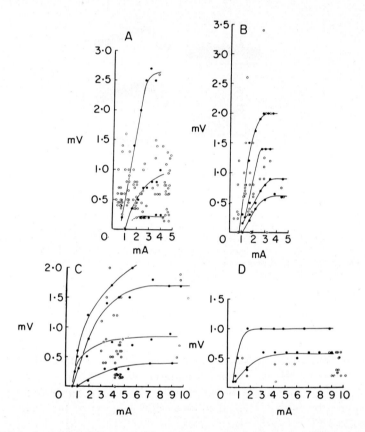

Fig. 5.2. A. Quantities of monosynaptic excitatory action (ordinates) at different strengths of cortical stimulation with single S+, 0.2 ms pulses (abscissae) in 94 motoneurones of the median nerve. Eleven other motoneurones gave no monosynaptic excitatory response at stimulus strengths of 4.5 mA. For three motoneurones, typical curves show growth of monosynaptic action with increasing volleys (filled circles). For remaining motoneurones, open circles show measurements at a single strength (the largest strength, or the only strength, used).

B. Results, plotted as above from 45 motoneurones of the ulnar nerve.

C. Results from 47 motoneurones of the musculocutaneous nerve.

D. Results from 21 motoneurones of the triceps nerves. No monosynaptic excitatory responses were obtained from 28 further triceps motoneurones. Of these, 15 gave early inhibitory responses.

(Phillips and Porter, 1964.)

The maximum quantity of EPSP that can be commanded in its target motoneurone by a whole colony also differs from one colony to another (Fig. 5.2) (Phillips and Porter, 1964; Clough et al., 1968). A larger maximal EPSP (greater 'preferential accessibility') suggests larger numbers of PTN in the colony, or more synapses contributed on average by each PTN to the motoneurone, or both. The evidence cannot distinguish between these possibilities.

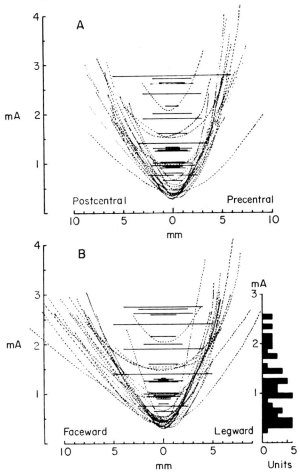

FIG. 5.3. Curves of pyramidal fibre thresholds against distances from lowest-threshold points on cortex. S+, 0.2 ms pulses. Horizontal lines show extent of outline maps drawn at the strengths indicated, for other fibres for which curves were not plotted.

A. At right angles to central fissure.

B. Along precentral gyrus. 'Faceward' means towards face area, and 'legward' towards leg area of cortex. Right, short-pulse S+ thresholds for 59 pyramidal fibres. Ordinates, threshold; abscissae, number of fibres.

(Landgren et al., 1962b.)

We can go no further unless we can estimate the physical spread of S+ pulses of the strengths used in mapping the colonies. We can do this by measuring the currents needed for direct excitation of single CST neurones when applied at their best points (i.e. vertically overlying the cell), and at different horizontal distances, measured along lines which intersect at the best point, running at right angles to the central fissure and 'parallel' to it (Fig. 5.3: Landgren et al., 1962b). That the spread is physical, and not physiological, is attested by the fact that the latency of the impulse (recorded from the axon in the LCST) is the same from every point stimulated, as explained in Chapter 3. Inspection suggests that the curves which relate threshold to distance from the best point are parabolas, as would be expected if the current strength had to be increased as a function of the square of the distance from the best point:

$$I = kr^2 + I_{min} \qquad (1)$$

where I is the threshold at any point, I_{min} is the threshold at the best point (vertically overlying the CST neurone) and r is the distance of the neurone from a point whose threshold is I (see Fig. 5.5).

If the curves of Fig. 5.3 are parabolas, the measured thresholds, if plotted against (distance)^2, should fall on straight lines. In Fig. 5.4 we have replotted representative curves from Fig. 5.3, which show that the fit is imperfect. Further, if the cortex were an isotropic conducting medium, the curves of Fig. 5.3 should be symmetrical about the vertical axis passing through I_{min}. Inspection shows that they are not, the deviation from symmetry being most obvious in the lateral ('faceward') direction (Fig. 5.3B; note outlying points in Figs 5.4A, B). An obvious anisotropic feature (apart from the cyto- and myelo-architecture of the cortex itself) is the curving central sulcus, filled with blood vessels and CSF. To a first approximation, however, we may accept the pairs of curves as symmetrical parabolas, and in Fig. 5.4, therefore, we have plotted all the points from the pair of curves for each of the CST neurones selected from Fig. 5.3 (postcentral to precentral, crossing the central sulcus; 'faceward to leg-ward', running parallel to it).

The threshold currents (I_{min}), and the proportionality constant (k) which determines the slopes of the lines of Fig. 5.4, are different for the different neurones, and are determined, in ways not yet explained in detail, by geometry (distance of the neurone from the surface; orientation of its long axis in relation to lines of current flow) as well as by the excita-bility of the neuronal membrane (cf. Armstrong et al., 1973). In their study of antidromic excitation of climbing fibres by stimulating the surface of the cerebellar cortex, these authors point out that the depth at which excitation occurs can be read off from plots such as those of Fig. 5.4, as the square root of the value of the intercept on the (distance)^2 axis. This is because the depth from the surface should be equal to the horizontal distance from the best point of any point at which the threshold $= 2I_{min}$. This is set out in Fig. 5.5 and its legend. The probable depths of the points at which a selection of CST neurones from Fig. 5.3 are stimulated,

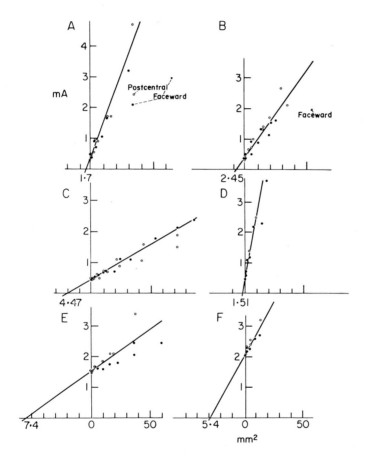

FIG. 5.4. Replotting of the experimental points of six representative parabolas from Fig. 5.3. Ordinates, mA; abscissae, (distance)^2. Open circles, postcentral to precentral curves (see Fig. 5.3). Filled circles, faceward to legward curves (Fig. 5.3). The straight lines have been fitted by eye.

A. Conduction velocity of CST axon 50 m s^{-1}. $k = 105$ μA mm^{-2}. Approximate depth of neurone (square root of intercept on x-axis), $\sqrt{3} = 1.7$ mm.

B. Conduction velocity 39 m s^{-1}. $k = 60$ μA mm^{-2}. Approximate depth, $\sqrt{6} = 2.45$ mm.

C. Conduction velocity 43 m s^{-1}. $k = 20$ μA mm^{-2}. Approximate depth, $\sqrt{20} = 4.47$ mm.

D. Conduction velocity 27 m s^{-1}. $k = 200$ μA mm^{-2}. Approximate depth, $\sqrt{2.3} = 1.51$ mm.

E. Conduction velocity 46 m s^{-1}. $k = 30$ μA mm^{-2}. Approximate depth, $\sqrt{55} = 7.4$ mm.

F. Conduction velocity 40 m s^{-1}. $k = 70$ μA mm^{-2}. Approximate depth, $\sqrt{29} = 5.4$ mm.

are indicated in Figs 5.4 and 5.6. These values are all within the anatomically possible range, none less than 1.5 mm and none exceeding 9.0 mm
from the surface of the precentral gyrus.

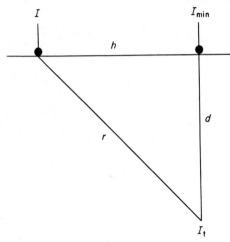

FIG. 5.5. I_{min} is the threshold at best point, vertically overlying the CST neurone at depth
d; I is the threshold at a point at horizontal distance h. Let I_t be threshold current density
at the neurone. Assuming medium is isotropic, $I_t = I_{min}/d^2 = I/r^2$. Since $r^2 = h^2 + d^2$,
$I/r^2 = I/(h^2+d^2)$. Therefore, when $I = 2I_{min}$, $2I_{min}/(h^2+d^2) = I_{min}/d^2$. Eliminating I_{min},
$h^2+d^2 = 2d^2$ so that h (which we can measure) $= d$ (which we wish to know). (R. J.
Harvey, personal communication.)

With regard to 'excitability' of the neurones, this should be related
to the conduction velocity of their axons. In the nature of microelectrode
recording from the LCST, it is not surprising that the samples collected
by Landgren et al. (1962b) and Phillips and Porter (1962) should have
belonged to the fast group; so that major differences in excitability would
not be expected. Figure 5.4D, however, illustrates one CST neurone
whose conduction velocity was slower than that of the others, and whose
slope was steeper, possibly because of a lower excitability to extrinsically
applied current. It is instructive to compare this neurone with that of
Fig. 5.4A. These are similar 'geometrically': both are located in the cortex
nearest the surface of the precentral gyrus, at about the same depth, and
with their apical dendrites presumably orientated at right angles to the
surface of the gyrus. But the two neurones seem to differ in excitability:
conduction velocities are 27 m s^{-1} and 50 m s^{-1} respectively; I_{min} 0.5 mA
and 0.3 mA; and slopes 200 μA mm^{-2} and 105 μA mm^{-2}. Figure 5.4B offers
another instructive comparison. This neurone is located about 2.5 mm
from the surface of the gyrus, which is where the cortex is curving into
the sulcus (cf. Fig. 5.12), so the long axis of the cell would be oblique

or horizontal. I_{min} is 0.3 mA, as low as that of any cell of the sample (Fig. 5.3B), and slope about 60 μA mm^{-2}.

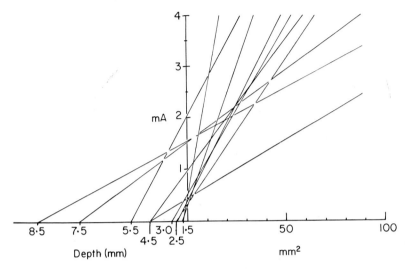

FIG. 5.6. Replotting of ten parabolas from Fig. 5.3, including those replotted in Fig. 5.4A–F. Approximate depths of the neurones range from 1.5 to 8.5 mm. I_{min} range from 0.3 mA to 2.05 mA.

The application of these results to the mapping of CM colonies can now be considered. To gain a first rough measure of spread, in the experiment of Figs 5.1 and 5.2 in which current strength was increased from threshold (0.8 mA) to maximal (about 3.0 mA) for a CM colony, we can draw a pair of arcs of equal radius, centred on the best point and marking off a length of precentral gyrus. The radius appropriate to any current can be read from Fig. 5.3 and represents its maximal horizontal spread. That currents of 3.0 mA also spread downwards, to stimulate CST neurones in the depth of the central sulcus, is attested by experiments such as that of Fig. 3.17I (p. 84) in which a single unit which responded at low threshold to deep intracortical stimulation was fired from the surface at 2.5 mA, and by experiments in which populations of deep-lying CST neurones were made refractory to intracortical stimulation when the surface stimulus reached 3.2 mA (Phillips and Porter, 1964, Fig. 5). Figure 5.7A is a hypothetical diagram of a section through the arm area at right angles to the central sulcus, with the row of large PTN cell-bodies indicated by dots. Figure 5.7B is at right-angles to A, so that we are facing the axonal poles of the vertically orientated sheet of PTN cell-bodies in the rostral wall of the sulcus. It illustrates how the threshold S+ stimulus (about 0.3 mA: Fig. 5.3B) would reach the PTN on the convexity of the precentral gyrus,

and evoke a minimal EPSP in a target motoneurone whose colony included any of these PTN; and how, with increasing strengths (successive
semicircles), the effective current (about 3.0 mA) would reach the depth
of the central fissure and would spread about 10 mm horizontally on either
side of the best point (cf. Fig. 5.3).

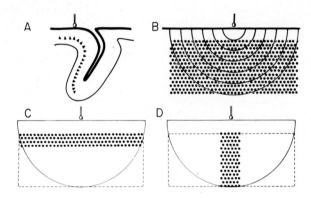

FIG. 5.7. A. Diagram of parasagittal section through arm area of right hemisphere of
baboon. Perikarya of PTN marked by triangles (not to scale). A ball-tipped anode is
resting on surface of precentral gyrus.

B. Rostral bank of central sulcus, seen from rostral view point looking caudally. Dots
(not to scale) mark perikarya of PTN. *Smallest semicircle*, centred on ball-tipped surface
anode, represents effective current spread at threshold for most superficial PTN (0.3 mA);
this current evokes a minimal EPSP in the target motoneurone. *Largest semicircle* represents strength of current which is needed to excite every PTN which belongs to the
colony which is monosynaptically connected to the target motoneurone, and evokes the
maximal CM-EPSP.

C. The colony cannot have this distribution; if it had, a minimal EPSP could be evoked
at any point along this length of precentral gyrus and not only at the best point.

D. The colony probably has this distribution. See text.

Figure 5.8 shows more precisely how CST neurones lying at the depths
of those presented in Fig. 5.4, and with their specific properties, would
have been involved in the spread. Those vertically below the best point
would have been fired when their I_{min} was reached. At 3.0 mA, their
fellows at the corresponding depths, and with the same specific properties,
would have been excited as far away as the arrowheads. The dotted lines
indicate the positions of the arcs that would have been drawn from Fig. 5.3
on the map of the cortical surface to indicate the maximum horizontal
spread at this current strength. Clearly an enormous population of CST
neurones is involved in the response. Estimates made for Landgren *et al.*
(1962b) by T. P. S. Powell showed that a cylinder of baboon's motor cortex
of area 1.0 mm² contains about 18 000 small and about 90 large pyramidal
cell bodies in the fifth layer. Not all of these are CST neurones, and of the
CST neurones not all can belong to the colony, since the best points of

other target motoneurones may be located at virtually the same electrode position (Fig. 5.10: Landgren *et al.*, 1962b). From such experiments, two things only can be asserted about a colony: first, that if it responds at a threshold of about 0.3 mA, some of its CST neurones must lie near to the best point; second, that others must lie along some part of the circumference of the largest semicircle in Fig. 5.7B, since they contributed only in response to the maximal stimulus. About the actual shape of the colony, nothing can be affirmed: its cells might be scattered through a large part of the semicircular population, or arranged in a vertical strip, as in Fig. 5.7D. They are not, however, arranged in a superficial horizontal strip (Fig. 5.7C), since the area, when mapped with weaker stimuli delivered at different points, measures much less than 20 mm along the mediolateral length of the precentral gyrus.

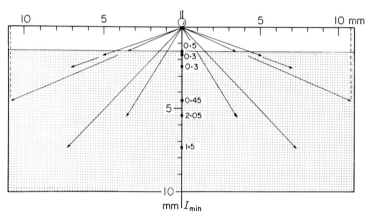

FIG. 5.8. The sheet of CST neurones in the anterior wall of the central fissure (orientation as in Fig. 5.7B) is represented by dots. Cells with the properties of those plotted in Fig. 5.4, and lying at depths indicated on scale, would be excited by pulses of duration 0.2 ms and strength 3.0 mA at different distances, marked by arrows, from the surface anode situated at zero on surface scale.

Further information can be gained by mapping with a roving focal anode, delivering submaximal stimuli (e.g. 0.4 to 1.4 mA). Figure 5.9 shows how the amplitude of the monosynaptic EPSP in the target motoneurone declines to zero as the anode moves in either direction away from the best point. The row of points which followed the curvature of the central sulcus has been omitted in order not to confuse the picture. Figure 5.10 shows, for four motoneurones, plots of amplitude of EPSP against distances from the best points along a line parallel to the sulcus. Since the amplitude of the constant current pulses was fixed at 1.3 mA, similar numbers of corticofugal neurones would have been excited from each point of contact; in spite of this, the curves of the four colonies differ in breadth and amplitude. The architecture of the four colonies must therefore differ, but the experiment cannot distinguish between such features as differences in shape and location (wider or narrower, deeper or more superficial), different numbers of CST neurones and of CM synapses, etc., and, above all, whether the colonies really overlap, as the curves at first sight suggest. The lower part of Fig. 5.10 shows how closely the best points of different colonies may be crowded together in the same brain. This map is for the motoneurones of distal muscles; best points for biceps and triceps are also found in the same area, but for some of these 'proximal' colonies there was no best point, the synaptic actions being evoked only with stronger cortical stimuli, and then with equal ease from all parts of a wide area (Phillips and Porter, 1964).

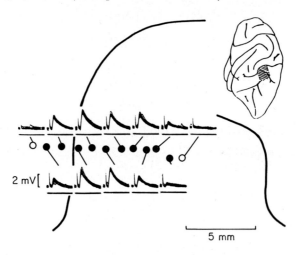

FIG. 5.9. Monosynaptic EPSPs evoked in a motoneurone of the ulnar nerve (membrane potential 67 mV) by surface-anodal stimulation at a series of points along a latero-medial axis which crosses the genu of the central sulcus at right-angles. Stimulating pulses 0.2 ms in duration, 1.35 mA in amplitude.

   Inset: dorsolateral view of baboon's brain to show location of parts of central and superior precentral sulci which are represented on left of Figure (Phillips, 1967).

From everything we have learned about the spread of surface stimuli in the cortex, we ought not to expect that there would be any possibility of being able to define the location, sizes and shapes of these colonies which are largely or wholly buried in the wall of the central sulcus, or of providing critical evidence about whether or not they overlap. We might hope, however, to be able to make statements about those projection areas which are located, in part or in whole, on the convexity of the precentral gyrus, and whether these parts or wholes overlap. This requires that we should concentrate on the results of mapping with the weakest pulses.

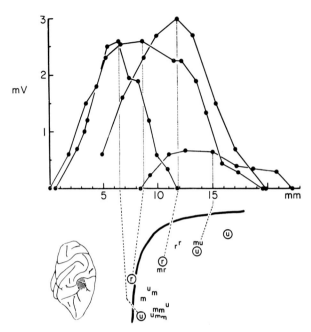

FIG. 5.10. *Above*: amplitudes of CM-EPSPs (ordinates, mV) evoked in four motoneurones by surface-anodal pulses (duration 0.2 ms, strength 1.3 mA), plotted against distances from best points (abscissae, mm). All membrane potentials exceeded 60 mV.

Below: Map of genu of right precentral gyrus, same scale. The best points are ringed; the distances measured along the abscissae in the graphs (*above*) are measured along lines passing through each best point and running parallel to the curvature of the central fissure. Best points are also indicated for 16 other motoneurones in the same preparation: u, ulnar, r, radial, and m, median motoneurones.

Inset: dorsolateral view of right hemisphere of baboon. Hatching indicates location of genu of central sulcus. (Phillips, 1967.)

Fig. 5.11A shows the results of an experiment on a motoneurone of the median nerve. From the outlying points (filled circles) no EPSP was evoked by 0.2 ms pulses, S+, strength 0.45 mA. A rough indication of the maximum effective spread of stimulating current is given by the arcs centred on the filled circles, whose radii are derived from Fig. 5.3. Since any advance of the roving anode towards the best point (open circle) evoked an EPSP, the projection area containing this colony would have extended at least 2 mm along the length of the precentral gyrus, and at least 3 mm forward on to the convexity of the precentral gyrus. Figure 5.11C shows how 0.45 mA would have spread downwards to excite CST neurones at the depths, and with the properties, of those of Fig. 5.4A, B, C. These support the conclusion that the rostral rim of this colony spreads forward on to the convexity of the precentral gyrus, but that some of it may also be near the top of the anterior wall of the sulcus. These are the only territories that would be reached by these weak pulses from points just within the filled circles of Fig. 5.11A. The amplitude of the EPSP evoked from the best point was 1.0 mV. The threshold at the best point was not determined, but was probably less than 0.45 mA. (For a 5.0 ms pulse it was >0.2, <0.25 mA). Since stronger pulses were not used, we do not know if larger EPSPs would have been evoked, which would have indicated that the projection area extended further downwards into the

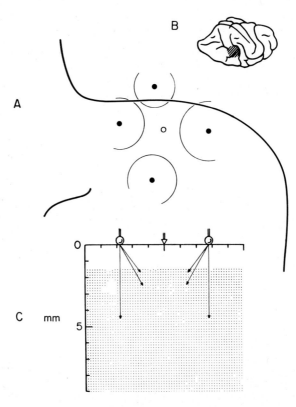

FIG. 5.11. A. Part of central sulcus and inferior precentral sulcus of right hemisphere of baboon. Orientation shown in B. Scale indicated by millimetres in C. In A, filled circles show points from which no EPSP was evoked in a median motoneurone by 0.2 ms pulses, 0.45 mA. Any advance towards the best point (open circle) evoked an EPSP. Arcs centred on filled circles indicate spread of current of 0.45 mA obtained from Fig. 5.3.

C. Spread of 0.45 mA indicated for three CST neurones (A, B and C of Fig. 5.4) lying at depths estimated at 1.7 mm, 2.45 mm and 4.5 mm. $I_{\min}$ for each neurone was 0.3 mA, 0.3 mA and 0.45 mA respectively. The anterior wall of the central sulcus is viewed from in front (cf. Fig. 5.7C, D, E), the sheet of PTN being indicated by dots. Arrow at surface marks best point.

Membrane potential of motoneurone -66 mV. EPSP amplitude at best point with 0.45 mA pulse was 1.0 mV. Threshold for 5.0 ms pulse at best point was >0.2 <0.25 mA.

(Unpublished observations of Landgren, Phillips and Porter.)

wall of the sulcus. The experiment shows only that the colony was superficially located in part or in whole, and gives an estimate of the minimal
extension of the superficially located part of its projection area.

Figure 5.12A shows the best point for an ulnar motoneurone (filled
circle) and the outlying points (open circles) from which the 0.7 mA
pulses just failed to evoke any EPSP. Arcs centred on the most medial
and most lateral points, and with radii measured from Fig. 5.3 for 0.7 mA,
suggest that the minimum width of the colony is about 4 mm. Figure
5.12B shows how the current of 0.7 mA would have spread in depth to
reach CST neurones at the depths, and with the properties, of those of
Fig. 5.4D, A, B, C. If these individual neurones were representative of
larger populations, one might conclude that the colony was narrowest at

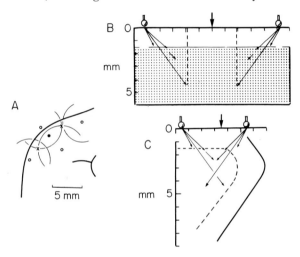

FIG. 5.12. Ulnar motoneurone. Membrane potential −60 to −64 mV.
   A. Filled circle, best point; open circles, null points for 0.7 mA, S+, 0.2 ms. Scale in
mm. Arcs indicate spread of 0.7 mA from null points.
   B. Spread in depth of 0.7 mA from null points to reach CST neurones at depths, and
with properties, of those of Fig. 5.4D, A, B, C. Dotted lines correspond to arcs centred on
null points in A. Arrow marks best point.
   C. Spread of 0.7 mA in depth, from pre- and postcentral null points, in parasagittal
plane. Arrow marks best point. See text.
   The longest arrows in B are 5.6 mm in length. Why may we not draw an arc of radius
5.6 mm to intersect the superficial Betz cells at a depth of 1.5 mm, and destroy the argument that this colony has a minimum faceward–legward extension of 4.0 mm?
   This argument can be rejected because no CST neurone so far encountered has shown
the necessary threshold–distance relationship. The cells which are most excitable in terms
of current density (i.e. those which have the lowest slopes in threshold–(distance)^2 plots,
e.g. that of Fig. 5.4) have invariably been found to be situated deep in the cortex. Thus, if
the cell of Fig. 5.4C were situated at a depth of 1.5 mm, then its I_{min} would be only 50 µA;
such a low I_{min} has never been observed with surface stimulation. Taking the lowest
observed I_{min} (0.3 mA), in combination with a cell as excitable as that of Fig. 5.4C, it
would be situated at a depth of 3.61 mm. Even if such cells existed, the minimum faceward–legward extension of the colony would still be approximately 2.5 mm.

a depth of 4.5 mm and broader more superficially, assuming that any of its CST neurones were located more superficially than 4.5 mm. That some are in fact located more superficially is suggested by Fig. 5.12C, which shows the usual morphology of the plane which, in this brain (which was not itself sectioned), contained the best point and the pre-and postcentral 'null points'. The only CST neurones that would not have been stimulated from the null points would have been those between the dotted lines, on the convexity of the gyrus. Figure 5.13 shows another colony whose minimum mediolateral extension, mapped with pulses of 1.0 mA, was about 6 mm. Although the complete architectural description of colonies such as those of Figs 5.12 and 5.13 cannot be derived from surface-anodal mapping, the fact of their overlap, at least in their more superficial parts, is established by the overlapping of their surface maps on the cortex of the same individuals.

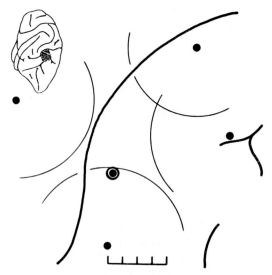

FIG. 5.13. The best point for a median motoneurone is shown by a ringed dot. The other black dots mark outlying points from which no monosynaptic responses could be evoked in the test motoneurone by surface-anodal shocks; strength, 1.0 mA; duration, 0.2 ms. Arcs, centred on these outlying points, show the maximum physical spread of stimulus at this strength, derived from curves such as those shown in Fig. 5.3. The area of precentral gyrus uncovered by these arcs measures approximately 6 × 3 mm, and is thus the minimal area that could contain the colony of pyramidal cells projecting monosynaptically to this test motoneurone. (Modified from Landgren et al., 1962b.)

Figure 5.14 is representative of 14 of 26 maps made by Landgren et al. (1962b). These differ from those we have been discussing in that they cannot exclude the possibility that the whole colony is confined within a cylinder of cortex, say of 1 mm diameter, on the convexity of the gyrus or in the wall of the sulcus. The curves of EPSP amplitude for 0.75 mA and 1.3 mA are practically symmetrical, and centred on the best point, which is effectively covered by 1.3 mA arcs centred on the null points. It may be thought more likely that the stronger stimulus should spread to excite CST neurones lying deep to those excited by 0.75 mA, than that it should increase the EPSP more than six-fold by exciting more neurones within the same cylinder of cortex. That such arguments can be multiplied inconclusively is inherent in the complex geometry of the arm area, that is, in the varying depth and orientation of its CST neurones in relation to a focal anode which explores only the exposed surface of the cortex, and in the nature of experiments in which pulses stronger than 0.5 mA have to be used.

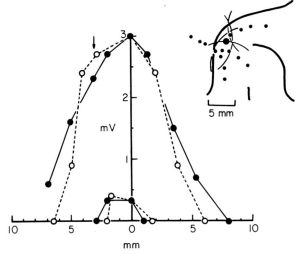

FIG. 5.14. Radial motoneurone. Map shows points stimulated along line at right angles to Rolandic fissure, and along a line parallel to it. S+ pulses, 0.2 ms, 1.3 mA; best point enclosed in circle. Arcs (radii measured from Fig. 5.3) show furthest limits of cell populations excited by stimuli applied at points of zero synaptic action on test motoneurone (see text). Scale in mm.

Below: peak amplitude of monosynaptic potentials, measured from superimposed records, plotted against distance from best point. Upper curves, stimulus 1.3 mA; lower curves, stimulus 0.75 mA; membrane potential −66 mV.

Dotted line, points along line at right angles to Rolandic fissure (point just in front of fissure marked by arrow); postcentral gyrus to left, precentral gyrus to right of arrow. Full line, points parallel to Rolandic fissure; to left, faceward from best point; to right, legward from best point.

(Landgren *et al.*, 1962b.)

By contrast, the leg area of macaque monkeys is unfolded at its medial end, so that its CST neurones are all equidistant from the surface and all orientated at right angles to the convexity of the brain; they thus form an ideal field for mapping by surface anodal pulses. Jankowska *et al.* (1975b) have taken full advantage of this simpler geometry in their mapping of the areas of origin of CST neurones projecting monosynaptically to moto-neurones of the main muscle-groups of the hindlimb. From computer-averaged records of action potentials of the LCST they confirmed Land-gren *et al.*'s (1962b) measurements of the lowest S+ threshold for firing CST neurones: 0.3 mA. The amplitude of these minimal CST volleys was similar to that of volleys evoked by intracortical stimulation with a microelectrode. The method of recording was sensitive enough to detect the action potentials of a single large axon within the tract. Jankowska *et al.* could therefore assume that the minimal EPSPs evoked in target motoneurones by 0.3 mA pulses were due to stimulation of CST neurones immediately underlying the focal anode. With 0.4 mA, the stimuli would spread to CST neurones within a radius of 0.5 mm, and with 0.5 mA, within a radius of 1.0 mm (cf. Fig. 5.3). Thus, in outlining the area containing CST neurones projecting to a target motoneurone, the true area would be 0.5 mm narrower with 0.4 mA and 1.0 mm narrower with 0.5 mA. The amplitudes of the EPSPs evoked from the edges of the areas by 0.4 mA were less than 30 per cent of those from the centres. For comparing the areas for different motoneurones, therefore, Jankowska *et al.* adopted an arbitrary standard, defining the 'total projection area' as being bounded by responses not less than 30 per cent of those from the centre (Fig. 5.15A, full line). Since the EPSPs were computer-averaged, very

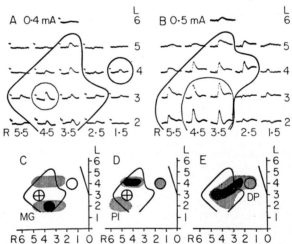

FIG. 5.15. Area of origin of pyramidal tract cells projecting to a lateral gastrocnemius motoneurone. A, B. Averaged records of postsynaptic potentials evoked from indicated electrode positions by 0.4 and 0.5 mA respectively. In C, D and E the total projection areas and the optimal projection areas (from which largest EPSPs were evoked at 0.4 mA strength) are compared for the illustrated lateral gastrocnemius motoneurone and for motoneurones to the synergistic muscles medial gastrocnemius, MG (in C), and plantaris, Pl (in D), and the antagonistic deep peroneal muscle, DP (in E). (Jankowska *et al.*, 1975b.)

small responses could be measured accurately. The 'total projection areas' thus defined would tend to be smaller than the true areas. Within the areas, 'optimal projection areas' (equivalent to the best points of Landgren *et al.*, 1962b) were drawn to enclose the points from which responses of 80–100 per cent were evoked (Fig. 5.15A, dotted line). 'As they were clearly submaximal, the amplitudes of these EPSPs are not given as a measure of the total cortical output to different groups of motoneurones. . . . They indicate only the relative density of pyramidal tract cells projecting to the impaled motoneurones, the strength of stimulation being constant.' The differential accessibility of the various muscle groups has been described already (Chapter 4, section 4.6).

The area of cortex containing the projection areas is adjacent to the midline, and is shown, for the right hemisphere, in Figs 5.15 and 5.16, in which OR represents the midline (R, rostral) and OL, the mediolateral line at right angles to it; distances along both lines are marked in mm. The central sulcus does not begin until 3 mm from the midline and then runs forward obliquely, so that the mapped areas are all on the convexity of the precentral gyrus (Fig. 5.15C–E). The points stimulated were on a grid of 1.0 mm (Fig. 5.15A) or 0.5 mm, as far as was permitted by the blood vessels. Figures 5.15 and 5.16 show that the areas containing the CST colonies projecting monosynaptically to the target motoneurones were of 'considerable size', the 'total projection areas' ranging from 1 to 13 mm². The differences between the sizes for the motoneurones of different muscles did not exceed those between motoneurones of the same muscles. The overlaps between areas for motoneurones of different muscle-groups were not confined to synergistic muscles, but were equally in evidence for the motoneurones of antagonists; the optimal projection areas, as well as the total projection areas, were overlapping. This can be seen in Fig. 5.15E, in which there is overlap between the 'total' and 'optimal' areas for a lateral gastrocnemius (LG) motoneurone and an antagonistic motoneurone from the deep peroneal group. The areas for different motoneurones of the same muscles are located in different places (Fig. 5.16). Finally, there are, in some cases, multiple areas projecting to single motoneurones, well separated by intervening points which yielded hardly any EPSP. Figure 5.15A shows a detached area for an LG motoneurone; C shows two areas for a single medial gastrocnemius motoneurone (overlapping its synergist, the LG motoneurone); and D shows three areas for a single plantaris motoneurone (overlapping the synergist LG motoneurone).

These experiments provide critical evidence that the minute localization of the elemental monosynaptic outputs from the leg area of the motor cortex is overlapping and not abrupt. These are some of the outputs that are available for selection in varying combinations by intracortical and thalamocortical patterns of activity. The evidently complete mapping of the colonies by pulses of <0.5 mA is in contrast with the experience from the forelimb (Landgren *et al.*, 1962b). It is now clear that some of the colonies for the forelimb have their rostral rims extending on to the convexity of the precentral gyrus, since minimal EPSPs can be evoked in some of them by equally weak pulses, and that they may here overlap; but it is equally clear that their main localization is in the wall of the central sulcus.

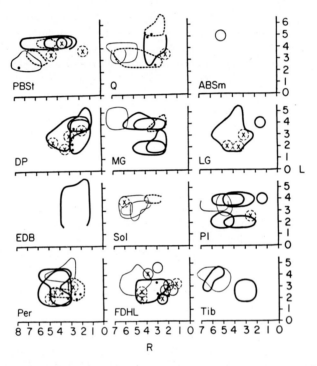

FIG. 5.16. Areas of origin of pyramidal tract cells projecting to motoneurones innervating different muscles. Thick and thin continuous lines encompass total projection areas from two most complete mapping experiments. Dashed lines encompass total projection areas from all other experiments. Large circles with crosses (x) and dots (•) indicate origin of EPSPs evoked by surface and intracortical stimulation when stimuli were applied at only one or two electrode positions. Breaks in the lines indicate that the areas outside them were not tested and that the total projection areas might extend beyond the breaks. (Jankowska *et al.*, 1975b.)

Their complete mapping by surface-anodal stimulation would therefore require removal of the postcentral gyrus. Tentative attempts to separate the walls of the central sulcus in baboons have convinced us that the pial circulation, whose integrity is essential for mapping of this degree of refinement, would be compromised unacceptably by such an operation.

5.3 Mapping of projection areas by intracortical microstimulation

The introduction of intracortical microstimulation by Asanuma and Sakata (1967), and its progressive refinement and elaboration in the important series of studies by Asanuma and his colleagues which we shall be citing in what follows, was a major advance in technique which has opened up quite new possibilities for investigating the microanatomy and microphysiology of the cerebral cortex. The precise modes of its action on PT neurones and axons, on incoming afferent axons and on cortical interneurones are now being energetically analysed and debated. We must review the main themes of this research before we shall be ready to consider the application of this powerful new technique to the mapping of corticomotoneuronal colonies.

The first experiments were made on cats (Asanuma and Sakata, 1967); the actions of brief high-frequency bursts of intracortical microstimulation were detected by the resulting facilitation of monosynaptic spinal reflexes. Since this is an indirect detector of corticofugal discharge (Chapter 4, section 4.2), we shall defer consideration of those experiments until we have looked at the two modes of action of single microcathodal pulses on single PTN: direct and trans-synaptic. Since we wish to use the method for the mapping of cortical projection areas, our primary interest is in the direct mode, and we shall be specially concerned with threshold as a function of distance between the tip of the microelectrode and the PTN. We need to be able to estimate the radius of a cylinder of cortex whose axially orientated PTN will be excited by a pulse of given strength.

5.3.1   MODES OF EXCITATION OF PTN BY MICROCATHODAL STIMULATION

5.3.1.1 *Direct stimulation*

Stoney *et al.* (1968) used a pair of glass-coated tungsten microelectrodes, one for microstimulation and the other for extracellular recording of the responses of the PTN. In each, the sharpened tungsten wire projected 10–15 μm from the glass. The pair were parallel and as close together as possible, and could be micromanipulated independently along parallel axes within the cat's motor cortex. PTN were identified by antidromic stimulation of the pyramid. The recording microelectrode was then left in a position nearest to the cell, and the stimulating microcathode was used to measure the threshold for single 0.2 ms pulses at different depths, superficial (+ in Fig. 5.17) and deep (− in Fig. 5.17) to the PTN. The success of direct stimulation was verified, when the impulse was obscured by the stimulus artefact, by collision between the orthodromic impulse and a suitably timed antidromic impulse. The latency of responses to direct stimulation was <0.5 ms. Figure 5.17 (filled circles) shows that the relation between threshold and distance for direct stimulation is roughly

oronparabolic. Figure 5.17 (open circles) shows that the amplitude of the anti-dromic spike potential, when recorded by the microelectrode used for stimulating, was greatest at the point (0 on abscissae) at which the threshold was minimal. This therefore would be the point at which the track passed nearest to the most excitable region of the PTN. The geometry can be represented by the diagram we have already used for considering stimulation of PTN from the surface of the cortex (Fig. 5.5); d now stands for the shortest distance from the PTN to the track, h stands for distances along the track (microdrive readings and histological reconstructions), and r stands for distances from points on the track to the electrically excited part of the PTN (soma, initial segment or first node).

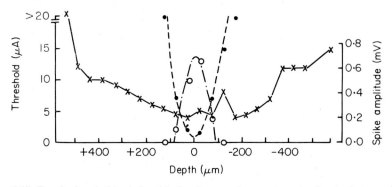

FIG. 5.17. Depth–threshold relationship for direct and synaptic activation by intracortical current pulses. Threshold current (left ordinate) for direct excitation (closed circles) and synaptic excitation (crosses) are plotted as a function of the relative depth of the stimulating microelectrode. Positive abscissae measure electrode depths at points lying superficial to point of lowest threshold, which is at zero; negative abscissae represent points lying deep to point of lowest threshold. Open circles and barred line show amplitude of the antidromic spike (right ordinate) at different depths. (Stoney et al., 1968.)

When the threshold was less than 10 μA, the tip of the stimulating microelectrode was always found, in histological sections (in which its position was marked by a small electrolytic lesion), to have been 'localized within the PT cell layers of the cortex'. The value of I_{min} was less than 20 μA in 13/39 cells: it ranged from 1.2 to 17.0 μA in 12 cells which were fully investigated. The lowest attainable value was probably about 1.0 μA, in a cell which was presumably very close to the track, since it began to give injury discharges after this measurement and then died. The stimulating tracks would not normally have passed so close to the stimulated cells, and some idea of the shortest distances (d, Fig. 5.5) can be gained from the curves of Figs 5.17 and 5.18 by noting the distance along the track at which the threshold was $2I_{min}$ (cf. Armstrong et al., 1973): in Fig. 5.17 about 40 μm; in the bottom wide curve of Fig. 5.18, about 50 μm if we take the superficial $(+)$ side and about 35 μm if we take the deep $(-)$ side; in the curve with $I_{min} = 10$ μA, about 100 μm or 75 μm; and in the curve with $I_{min} = 15$ μA, about 150 μm.

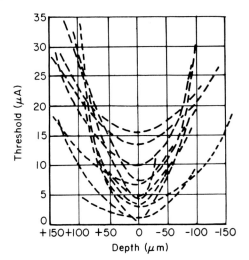

FIG. 5.18. Relationship between threshold for direct excitation by cathodal current pulses and depth of the stimulating electrode for 12 PT cells (Stoney *et al.*, 1968.)

The curves collected in Fig. 5.18 are of different widths, and in order to estimate the effective spread of currents of different strengths, a choice must be made of a representative value for k in the equation $I - I_{min} = kr^2$. Such a choice is bound to be arbitrary. It is necessary first to test whether the curves are parabolas. We should not expect perfect parabolas, since the cortex is unlikely to be an isotropic conducting medium: spread of current in the direction of the radially orientated apical dendrites and corticopetal afferent axons should be more extensive than at right angles to these. A model is provided by the dorsal spinocerebellar tract, in which Roberts and Smith (1973) stimulated single nodes with a microcathode and found that effective spread of current was greater in the axial than in the transverse direction. Stoney *et al.* (1968) plotted their threshold-distance measurements for 12 PTN as $I - I_{min}$ against (distance)^2. The points did not fall on straight lines, but were fitted with straight lines by a least-squares analysis; for each cell, the value of k was read off as the slope of the line. In Fig. 5.19A we have drawn the line for one of the 12 cells (slope 1990 μA mm^{-2}), and have marked the experimental points, and in Fig. 5.19B we have plotted the theoretical parabola of $I - I_{min} = kr^2$ when $k = 1990$, again marking the experimental points. Values of k in the 12 cells ranged from 272 to 3460 μA mm^{-2}. Estimates of effective spread of pulses of 5 μA would therefore range from about 35 μm ($k = 3460$) to about 140 μm ($k = 272$). For the 12 cells, Stoney *et al.* (1968) adopted a mean value of 1292 μA mm^{-2} (about 1300), giving an effective spread of 5 μA across about 65 μm. Figure 5.19B shows the theoretical parabolas drawn with the largest, smallest, and mean values of k, and Fig. 5.19C shows the theoretical curve for 1292 μA mm^{-2}, with shaded area to mark the 95 per cent confidence interval, as plotted by Stoney *et al.* (1968). The factors determining the value of k for any individual PTN are complex, and are dependent on factors of geometry and excitability. Stoney *et al.* (1968) estimate that 45 per cent of the observed variation in k is related to conduction velocity (and hence to the 'size' and 'excitability') of the PTN.

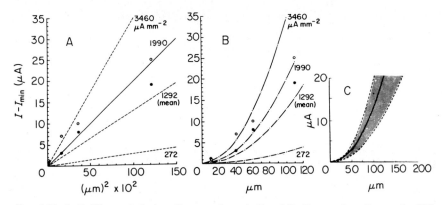

FIG. 5.19. A, B. Theoretical plots, linear and parabolic, of $I - I_{min}$ against distance for PT neurones with different values of k (maximum 3460, minimum 272 μA mm^{-2}). For the plots of the PTN with $k = 1990$, the experimental points of Stoney *et al.* (1968) are included: open circles, deep, and filled circles, superficial to lowest-threshold point in track.

C. Theoretical curve for mean value of k (1292 μA mm^{-2}), reorientated from Stoney *et al.* (1968). Shaded area marks 95 per cent confidence interval.

It is interesting to compare these results with those of microstimulation of the axons of spinal interneurones by Jankowska and Roberts (1972). For their estimates of current spread they selected only those axons whose I_{min} was between 0.1 and 1.0 μA 'in order to compare similar populations'. Linear replotting of their broadest and narrowest curves (from axons with conduction velocities of 85 m s^{-1} and 9 m s^{-1} respectively) gave approximate values of 80 μA mm^{-2} and 500 μA mm^{-2} for k (Andersen *et al.*, 1975). Jankowska and Roberts commented that the spreads estimated by themselves 'are 2–3 times higher than those calculated by Stoney *et al.* (1968) for pyramidal tract cells'. Thus, 5 μA would spread from about 80 μm ($k = 500$) to >200 μm ($k = 80$). It would seem prudent, therefore, to be prepared to test the possible spread of current in microstimulation experiments with a range of values of k and not only with a single averaged value, and to consider the possibility that many cortical cells and axons would have lower values so that the currents would directly excite some, if not all, of the structures enclosed within spheres with radii larger than the average.

5.3.1.2 *Indirect stimulation : the problem of horizontal spread*

So far we have been considering microstimulation as if the output pyramidal neurones were the only structures responding to it. Their recurrent axon collaterals, which spread excitation and inhibition orthodromically (Chapter 3), may be 0.5 to 1.0 mm long (T. Tömböl, cited by Jankowska *et al.*, 1975b), and can be excited directly (Asanuma *et al.*, 1976b). The intracortical microcathode must also excite clusters of stellate and basket cells and their axons and bundles of afferent axons streaming radially into the cortex, distributing synaptic excitation and inhibition amongst the pyramidal cells. Figure 5.17 (crosses) shows synaptic excitation of a PTN from points up to 0.5 mm superficial and deep to it along the stimulating track. The synaptically evoked responses were distinguished by their longer latency, from 0.8 ms up to 6.0 ms, generally 2.0 to 4.0 ms. Such a physiological spread of excitation across horizontal distances considerably greater than those involved in physical spread (Fig. 5.17) would introduce error into the mapping of projection areas by microstimulation. There is, however, some evidence that the spread tends to be greater in the radial than in the horizontal direction. In 5/6 PTN which were excited indirectly by 10 μA or less in experiments in which the tracks were reconstructed histologically, spread ranged from 1050 μm with a track at 40° to the radial architecture to 350 μm at 80° to it (Stoney *et al.*, 1968).

Jankowska *et al.* (1975a) stimulated fast CST neurones in the leg area of cats and monkeys with saline-filled micropipettes, the tip being placed very close to the soma, and found that near-threshold cathodal stimulation generally excites the cells trans-synaptically and not directly. The discharges were detected in computer-averaged records from the LCST; the method was sensitive enough to record impulses in single large CST axons. The evidence for indirect (trans-synaptic) excitation was derived from systematic discrepancies between the latencies of orthodromic responses to microcathodal stimulation, of orthodromic responses to S+ stimulation, and of the antidromic response of the CST neurone to stimulation of the LCST. Thus, the latency of orthodromic LCST volleys evoked by S+ stimuli in the range 0.2 to 1.0 mA was constant (Fig. 5.20B). The cortical microcathode was first switched to the recording mode and adjusted until it recorded a large unitary extracellular action potential when the LCST was stimulated antidromically (Fig. 5.21B, F). It was then switched to the stimulating mode. The latency of the start of the orthodromic response to microstimulation (0.5 ms pulses, about 7–18 μA) was about 1.5 to 1.7 ms longer than that of the start of the orthodromic response to S+ stimulation (Fig. 5.20B–E). In Fig. 5.21, at threshold, it was about 1.4 ms longer than the antidromic latency of the CST neurone in a monkey (Fig. 5.21E) and about 1.7 ms longer in a comparable experiment in a cat (Fig. 5.21I). The microcathodal threshold was about 7 μA in the monkey and about 5μA in the cat. These systematic differences between axonal conduction time and total orthodromic conduction time can be explained only by the addition of intracortical synaptic delays (cf. action of surface cathodal stimulation, Chapter 3).

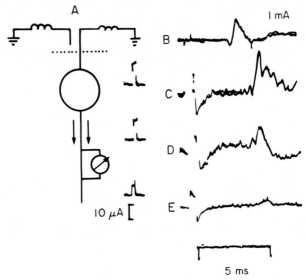

FIG. 5.20. Latencies of the descending volleys evoked by intracortical stimulation in relation to the latency and total duration of the descending volleys evoked by surface-anodal stimulation in a monkey. A. Diagram of the experimental arrangement for intra-cortical (right) and surface (left) stimulation. B. Descending volleys evoked by S+ pulses, strength 1.0 mA. C-E. Descending volleys evoked by intracortical stimulation with decreasing strengths; the amplitudes of the corresponding stimulus pulses (shown to the left) are calibrated by the 10 μA scale below. (Modified from Jankowska et al., 1975a.)

The tip of the stimulating microcathode was judged to be very close to the soma of the CST neurone because it was situated at that point along the track at which the amplitude of the antidromic action potential was largest, and because 'the cells were often impaled with a further movement of the electrode' (Jankowska et al., 1975a). If stimulation with pulses up to 30μA is then found to be indirect, some closely adjacent membranes must have a lower electrical threshold: incoming afferent axons travelling radially to excite stellate cells which would monosynaptically excite the PTN dendrite; recurrent collaterals of small PTN which would mono-synaptically excite the large PTN (Chapter 4), etc. All this, when the pulses are near threshold, could be fairly narrowly confined within the radially organized synaptic apparatus surrounding the PTN (Szentágothai, 1969; see Chapter 6). When the strength is increased above threshold, however, as in Fig. 5.20E–C, the amplitude and duration of the CST discharge is increased. The increase in amplitude can only be due to the discharge of CST neurones surrounding the cell nearest to the micro-cathode—that is, to *horizontally*-spreading excitation; but the experiment cannot tell us the radius of spread. Measurement of that radius requires the independent manipulation of two microelectrodes at different tangen-tial (horizontal) distances within the cortex.

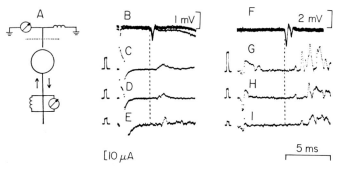

FIG. 5.21. Comparison of the latencies of antidromic activation of pyramidal tract cells and of the earliest components of the descending volleys evoked by intracortical stimu-lation, in monkey (B–E) and cat (F–I). A. Diagram of experimental arrangement. B, F. Extracellular records of antidromic potentials in pyramidal cells. C–E, G–I. Descending volleys recorded at L 1–2 from the surface of the lateral funiculus in monkey and at Th 11–12 from a dissected fascicle of the dorsolateral part of the lateral funiculus in cat, respectively. (Note higher amplification in E than in C, D.) Stimulation of the same sites from which spike potentials of PTN in B and F were recorded. Averaged records of descending volleys. Amplitudes of the stimulating intracortical pulses are given to the left of corresponding records, with the calibration under E. (Jankowska *et al.*, 1975a.)

A few such measurements have been published by Asanuma and Rosén (1973). They recorded intracellularly with a citrate-filled micropipette from 9 antidromically labelled PTN in cats. These cells responded trans-synaptically to 4 µA pulses from a tungsten microcathode which could be manipulated independently in the cortex. The 7 stimulus sites from which PTN could be influenced were all deeper than 0.7 mm and within 0.4 mm tangentially. Three sites gave monosynaptic excitation, 2 gave polysynaptic excitation, one gave monosynaptic inhibition and one gave polysynaptic inhibition. The extent of tangential spread of excitation with stronger stimulation has yet to be measured by the use of two microelectrodes.

Repetitive stimulation favours tangential spread of trans-synaptic excitation of CST neurones. In Fig. 5.22 (Jankowska *et al.*, 1975a), three pulses were delivered at about 285 Hz. In C (about 5 µA), there was no discharge in response to the first pulse, but a small discharge to the second and third. With about 8 μA (D), every pulse evoked a discharge, each one larger than its predecessor. In view of their anatomical arrangement in the cortex, such recruitment of CST neurones can be explained only by invoking tangential spread; but the extent of this spread remains to be measured by the two-microelectrode technique.

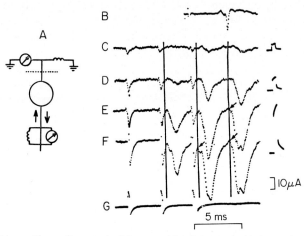

FIG. 5.22. Descending volleys evoked by repetitive intracortical stimulation. A. Experimental arrangement. B. Antidromic potential from a pyramidal tract cell in a monkey. C–F. Descending volleys evoked by increasing strengths of intracortical stimulation at the same microelectrode position as in B, recorded from a fascicle of the lateral funiculus dissected at L 1–2. F. Intracortical stimulation 300 μm deeper. Averaged records. The amplitudes of the stimuli are shown to the right and their timing in G. Arrows indicate descending volleys with the same latencies as the latencies of the antidromic potentials. In all the records, negativity is downwards. (Jankowska *et al.*, 1975a.)

Asanuma *et al.* (1976a) have found that repetitive microcathodal stimulation in lamina V of cats (10 μA, 200 to 250 Hz) excites single CST neurones directly and trans-synaptically, with recruiting I waves which must indicate some degree of tangential spread. Similar stimulation in lamina III evokes I waves only, with less recruitment.

Jankowska *et al.* (1975a) found that direct excitation of those CST neurones in which they observed it was most readily obtained when the microcathode was inserted 200 μm to 400 μm deeper than the cell-bodies (300 μm in Fig. 5.22F). In the second and third response in Fig. 5.22F, and marked by arrows, the earliest component of the orthodromic response has the same latency as the antidromic response, indicating direct excitation of some CST cells (B; in C–F, the intervals between the stimulus artefacts and the vertical lines mark the axonal conduction time).

There remains, therefore, some uncertainty about the conditions in which CST neurones will be stimulated directly at lowest threshold. It is possible that a relatively coarse metal microcathode of the type used by

Stoney *et al.* (1968), thrust in amongst the initial segments of the PT axons, 'where the extracellularly recorded spikes may be smaller but the excitability higher' (Jankowska *et al.*, 1975a), will usually excite the output axons, either directly, or by exciting their recurrent collaterals antidromically (Asanuma *et al.*, 1976a). In spinal motoneurones, Gustafsson and Jankowska (1976) found that the threshold for direct excitation was lowest when their saline-filled microcathode was close to the initial segment of the axon; when it was close to the soma the threshold was higher.

5.3.2 MICROMAPPING OF CORTICOMOTONEURONAL PROJECTION AREAS IN MONKEYS

A complete description of the architecture of a CM colony would include (1) the size, shape and location of the projection area which contains it; (2) the maximum quantity of monosynaptic depolarization it can evoke in its target motoneurone, which is a function of the total number of its cells and of the number of synapses they contribute to the motoneurone; (3) its texture, that is to say, the varying density of the output from different parts of the projection area; and (4) the extent of its overlap with the projection areas of other colonies. The ideal experiment would therefore measure the EPSPs evoked in the target motoneurone by single microcathodal pulses of a range of standard strengths, delivered at every effective intracortical locus, and would try to relate the sum of the separate quantities to the amplitude of the maximal EPSP that could be evoked by a single S+ pulse. In this way, the architecture could be pieced together from the separately stimulated spheres of tissue, whose radii, at each of the standard strengths, could be estimated by the methods we have already presented in section 5.3.1. This assumes that the microstimuli act directly on the corticofugal cells. The assumption would be justified if the latency of the EPSP evoked by S+ stimuli was found to be the same as that of the EPSPs evoked by microstimulation (cf. Jankowska *et al.*, 1975a).

The mapping of projection areas would be subject to error if the microcathode were to excite the recurrent axon collaterals of CST neurones lying at a distance from its tip, as well as the initial segments of CST axons in its immediate proximity: impulses would then travel antidromically to the branch-points and thence orthodromically to the spinal cord. Tömböl (cited by Jankowska *et al.*, 1975b) measured the spread of recurrent collaterals as 0.5 to 1.0 mm, and Asanuma *et al.* (1976b) found that PT cells could be excited, without synaptic delay, by microstimulation as far as 1.0 mm horizontally from the recording site. There was no difference in the range of thresholds (0.4 to 4.5 μA). These measurements set limits to the magnitude of two possible errors: (1) spurious enlargement of the boundaries of the maps, by antidromic stimulation of collaterals spreading up to 1.0 mm beyond the true boundaries of the projection areas; (2) spurious smallness of the areas mapped by stimuli <10 μA—such 'hot spots' might be the centres of networks of collaterals which would enlarge the field of corticofugal discharge by up to 1.0 mm beyond the apparent dimensions of the 'spot'.

If, in addition, trans-synaptic excitation of the corticofugal cells were to occur to a significant extent, there would be another source of error in the mapping. Such physiological spread is more extensive than physical spread (Fig. 5.17). Thus, the apparently large size of a projection area might be spurious; the cells and axons stimulated within it might all be 'presynaptic' to a more limited projection area, upon which they all converge, and which constitutes the sole output from the cortex to the target motoneurone. Equally, the apparently small size of another projection area might be spurious: such a hot spot might not only be the focus of a dense cluster of CST neurones, but also the centre of a radiating intracortical network through which excitation would spread orthodromically to less dense parts of the projection area surrounding the hot spot. Only by intracellular recording would one be able to detect the occurrence of trans-synaptic excitation of corticofugal cells by lengthenings of the latency of the EPSP in the target motoneurone, and by rufflings of its contour by delayed synaptic impacts resulting from the excitation of different CST neurones after different intracortical delays.

Unfortunately, spinal motoneurones cannot survive impalement by intracellular microelectrodes for periods long enough to permit a full investigation of this exacting kind. In the leg area, Jankowska et al. (1975b) were able to evoke EPSPs from several motoneurones with currents of 3 to 20 μA, applied at a single intracortical stimulus site at which an antidromic CST impulse could always be recorded. In a few cases they could evoke EPSPs in a single motoneurone from more than one site, but the cells did not last long enough for them to produce any complete maps. The CM projection areas to motoneurones of leg muscles can be accurately mapped with liminal S+ pulses (Fig. 5.15), so that for the mapping of outputs (as distinct from the analysis of intracortical circuitry) microstimulation offers no advantages. For mapping projection areas in the buried cortex of the arm area, however, microstimulation remains essential, but it is so time-consuming that there seems no possibility of using EPSPs as the quantitative detectors of output from different parts of the colonies. Thus as many as 20 tracks might be required, each penetrating to a depth of 10 mm, with microstimulating pulses of a range of strengths needing to be applied at each of 50 points along each track.

It is necessary therefore to fall back on the recording of EMGs of single motor units, or of small aggregates of motor units, and to depolarize the target motoneurones to a degree sufficient to make them discharge at least one impulse. Unfortunately this requires repetitive microstimulation. In so far as repetitive stimulation acts directly on the CST neurones and antidromically on their recurrent axon collaterals, we have no grounds to fear that its physical spread within the cortex will be increased by repetition. The need for repetition is explained, not by the need for intracortical spread, but by the need for presynaptic facilitation at the CM synapses (Chapter 3) to bring an EPSP to the firing level. But insofar as repetition has been shown to increase the extent of physiological intracortical spread by orthodromic actions of CST collaterals, thalamocortical axons and stellate cells, etc. (Jankowska *et al.*, 1975a), and since the extent has yet to be measured for different frequencies, current strengths and numbers of pulses, there is, as we have seen, an inescapable and unknown element of error in all such mapping experiments. Regrettably, EMG recording does not give sufficiently accurate timing of the excitatory effects on moto-neurones to provide critical evidence of the presence or absence of in-directly evoked corticofugal discharges.

Mapping of the buried arm area was first performed in Cebus monkeys by Asanuma and Rosén (1972). The animals were tranquillized with small doses of pentobarbitone, but could move spontaneously and could accept food and juice. Operative preparation was completed under inhalation anaesthesia (N_2O, O_2 and halothane), followed by infiltration of long-lasting local anaesthetic. Responses to cortical stimulation were recorded electromyographically from forearm muscles. Since there was so much spontaneous movement, the EMGs were averaged in order to reveal the responses. Responses of the digits were recorded by stroboscopic photo-graphy, on account of the difficulty of recording EMGs from intrinsic muscles of the hand. These responses could not therefore be associated with specific muscles, and certainly not with individual motor units, i.e. with single target motoneurones. The cortex was first mapped with trains of 0.5 mA S+ pulses to find the thumb and finger area, and this area was then probed with a tungsten-in-glass microcathode of the dimensions used by Stoney *et al.* (1968), and stimulated with trains of 11 pulses at 333 Hz, duration 0.5 ms. Motor thresholds at different points ranged from 2 to 10 µA. The positions of the tracks and stimulated points were reconstruc-ted histologically. Thresholds were lowest in the inner cortical layers. 'Effective spots' were confined to 8 mm of the mediolateral length of the precentral gyrus and to a depth of 4 mm. The majority of responses were of thumb and fingers; fewer were from wrist and fewer from elbow. There were no responses from other peripheries. The preferential accessibility of distal parts that is seen in surface stimulation (Chapter 2) is thus equally striking with microstimulation. A greater variety of responses from thumb (flexion, extension, adduction and abduction) was obtained with micro-stimulation than with S+ stimulation.

Microstimulation with 10 μA and 5 μA often evoked effects in two or more muscles. Thus there was 'constant overlap' of zones for extensor digitorum communis and flexor digitorum sublimis and profundus. In the case of the thumb movements the relationship to the action of particular muscles could not be specified. Figs 5.23 and 5.24 shows the points that were stimulated in a single para-sagittal plane in one experiment with 5 μA (5.23) and 10 μA (5.24), and the thumb movements that were obtained from the effective points. To each Figure we have added a circle to indicate the maximum possible physical spread of the stimulus centred on any point: its radius represents the lowest value of k, 272 μA mm^{-2}, determined by Stoney et al. (1968). The maximum possible physiological spread remains unknown. The Figures show the general direction of the radially orientated architecture of the cortex, and Fig. 5.24 suggests strongly that the effective points for thumb extension (open squares) are disposed along the axis of the radial bundles in 'a columnar arrangement'.

Motor cortex

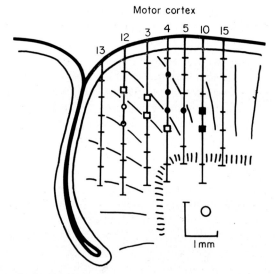

FIG. 5.23. Parasagittal section of precentral gyrus of cebus monkey, showing effective spots located by microstimulation (strength 5 μA) within the depth of the cortex. Points marked by horizontal bars along tracks evoked no responses. Open circles, flexion of thumb; open squares, extension of thumb; filled circles, adduction of thumb; filled squares, abduction of thumb. Within the millimetre scales we have drawn a circle whose radius indicates maximum probable physical spread of 5 μA ($k = 272$ μA mm^{-2}). (Asanuma and Rosén, 1972.)

That 'the remaining effective spots did not show a columnar arrangement as clearly as those for thumb extension' was ascribed to the possibility that the section of Figs 5.23 and 5.24 was not coplanar with the rostro-caudal plane which included the axes of the other 'columns'. Very rarely, 'a double cortical representation for one movement' was observed. In Fig. 5.24, thumb abduction (solid squares) was elicited by 10 μA from two separate zones, but by 5 μA (Fig. 5.23) from one zone only. 'This double representation may be interpreted as due to stimulus spread from two different regions to one common zone or as a true double representation. A third possibility would be that thumb abduction was a net movement caused by simultaneous activation of neighbouring extension and flexion zones produced by current spread or synaptic transmission.' The circle we have added to Fig. 5.24 shows that current would not have spread from tracks 3 or 4 to track 10, the lowest-threshold track, which gave thumb abduction with 5 μA (Fig. 5.23). Co-activation, by current spread, of flexion (tracks 12 and 13) and extension (tracks 3 and 4) seems hardly possible even with $k = 272$ μA mm^{-2}, at least in the plane of section (Fig. 5.24). If, with Asanuma and Rosén, we assume the mean value of $k = 1300$, the spread will be still less.

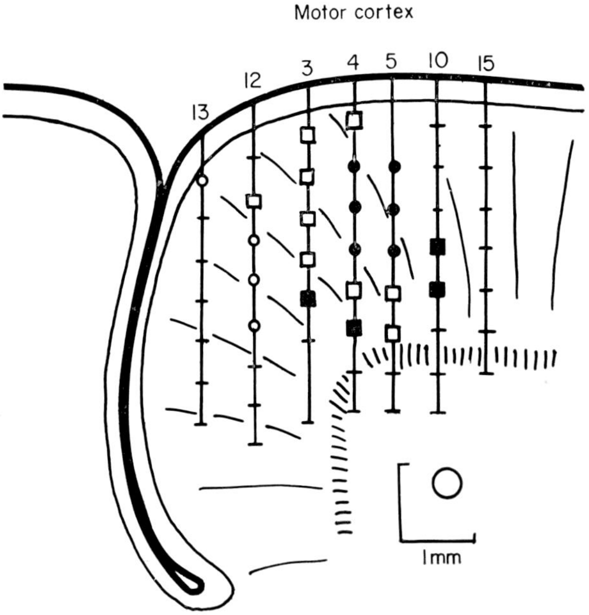

Motor cortex

Fig. 5.24. Microstimulation of effective spots within the depth of the cortex, strength 10 μA. Same experiment and symbols as in Fig. 5.23. Circle within millimetre scales has been added to indicate maximum probable radius of physical spread of 10 μA ($k = 272$ μA mm^{-2}). (Asanuma and Rosén, 1972.)

In spite of the uncertainties about spread of stimulus and about which specific muscles were responding, Asanuma and Rosén (1972) did well to propose a firm and clear interpretation, based on the majority of their admirably clear-cut results, which shares with other productive hypotheses the merit that it can be submitted to further experimental tests. This interpretation states that 'effective spots for a particular movement were confined within a cortical volume arranged in a columnar fashion along the direction of the radial fibers', and that 'each efferent zone is confined to a small cortical volume and projects to a specific motoneurone pool'. They state also that 'each efferent zone had a sharp boundary', but that it 'frequently overlapped with another efferent zone which produced an opposite movement'. This last statement needs special emphasis, since the word 'mosaic' occurs elsewhere in the paper, a word which, in its strict sense, implies that the *sharp boundary* of each efferent zone actually *separates* it from adjacent zones (Fig. 5.25A). Asanuma and Arnold (1975) have since introduced the term 'overlapping mosaic', an oxymoron which makes the conception perfectly clear. Figure 5.25B illustrates that there is no essential contradiction; zones may 'overlap' and yet each may still have a 'sharp boundary'.

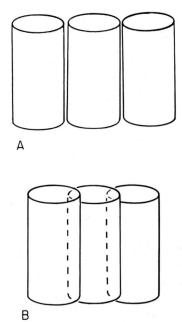

Fig. 5.25. A. An unlikely hypothesis: a mosaic of columnar efferent zones, separated from one another, each with a sharp boundary.

B. An 'overlapping mosaic' of columnar efferent zones each with a sharp boundary; to illustrate the conception of Asanuma and Rosén (1972) and Asanuma and Arnold (1975). See text.

Figures 5.23 and 5.24 tell us nothing about the extension of the 'efferent zones' along the mediolateral axis of the precentral gyrus. Figure 5.26 illustrates one of the two experiments in which this was investigated with microcathodal pulses of 5 μA. The five most laterally situated tracks gave different responses of thumb, the remainder of the tracks gave responses of the second and third digits. Flexion and extension of wrist were evoked from tracks in a more rostral plane. The circle we have added to the drawing shows the spread of 5 μA when $k = 272$ μA mm^{-2}. The areas for the different responses do not show overlap.

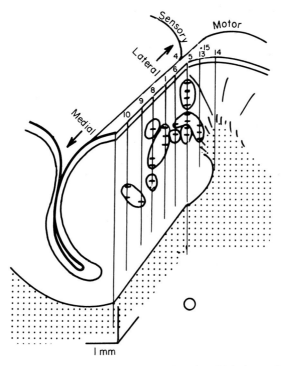

FIG. 5.26. Effective zones in one of two cebus monkeys in which the mediolateral extent of the zones was mapped by microstimulation (strength 5 μA) at intervals of 0.25 mm along the tracks. Crosses on tracks mark spots where effects appeared; no effects were obtained from tracks 4, 14 and 15. Two representative planes are shown, crossing perpendicularly. Regions which produced thumb movements were located close together and the rest of the areas were located medially within the same plane. The eight zones (from lateral to medial) were: 1, thumb adduction; 2, thumb extension; 3, thumb abduction; 4 and 5, thumb flexion; 6, digit II flexion; 7, abduction of digits II and III; 8, extension of digits II, III. Regions which produced wrist movements were found in a plane rostral to that shown in this figure. As in Fig. 5.23 we have added a circle whose radius measures maximum probable physical spread of 5 μA ($k = 272$ μA mm^{-2}). (Asanuma and Rosén, 1972.)

Andersen *et al.* (1975) have raised the question whether the eight hot spots which have been so clearly demonstrated in this experiment really constitute the sole output from area 4 to these peripheries (the first three digits), or whether the spots are merely the densest cores of wider, over-lapping projection areas. They investigated the arm area of baboons with a combination of surface positive and microcathodal stimulation. Their experiments were performed under nitrous oxide–oxygen anaesthesia, supplemented by minimal doses of pentobarbitone which were injected intravenously whenever small spontaneous movements occurred, every 30 to 60 min. Fine EMG electrodes were placed in three muscles: first dorsal interosseus, thenar eminence (adductor or flexor brevis or opponens pollicis), and extensor digitorum communis, which were chosen because their motoneurones receive, on average, the largest quantities of mono-synaptic excitation from their cortical colonies (Clough *et al.*, 1968). These specially designed electrodes could maintain contact with the same motor units for as many hours as necessary, in spite of the occasional spontaneous movements. For most of the time, however, the motoneurones were silent except when the cortex was stimulated. Stimulation, whether S+ or microcathodal, was with six pulses, duration 0.2 ms at 500 Hz. The micro-cathodes were of silver wire, protruding about 30 µm from a glass pipette of about 15 µm internal diameter at its tip. The fine tracks made by these pipettes were difficult to find in the serial sections, and the making of electrolytic marker lesions would have interfered with the responsiveness of the cortex, so every pipette in some experiments, and some pipettes in every experiment, were cut off at measured final depths and left *in situ*. The presence of 21 pipettes, all driven in to 10 mm depth, did not affect the thresholds for S+ stimulation, which were measured at intervals throughout the experiments as a control for possible cortical unresponsive-ness or injury. The pipettes were withdrawn after fixation of the brain, so that every track could be readily seen and measured in the serial sections, and the points along it related to the cortical laminae. At every stimulated point, the threshold for discharge of a single impulse by one or a few motor units was measured for each of the three muscles. The muscles were not manipulated while the thresholds were being measured, 'so that stretch-evoked discharges were just beginning to appear in the muscles undergoing examination' (Asanuma *et al.*, 1968); although such manipulation was used by them to minimize the threshold for cortically evoked EMGs in cats, Andersen *et al.* (1975) had no difficulty in discovering hot spots with thresholds below 10 µA in baboons.

Figure 5.27A shows the thresholds for a single motor unit of extensor digitorum communis at different depths along a track. The simultaneously recorded units from 1st dorsal interosseus and thenar muscles gave no responses from this track. There was a sudden fall of threshold from >80 µA to a first minimum of 16 µA at about 3.5 mm, where the track runs tangential to Betz cell-bodies in the outer border of lamina V, and a second minimum of 27 µA at about 5.0 mm, in lamina III, after which the threshold suddenly rose to >80 μA. Since the lowest thresholds in these experiments were about 5 μA (Figs 5.29 and 5.30), it is possible that the mediolateral location of this track was such that it by-passed the 'hottest spots'. Alternatively, those spots might have been in lamina VI, amongst the CST axons more rostrally. The sharp boundaries suggest that this projection area measured about 3.0 mm dorsoventrally, but this makes no allowance for current spread. Admitting the possibility that k may be as low as 300 μA mm^{-2}, we have drawn circles on the track, centred on the points of threshold 60 μA (radius 450 μm). These would reduce the minimum dorsoventral extension of the projection area to 2.0 mm. The shape of the curve shows that the colony was not homogeneous in its texture.

There is evidence that the strongest microcathodal stimuli used by Andersen et al. (1975), as well as the weakest, were not able to excite more

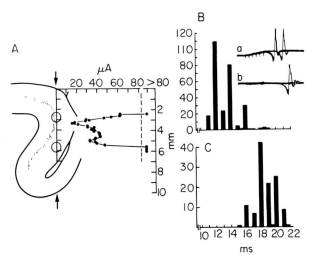

FIG. 5.27. A. Tracing of parasagittal section of right arm area of baboon, showing track of stimulating microcathode. Positions of some Betz cells are marked by dots. *Right*: plot of threshold (six 0.2 ms pulses at 500 Hz) against depth for a single motor unit of extensor digitorum communis. Vertical broken line indicates maximum current passed by the microelectrode. Filled circles to right of this line indicate no response to maximum current. Circles, centred on points of track at which threshold was 60 μA, indicate physical spread of this current if $k = 300$ μA mm^{-2} (radius 450 μm).

B. Histogram showing latency of 277 responses of same motor unit as in A, to near-threshold surface-anodal stimulation of best point and other points (six 0.2 ms pulses at 500 Hz). *Inset a*: three superimposed sweeps showing two responses of the unit at latency 12 ms from first pulse of train, and one response at 16 ms.

C. Histogram showing latency of 119 responses of same unit to near-threshold micro-stimulation in three tracks (one of which is shown in A). *Inset b*: three superimposed sweeps showing one response of unit to stimulation with 16 μA at depth 3.4 mm in track shown in A.

(Andersen et al., 1975.)

than a fraction of the cells of the colony. This evidence is presented in Fig. 27B, C. The range of latency of response of the same motor unit to near-threshold S+ stimulation of its colony was considerably shorter than the range of latency to microcathodal stimulation, pooled from all points in the three tracks in which microstimulation was effective. The probable explanation of this result is that even the strongest microstimuli were unable to excite as many cells as the weakest effective S+ stimuli. This explanation assumes that each pulse directly excites a constant number of CST neurones, and that presynaptic facilitation at the CM synapses (Chapter 3) results in growth of the successive EPSPs. The fewer cells excited by the microstimuli would evoke smaller EPSPs in the target motoneurone; a larger number of CM volleys would then be needed to reach the firing level. The more numerous cells excited by liminal S+ stimuli would evoke larger EPSPs, and fewer CM volleys would be needed to reach the firing level. This explanation is supported by the firing of the motor unit action potentials at preferred times in relation to specific pulses in the stimulus-trains, so that in successive records they were some-times exactly superimposed (Fig. 5.27, inset (a)); these muscle impulses would have been related to the crest of a specific EPSP. Transmission from cortex to muscle fibres of extensor digitorum communis takes about 10 ms. The two superimposed spikes of inset (a) were fired about 10 ms after the second S+ pulse, the later spike, about 10 ms after the fourth S+ pulse. The single spike in inset (b) was fired about 10 ms after the fifth micro-cathodal pulse (16 μA, depth 3.4 mm; Fig. 5.27A). The commonest latency of response to the liminal S+ pulses was 12 ms (Fig. 5.27B; impulse probably fired by the second pulse of the train); the commonest latency to microcathodal pulses was 18 ms (Fig. 5.27C; impulse probably fired by the fifth pulse).

It is difficult to reconcile these results with any notion that the whole colony of this target EDC motoneurone was concentrated at a depth of about 3.4 mm, within a single focus situated a little lateral or medial to the plane of section of Fig. 5.27A. They are, however, readily intelligible if we suppose that the density of the CST neurones (the 'texture' of the colony) varies from place to place within a 'total projection area' (cf. Jankowska et al., 1975b). At the hot spot the texture would be so dense that a small sphere of tissue (excited by weak microstimulation) would contain enough cells to depolarize the motoneurone to its firing level. In outlying, thinner-textured parts of the area, larger spheres would have to be excited, each containing enough cells of the colony to fire the target motoneurone. In the thinnest-textured regions the few cells included in the larger spheres excited by still stronger microstimulation could never produce enough depolarization to fire the motoneurone, though their discharge would evoke a subliminal EPSP. If this interpretation is correct, the projection area, as mapped with the discharge of a single motoneuronal impulse as detector, would always be smaller than the total projection area that would be mapped with a minimal motoneuronal EPSP as detector. Thus, liminal S+ stimulation of the convexity of the precentral gyrus can evoke an EPSP (Fig. 5.11), but microstimulation of the convexity never elicited any firing of preferentially accessible classes of motoneurones (Fig. 5.30), though Betz cells are plentiful in this region.

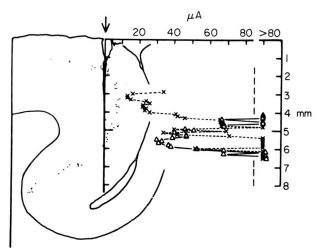

Fig. 5.28. Threshold-depth plot for a single motor unit of the first dorsal interosseus muscle (crosses and broken line) and for a few units of the flexor pollicis brevis/opponens pollicis/adductor pollicis region of the thenar eminence (triangles and full line). Same baboon as in Fig. 5.27. Conventions as in Fig. 5.27. (Andersen *et al.*, 1975.)

The projection areas of the colonies in the arm area, as mapped by microstimulation, overlapped as extensively as those mapped by liminal S+ stimulation in the leg area (Jankowska *et al.*, 1975b). Figure 5.28 (crosses and broken line) shows the threshold-depth curve for the colony of a target motoneurone of the first dorsal interosseus muscle. Its projection area has three separate concentrations of output. In its deeper parts its overlaps with colonies of thenar motoneurones (triangles and full line).

Some of the experiments of Andersen *et al.* (1975) were concerned not with single colonies but with small aggregations of colonies, whose discharges were detected by EMGs of several motor units. Figure 5.29 shows a map of the points of entry of the tracks in one such experiment; six of these are shown in the sections of Fig. 5.30. The EMGs of Fig. 5.29 are from the first dorsal interosseus (Io) muscle. The motor unit which responded at threshold from points along tracks D, E and F (and also from tracks K, J and P) did not respond at threshold from points along tracks

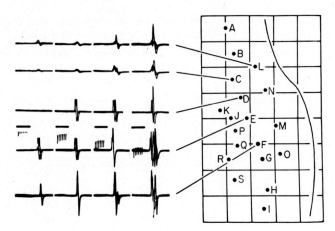

FIG. 5.29. *Right*: map of right arm area of another baboon, showing central fissure and points of entry of microelectrode tracks superimposed on millimetre grid. *Left*: responses of motor units of first dorsal interosseus muscle to stimulation (six pulses, 0.2 ms, 500 Hz) in:

Track *L*, at depth 4.7 mm, strengths 42, 48, 56 and 80 μA.

Track *C*, at depth 5.5 mm, strengths 22, 26, 40 and 50 μA.

Track *D*, at depth 3.8 mm, strengths 50, 58, 75 and 75 μA.

Track *E*, at depth 4.6 mm, strengths 23, 40, 57 and 70 μA.

Track *F*, at depth 6.0 mm, strengths 28, 32, 55 and 80 μA.

No responses were obtained from tracks A, B, N, O and I. (Andersen *et al.*, 1975.)

L and C. In track D (Fig. 5.30) it responded at threshold at depth 3.8 mm (first minimum) but took no part in the responses from deeper than 4.0 mm. Thus the areas from which microstimulation can evoke minimal EMGs in a single hand muscle are more extensive than the areas from which single motor units can be made to respond. The dorsoventral overlap of the projection areas containing aggregations of colonies of the three muscles is obvious in Fig. 5.30. Mediolaterally the Io area measures at least 3.0 mm; it overlaps EDC medially (tracks F and P) and Th laterally (tracks D, C, L).

An alternative way of visualizing the projection areas containing the aggregations of colonies is by drawing contour maps. This is shown in Fig. 5.31, from another experiment. As in Fig. 5.7B, we are facing the axonal poles of the Betz cells. To simplify the picture, the contour maps of the projection areas for the three target muscles are separated, but reference to the lettering of the tracks will reveal the degree of their overlap. In their rostro-caudal position, all these tracks correspond, approximately, to that of track C in the experiment of Fig. 5.30. In Fig. 5.31 the horizontal zero line marks the approximate intersection of the tracks with the layer of Betz cell-bodies, about 6 mm below the convexity of the precentral

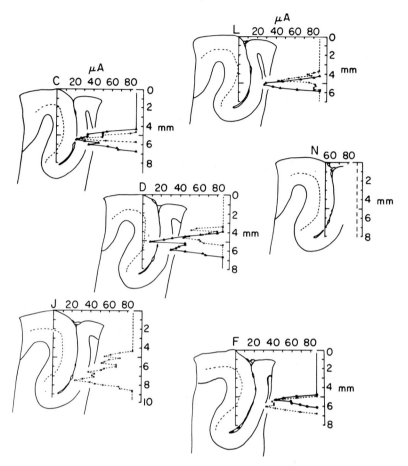

FIG. 5.30. Parasagittal sections displaying tracks L, C, N, D, J, F of Fig. 5.29. Conventions as in Fig. 5.27A except that no individual Betz cell-bodies are marked, their general level being marked by dotted line. No responses were obtained with >80 μA from track N. Crosses and broken line, units of 1st dorsal interosseus muscle. Triangles and full line, units of flexor brevis/opponens pollicis/adductor pollicis. Filled circles and full line, units of extensor digitorum communis. (Andersen *et al.*, 1975.)

gyrus. Above this line, which is labelled 0 mm in the figure, the tracks are amongst the axons of the Betz cells in the inner layer of lamina V and in lamina VI; below the line, amongst the shafts of their apical dendrites in lamina III. The contour lines show that the texture of the aggregations is not homogeneous. If it were possible to record EPSPs from the target motoneurones for long enough periods, one would expect to find that the maps of discharge thresholds would be surrounded by fringes from which subliminal EPSPs could be evoked.

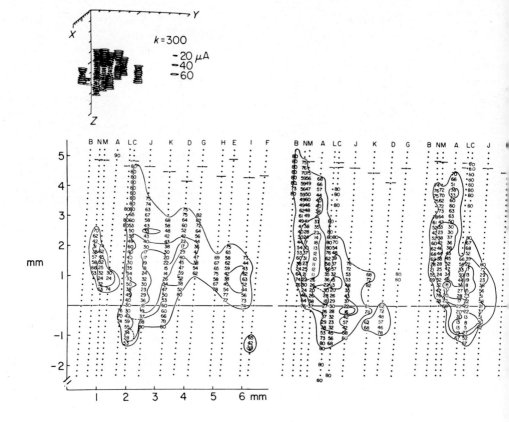

FIG. 5.31. *Below*: 14 of the 21 tracks in another baboon, selected because they all crossed the Betz cell bodies in roughly the same rostro-caudal position (illustrated in Fig. 5.30, track C, for another brain), and here viewed from the rostral aspect (as in the diagram of Fig. 5.7B): lateral to left, medial to right of figure. Tracks intersect Betz cell profile along horizontal zero line: points above this line are in laminae V or VI, points below it are in lamina III. Dots along each track mark points stimulated with >80 μA without EMG response from test muscle; numbers give thresholds for each muscle in μA. The three projection areas overlap extensively (note lettering of tracks) but are shown separately.

Left: thresholds for motor units of extensor digitorum communis. Contour lines have been drawn by eye to enclose points with thresholds <20 μA, <40 μA and <80 μA.

Above: computer-graphic display of physical spread of threshold currents at points along selected tracks, indicated by radii of horizontal circles (= equators of spheres) centred on each point. Currents >79 μA not displayed. Calibrations for 20, 40 and 60 μA, $k = 300$ μA mm^{-2}.

Middle: thresholds for motor units of flexor brevis/opponens/adductor pollicis. Contours drawn as for EDC units.

Right: thresholds for motor units of 1st dorsal interosseus. Contours drawn as for EDC and thenar units.

(Andersen *et al.*, 1975.)

The sizes and shapes of these maps cannot be explained by physical spread of stimulating current from the edges to the centres of the areas. Figure 5.31 includes a computer-graphic display of some of the points along some of the tracks from which the contour map for EDC was constructed. The radii of the circles (= equators of spheres) represent the largest probable spread of the currents used at each point, determined by choosing a low value of $k = 300$ (Andersen et al., 1975). Piecing the spheres together reveals something of the size, shape and texture of the projection areas. Even the largest spheres are small in relation to the size of the projection area, and each thus contains no more than a fraction of its CST neurones. An examination of Fig. 5.31 will show that the largest distances from the fringes of the projection areas to their lowest-threshold zones are six to seven times greater than the radii of the largest spheres.

Recalling the estimate of 90 large and 18 000 small pyramidal neurones in lamina V of a cylinder of baboon's motor cortex of area 1.0 mm² (Landgren et al., 1962b) it is interesting to calculate the numbers of cortical pyramids that would be contained within the spheres of tissue centred on lamina V, whose radii are determined by the excitability of large PTN, $k = 300$ μA mm⁻², and by strength of current (Table 5.1).

TABLE 5.1

Current μA	Number of large pyramids	Number of small pyramids
5	5	900
20	19	3780
40	39	7750
60	58	11 500

It seems certain that excitation will spread horizontally beyond the confines of the spheres, and thus introduce error into the mapping of the projection areas. One mode of spread will be by antidromic excitation of recurrent axon collaterals of CST neurones. If future experiment shows the effect of such spread to be quantitatively significant, maps such as those of Fig. 5.31 may have to be shrunk by as much as 1.0 mm all round. Such shrinkage would not be sufficient to explain the responses obtained from the most distant fringes of the projection areas in terms of spread to the lowest-threshold zones. And it could no longer be assumed that the response to near-threshold stimulation of a 'hot spot' is due to the discharge of a few CST neurones near to the tip of the microcathode; it may prove to entail the discharge of every CST neurone within a cylinder of cortex of radius 1.0 mm. The second mode of horizontal spread will be trans-synaptic. The magnitude of such spread, with different numbers, strengths and frequencies of stimulating pulses, awaits its measurement in future experiments. It is certain that spreading inhibition will be competing with spreading excitation.

But even if some reduction in the size of the projection areas that have been mapped by microstimulation turns out to be necessary, their most important feature, namely the overlap of the areas projecting to the moto-neurone pools of different muscles, will remain valid. Using the alternative technique of minimal surface-anodal stimulation, Jankowska *et al.* (1975b) confirmed the existence of patchy, overlapping projection areas in the leg area; their sizes were comparable to those mapped by Andersen *et al.* (1975) in the arm area. In both arm and leg areas, the numbers of CST neurones which project monosynaptically to a single spinal motoneurone are likely to be large, and the contribution of a single CST neurone to motor output is likely to be correspondingly small. This point will be pursued further in Chapter 7.

Independent evidence of overlap comes from experiments which do not involve electrical stimulation, and which will be described in detail in Chapters 6 and 7: when recording with microelectrodes from PTN in monkeys which were trained to perform motor tasks in order to earn rewards, it was quite common to find adjacent neurones whose discharges were regularly associated with active movements in different directions at the same joint, or with quite different movements at separate joints (Evarts, 1968; Lemon and Porter, 1976).

In considering spread of stimulus in the radial direction, it is instructive to compare tracks N and D in Fig. 5.30. In track D, at a depth of 5.0 mm, where the microcathode was among CST axons, the threshold for Th was 5.0 μA; from a point at the same depth in track N, about 1.0 mm 'radial' to D (i.e. nearer the cortical surface deep in the sulcus), there was no response, even when the current was increased to >80 μA. Physical spread to the inner cortical laminae across 1.0 mm can thus be ruled out: even if we choose $k = 250$ μA mm^{-2}, 90 μA would spread only 0.6 mm. Some synaptically evoked discharge of CST neurones might well have occurred, but if so, its quantity was insufficient to fire any of the small aggregation of target motoneurones. (In the cat, pulses <10 μA, delivered at a point 1050 μm superficial to a PTN and at an angle of 40° to the radial architecture, were effective in discharging that PTN: Stoney *et al.*, 1968.)

The lack of lowest-threshold spots in the outer cortical laminae in the work of Andersen *et al.* (1975), and their presence in that of Asanuma and his colleagues, marks an important difference between the techniques and objectives of the two groups of workers. The former were directed essentially to the mapping of projection areas and thus to the inner laminae, and, for this purpose, a relatively quiescent background was appropriate. The latter were directed essentially to the input–output structure of the cortex, and in these, the background of excitation that was generated by manipulation of the limbs of tranquillized animals was evidently necessary for the finding of hot spots in the outer as well as the inner laminae (Asanuma and Arnold, 1975). The question of input–output structure will be considered in Chapters 6 and 7.

Asanuma and Arnold (1975) have drawn attention to the harmful effects of six cathodal pulses, 0.2 ms, 500 Hz, when their amplitude exceeds 40 μA. Their experiments demonstrated that 40 μA caused reversible block of a PTN in close contact with the microcathode, and that 60 μA caused gas bubbles to form at the electrode's silver tip. The warning is useful and should be heeded. Most of the points stimulated by Andersen *et al.* (1975) received currents well below 40 μA, and no difficulty was experienced in finding 5 μA spots in the inner laminae. There was therefore no sign that the cortex had suffered significant damage, at least as far as these laminae were concerned.

5.3.3 MICROSTIMULATION OF CORTIFUGAL PROJECTIONS IN THE CAT

Of the many neuronal targets to which clusters of corticofugal neurones in the cat can directly project, none can yet be characterized in such unequivocal functional terms as the motoneurones of the different muscle-groups of primates. Since the cat has no corticomotoneuronal synapses (Chapter 4), the monosynaptically excited interneurones of Illert *et al.* (1974), which distribute monosynaptic excitation to motoneurones, will probably come closest to the ideal. Unfortunately, interneurones survive impalement much less well than motoneurones, so that quantitative work on EPSPs and IPSPs evoked by systematic tracking with an intracortical microcathode is impossible with present-day technique. Nor can extracellular recording of the discharges of interneurones which have been characterized in terms of their peripheral inputs (or lack of inputs) be kept up for long enough for a complete intracortical mapping to be achieved. To evoke any sublimal action on motoneurones, intracortical microstimulation must actually discharge the interneurones. Their actions on motoneurones of particular muscle-groups can be detected by intracellular recording, when microcathodal exploration of the cortex is limited by the lifetime of an impaled motoneurone, or by plotting curves of the facilitation and inhibition of monosynaptic reflexes, when the exploration is limited only by the lifetime of the preparation. Thus one could hope to map the cortical projection areas whose clusters of CST neurones were coupled to the motoneurones by a dense disynaptic linkage. Less densely coupled synaptic pathways, and *a fortiori* polysynaptic pathways, would be more at the mercy of background drifting of interneuronal responsiveness, and would be likely to give inconstant results. And any experimental design which depended on an actual discharge of motoneurones would fail to detect the patterns of subliminal excitation and inhibition that might be distributed amongst the motoneurone pools of other muscles.

Asanuma and Sakata (1967) used 11 pulses at 400 Hz for microcathodal stimulation of the motor cortex in cats under light barbiturate narcosis. It is sometimes stated that this paper reported *contraction* of single muscles of the forelimb in response to these stimuli, but this was not the case: the actions on the motoneurone pools of different muscles were detected by monosynaptic testing of subliminal changes in their excitability. Single submaximal group Ia afferent volleys were sent in along muscle nerves, and the amplitude of the reflex motor volleys was recorded. The conditioning microcathodal stimulation caused facilitation of the testing monosynaptic reflexes in 39 cases, and inhibition in 18 cases. The effects of the brief high-frequency corticofugal bursts were obtained at very low thresholds. Figure 5.32 shows three tracks which were made at the lateral end of the anterior sigmoid gyrus, and the threshold currents at points which gave facilitation of the monosynaptic reflex of a pronator muscle of the forearm. The lowest-threshold points (2.5 to 3.0 µA) were orientated radially in the cortex. Adjacent tracks 1, 2, 5, 7 (Fig. 5.32B) gave no facilitation at strengths <20 µA. Such 'efferent zones' measured 0.5 mm to a few mm across, 'and the fringes overlapped'.

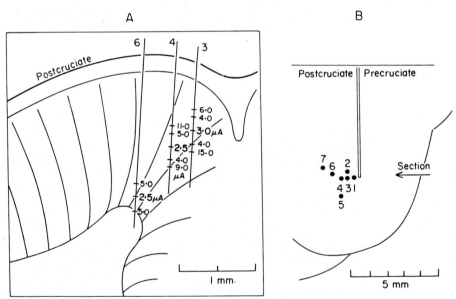

Fig. 5.32. A. Low-threshold points along tracks 3, 4 and 6 (map in B shows points of entry and plane of section) for facilitation of monosynaptic reflex of a pronator muscle of the cat's forelimb, by trains of 11 pulses, duration 0.2 ms, at 400 Hz (Asanuma and Sakata, 1967).

The impression of a very narrowly circumscribed, radially orientated efferent zone is certainly very striking, but the uncertainties related to physiological spread of excitation with repetitive stimulation, which we have already considered, need to be kept in mind. By itself, the existence of such a low-threshold zone does not prove that the entire corticofugal output is discharged from a cylinder of cortex whose radius is defined only by physical spread (e.g. 90 μm for 10 μA if $k = 1300$ μA mm^{-2}). If the lowest-threshold zone is the densest core of the total projection area, and also its geometrical centre, the disynaptic or polysynaptic breakthrough to the motoneurones may still require the additional spatial summation that would be provided by excitation spreading physiologically (trans-synaptically, or antidromically along recurrent collaterals of CST axons) to the fringes of the projection area. The actual area of output excited by 11 pulses at 400 Hz, strength 3.0 μA, remains to be measured.

Figure 5.32 does not show whether the motoneurone pools of any muscles other than the pronator were influenced by the discharges that were evoked by stimulation of this low-threshold zone. Figure 5.33 shows plots of threshold against depth along a single track (inset) for facilitation or inhibition of the motoneurone pools of four muscles supplied by the radial nerve. The overlap is evident. In nineteen experiments, of which

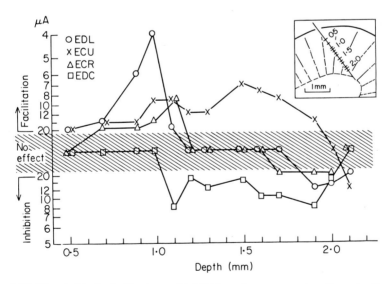

FIG. 5.33. Thresholds for facilitation and inhibition of monosynaptic reflexes (ordinates, logarithmic scales) of four muscle-nerve-branches of cat's radial nerve at different depths (abscissae) along track figured in inset. Labelling of plots is indicated on the Figure. EDL, extensor digitorum lateralis; ECU, extensor carpi ulnaris; ECR, extensor carpi radialis; EDC, extensor digitorum communis. Cortical stimulus trains as for Fig. 5.32. (Asanuma and Sakata, 1967.)

this was one, the monosynaptic reflexes of muscles supplied by the ulnar and median nerves were not tested, so the extent of overlap with these has not been, and perhaps cannot be, fully worked out. It would be impracticable to record monosynaptic reflexes from the motoneurone pools of all the muscles in the limb; and Asanuma and Sakata (1967) found that monosynaptic reflexes could not, in any case, be obtained in some of the muscle nerves of cat's forelimb. The combinations of overlapping foci that were observed for excitation and inhibition of groups of muscles showed no 'meaningful correlation between the overlappings and the functions of the muscles'. The foci for different muscles were in different places in the brains of different cats.

Not much headway has been made in the very difficult task of combining microcathodal stimulation of the cortex with the recording of synaptic potentials and impulses from interneurones of the cat's cervical enlargement. Systematic microprobing of the cortex being impracticable, Asanuma et al. (1971) placed four microcathodes, 1.0 mm apart, in the cortex, and left them in positions at which one or more of them would give facilitation or inhibition of monosynaptic reflexes of muscles supplied by the radial nerve. Stimulation was with 10–11 pulses, usually 10 µA (sometimes 100 µA) at 400 Hz. Intracellular records were obtained from 6 interneurones in which EPSPs could be evoked from one cortical site, and from 4 in which EPSPs could be evoked from two or more sites. Some EPSPs were followed by IPSPs. There was no evidence of possible monosynaptic excitation by single corticofugal volleys. To the bursts of 11 pulses, the minimum latency of the slowly rising EPSPs was 5 ms and the maximum 15 ms. In extracellular records from 52 interneurones, the maximum impulse activity occurred 20–24 ms after the onset of the stimulating burst. Thus this sample of interneurones, unlike that of Illert et al. (1974), was not tightly coupled to the CST. Some were influenced from more than one cortical site (maximum separation 3.0 mm).

We come finally to the recording of actual contractions of forelimb muscles. Asanuma and Ward (1971) connected the tendons of extensor digitorum communis and palmaris longus to myographs, and stimulated the cortex with 60 to 1500 microcathodal pulses at 300 Hz, in cats under light thiopentone anaesthesia. The lowest threshold was 4.0 µA. The muscles sometimes contracted simultaneously, sometimes reciprocally. Sustained contractions were evoked only by stimulation in the deeper layers. The summation period was long: minimum 40 ms. With so many pulses, the uncertainty about horizontal physiological spread becomes greater; and the long latency may indicate temporo-spatial summation within the cortex as well as at interneuronal and motoneuronal levels. After 900 pulses, there was 'spontaneous rhythmic contraction of the muscle'—presumably a minimal epileptic discharge.

Shorter trains of microcathodal pulses are effective in eliciting minimal EMG responses in preferentially accessible muscles in the cat if sedation and local analgesia are substituted for general anaesthesia. At threshold, e.g. 5 µA, 14 pulses at 400 Hz were needed for extensor digitorum communis (Asanuma et al., 1976a). For comparison, surface-anodal stimulation (at threshold, 0.34 mA) required 8 pulses at 400 Hz to elicit an EMG in extensor carpi ulnaris. Averaged values for microstimulation at 1.5 × threshold 'from superficial (III) as well as from deep (V and VI) layers' in 7 experiments were 11 pulses at 400 Hz (range 8 to 13). For S+ at 1.5× threshold in 5 experiments, the averaged requirement was >4<5 pulses (range >3<4 pulses to >7<8 pulses).

Asanuma et al. (1968) made EMG records from eight muscles of the forelimbs of cats which were sedated with small doses of pentobarbitone. As their primary interest was in the mapping of input-output structure (Chapter 6), they did not stimulate in a systematic grid of points, but searched the pericruciate cortex with a microelectrode for neurones which responded to natural stimulation of the limb, and then applied microcathodal stimulation at each neuronal locus. Stimulation was with 11 pulses, 0.2 ms, at 400 Hz; the limbs were constantly manipulated to keep the thresholds as low as possible. Motor responses were obtained with stimuli < 10 µA from 156 loci in 13 animals: of these, 94 loci gave responses which were confined, at threshold, to single muscles ('single effect zones'), and 62 loci gave responses of two or, rarely, three muscles ('multiple effect zones'). Latency of response was 20–40 ms. In 'high-threshold regions', which were 'intermixed with low threshold zones in mosaic fashion', more than 67 loci were stimulated with >15 µA without motor effect, though the neurones at these 67 loci shared a similar range of inputs with those within the low-threshold zones (Chapter 6). The degree of separability of the projections to the eight muscles, and the differential accessibility of those muscles to microstimulation with 10 A, is illustrated in Table 5.2.

A technical problem was that a contraction was sometimes seen in the absence of any EMG record. When the threshold for such a contraction was lower than the threshold for any of the muscles containing EMG electrodes, 'we either attempted to insert EMG electrodes into that muscle or abandoned the track and inserted the microelectrode into a different cortical area'. In such a case a possible single-effect zone might have been lost. The occurrence of a contraction at a threshold higher than the threshold for any of the electrode-containing muscles posed a different problem. If the contraction was visible in a region that was well separated anatomically from the electrode-containing muscles, it was possible to insert EMG electrodes into it; but if such a contraction had been invisible, in the depths of the forearm, or in a muscle that was closely adjacent to an

TABLE 5.2

Muscle	Number of loci for:	
	Solitary response at threshold (Single effect zones)	Response at threshold inseparable from another muscle (Multiple effect zones)
Extensor digitorum comm. & lat.	21	18
Palmaris longus	23	15
Triceps	32	28
Extensor carpi radialis	4	31
Extensor carpi ulnaris	10	21
Flexor carpi ulnaris	0	8
Flexor profundus digitorum	1	6
Biceps	3	6

electrode-containing muscle, 'it was nearly impossible to detect it unless EMG electrodes were already inserted into the second muscle. Therefore, there is a possibility that some multiple-effect zones were counted as single-effect zones. Since our electrodes were routinely inserted into most of the neighbouring, superficial forearm muscles, we feel that the frequency of such miscounting was very small for these muscles. However a combination of a superficial and a deep forearm muscle might have escaped observation.' (Asanuma *et al.*, 1968.) The occurrence of subliminal excitation of the motoneurone pools of other muscles from the single-effect zones would, of course, have gone undetected. The high-threshold regions may well have been inhibitory, as the authors rightly suggest, but they may also have been regions of lower output density belonging to the same projection areas as the hot spots. We have already cited more recent experiments which make it necessary to suspend judgement on the originally reasonable estimate that repetitive stimulation with 10 μA excited only neurones within a radius of 90 μm, and on the originally reasonable suggestion that at the lowest effective threshold, 2 μA, 'repetitive activity of one or two cortical neurons within an efferent colony can lead to muscle contraction'.

We hope that in this chapter we have been able to communicate something of the excitement that has been aroused by the pioneering discoveries of Asanuma and his colleagues, and by the application of his powerful techniques to the elucidation of the structure of cortical projection areas. The time of writing is also a time of rapid advance, so that some of the problems of interpretation we have been raising may well have been solved by the time these lines have appeared in print. We hope nevertheless that our introduction to these problems may retain some interest as a study in neurological discovery, even after they have been solved by fresh experiments.

5.4 Summary

In Chapter 4 we reviewed the different destinations of the outputs from
the motor cortex of cats and monkeys. These are the outputs which would
be available for selection and recombination by cerebro-cerebellar motor
programmes, and the problem we have considered in this chapter is
whether their cortical projection areas are isolated from one another, like
the stones of a mosaic, or whether they are overlapping. The first case to
be investigated has been that of the monosynaptic corticospinal projection
to the motoneurones of different groups of muscles of the fore- and hindlimbs of primates. These motoneurones can be readily identified by antidromic stimulation of their axons in the nerves going to the muscles. The
areas of origin of corticofugal projections to other classes of targets are
likely to be more difficult to map with an equal degree of precision.

The most favourable experimental conditions are found in the hindlimb
area of monkeys, where the cortex is unfolded (medial to the origin of the
central fissure). After each motoneurone has been impaled with an intracellular microelectrode, the cortical surface can be rapidly mapped with
a roving focal anode delivering pulses which are near-threshold for the
direct excitation of the CST axons, so that the maps are subject to little
error due to physical or physiological spread. It is found that the projection areas to single motoneurones are extensive (up to 13 mm²), that
they are sometimes multiple, and that they overlap with the areas for the
motoneurones of antagonistic as well as of synergic muscles.

In the arm area of baboons the central fissure is about 10 mm deep,
and the projection areas to motoneurones of distal muscles turn out to be
buried in the cortex of its anterior wall, though the rostral rims of some
of them extend on to the convexity of the precentral gyrus where they can
be mapped by S+ pulses which are near-threshold for the CST neurones
there. In this region the projection areas are found to overlap; but nothing
can be asserted decisively about the size, shape and probable overlap of the
buried parts of the areas.

For the mapping of the buried areas, Asanuma's method of intracortical
microstimulation is essential. Unfortunately it can hardly be combined
with the sensitive, quantitative detection of corticomotoneuronal discharge
that is provided by the intracellular recording of postsynaptic potentials
in the target motoneurones, which cannot survive impalement for the
necessary length of time. The detector of discharge has to be a minimal
EMG response, involving one or a few motor units. Firing of target
motoneurones requires repetitive stimulation of the cortex to produce the
necessary presynaptic facilitation of corticomotoneuronal synapses (Chapter
3). The largest possible limits of physical spread of microcathodal stimuli
do not introduce appreciable error into the mapping, but there is an
unknown error due to physiological spread of excitation across the cortex.

The areas which are connected monosynaptically to the target motoneurones are presumably larger than the maps, since these would be surrounded by less dense fringes which would only be detected by the intracellular recording of EPSPs. Thus no discharges of EDC, thenar or 1st
dorsal interosseus motoneurones were evoked by microcathodal stimulation of the cortex of the convexity of the precentral gyrus, although
EPSPs could be evoked from the surface in a separate series of experiments.
The buried areas are shown to overlap; their maps appear to be comparable
in size to those of the leg area.

These experiments have not yet been extended to the frontiers between
arm and leg or arm and face areas to see if there is any overlap between
their projection areas.

In experiments on cats, in which there is no direct corticomotoneuronal
projection, microcathodal intracortical mapping finds that the areas of
origin of projections which produce disynaptic or polysynaptic subliminal
excitation or inhibition of motoneurone pools (detected by the facilitatory
or inhibitory effect on their monosynaptic reflexes) are also overlapping.
In this example, repetitive stimulation, with its liability to physiological
spread, was necessary to *discharge* the interneurones (the primary target-
cells of the projection) which then produced the subliminal synaptic
actions on the motoneurones, or led to their discharge in some experiments.

There is no experimental basis for any suggestion that the motor cortex
might be built up of isolated cylindrical output columns of equal radius,
one for every muscle in the body.

In future work on other neuronal targets, surface-anodal mapping of
the monkey's leg area, combined with intracellular recording from well-
characterized interneurones and cells of origin of ascending tracts, seems
likely to be profitable. If it were technically feasible, microstimulation of
a few PT units, combined with intracellular sampling of the actions
produced in a large number of potential targets for this cortical output,
could provide valuable information about the divergence of influences
from a localized cortical efferent zone.

6
Electroanatomy of inputs to PT neurones and cortical projection areas

6.1 Introduction

Interest in the sources of nerve impulses which excite and inhibit the pyramidal neurones of the 'motor' cortex is of surprisingly recent growth. If we return to Fig. 1.4 (p. 18) as our starting-point, it seems sensible to divide these inputs into two main classes: those descending from higher functional levels and those ascending from lower levels. The sources of the former would include the whole of the neocortex, the lateral cerebellum, the basal ganglia and the ventrolateral thalamus. These can be loosely described as sources of 'command' derived from 'programmes for movement', both inborn and learned, whose nature and location still elude us, as their engrams eluded Lashley (1950), and whose activities are believed to be subject to continuous or intermittent correction by sensory information of progress towards the attainment of the overriding behavioural goals (Chapter 8). The signals ascending to the motor cortex would be mainly, if not exclusively, aroused as responses to its own projected activity. They can be classified as *internal feedback,* arising in the intermediate region of the cerebellum, in sensory relay nuclei, etc. (Chapter 4), as patterned responses to the patterned discharges of PT impulses, and *external feedback*, originating in the muscles, joints and skin of the moving parts. These internal and external feedbacks may be important in adjusting the sub-routines of ongoing movement and in compensating for the effects of perturbations imposed on the movements by 'unexpected' external forces.

6.2 The radial input–output architecture of the motor cortex

The thalamocortical, corticocortical and callosal afferents which bring these inputs into the motor cortex enter it obliquely but their predominant orientation is radial. The long, parallel dendritic shafts of the pyramidal neurones whose axons project its outputs to their various targets are all orientated at right angles to the pia-covered surface of the cortex. This preponderantly radial structuring is illustrated in the generalized diagram of Fig. 6.1 (Szentágothai, 1969), which portrays features which are present, though with considerable local variation in all areas of neocortex. The diagram owes much to the classic discoveries of Ramón y Cajal which have been extended by application of the Golgi and Nauta methods and

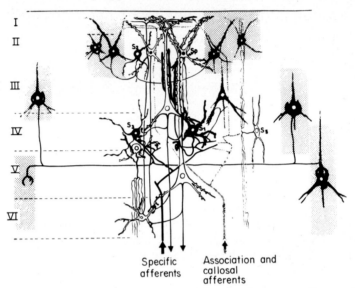

Specific afferents   Association and callosal afferents

FIG. 6.1. Szentágothai's generalized diagram of the most important cell types that are present in the six laminae of the neocortex, to illustrate the predominantly radial and the less dense horizontal interconnexions. The diagram is centred upon two pyramidal neurones, one in lamina III and one in lamina V.

Radial interconnexions. 'Specific afferents' form synapses upon large stellate interneurones (S_1) in lamina IV; these apply their special 'cartridge-type' synapses (?excitatory) to the radially oriented dendritic shafts of the pyramidal neurones. 'Association' and 'callosal afferents' ascend into the 'relatively loose synaptic neuropil' of lamina I, which also contains horizontally ramifying fine terminal branches of pyramidal dendrites, of ascending dendrites of lamina II neurones, and of ascending axons of stellate interneurones: note axon of interneurone in lamina VI, which receives synapses from recurrent collaterals of pyramidal axons; note also interneurone in lamina IV (S5: Cajal's 'cellule fusiforme à double bouquet dendritique'), whose branched axon extends radially across the whole thickness of cortex. Finally, there are stellate interneurones (S_4) with descending radially oriented axons endings in 'horsetail-shaped terminal arborizations' in laminae V and VI.

Horizontal interconnexions. In lamina I by horizontal (tangential) spread of apical dendrites of pyramidal neurones and of incoming axons—associative, callosal, and of stellate interneurones. *In lamina II* by stellate interneurones or basket cells (S_2) with horizontal axons which form basket-type endings (? inhibitory) on perikarya of star pyramids, as as far distant from S_2 as stippled areas. *In laminae III and V* by larger basket cells in lamina IV whose longer horizontal axons form baskets (? inhibitory) on perikarya of pyramidal neurones of laminae III and V. These axons may extend for 0.5 mm or more. (Szentágothai 1969.)

electronmicroscopy to normal and experimental material. 'Specific afferents' from the thalamus form synapses on large stellate interneurones in lamina IV (S_1) whose axons form special 'cartridge' synapses (or 'climbing' contacts: Colonnier, 1966) with the spines of the apical dendritic shafts of pyramidal neurones whose perikarya are situated in laminae III and V. These axospinous synapses are asymmetrical (type I of Gray, 1959), and would be presumed, on Uchizono's (1965) hypothesis, to be excitatory.

The apical dendrites of the pyramidal cells reach the surface of the cortex where they ramify horizontally in lamina I. 'Association afferents', which would presumably include the short U-fibres which interlink adjacent sub-areas of cortex as well as the longer fibres which interconnect more distant areas, and the callosal afferents which interconnect corresponding areas of the two hemispheres, ascend as far as lamina I, where they spread horizontally in the 'relatively loose synaptic neuropil' which also contains the apical dendrites of pyramidal neurones, the ascending dendrites of the star pyramids of lamina II and the terminal arborizations of the ascending axons of stellate interneurones. Thus lamina I would be a possible site of horizontally spreading activity, but whether of excitation or inhibition or both, and over what maximum distance, is uncertain—possibly for several mm (Colonnier, 1966). This estimate is supported by the range of spread of surface-negative waves across the cortical surface (Adrian, 1937; Burns, 1958).

A second structural basis for horizontal spread is provided by small stellate interneurones of lamina II whose horizontally running axons end in synaptic baskets around the perikarya of the star pyramids; and by larger interneurones whose perikarya are found in lamina IV and whose horizontal axons form synaptic baskets around the perikarya of pyramidal neurones in lamina III and V. These longer axons may reach across 0.5 mm or more. By analogy with the basket cells of the cerebellum and hippocampus, Colonnier (1966) suggested that these neurones would act as spreaders of 'lateral' or 'surround' inhibition.

A third possibility of spread depends on the horizontal extension of the richly branched terminal arborizations of thalamocortical afferents for >0.5 mm, particularly in lamina IV; these would form synapses on many stellate interneurones (S_1 in Fig. 6.1) and these in turn would contribute cartridge (climbing) synapses to many pyramidal cells. If we assume, with Colonnier (1966) and Szentágothai (1969), that these synapses are excitatory, we would then have a means for spreading excitation horizontally as well as radially. In the monkey's motor cortex, thalamocortical axons form a majority of their synapses on dendritic spines of pyramidal neurones, presumably on horizontal branches of apical and basal dendrites as well as on dendritic shafts (Sloper, 1973); these horizontally ramifying dendrites could increase the spread by a further 0.5 mm (Fig. 3.1B, p. 54).

A final possibility of horizontal interaction is provided by the recurrent collaterals of pyramidal axons. These may spread 1.0 mm (Tömböl, cited by Jankowska *et al.*, 1975b). In the motor cortex they mediate monosynaptic excitation of large PTN by small, and disynaptic inhibition of large PTN by large (Chapter 3).

The clear functional inference which has to be drawn from these structural features is that excitation which enters any area of the neocortex along a circumscribed packet of thalamocortical axons will be distributed in a preponderantly radial fashion throughout the thickness of the cortex, and that any resulting corticofugal discharge will be likely to emerge along the axons of those pyramidal neurones which are more or less coaxial with the afferent packet. This was perceived and stressed by Lorente de Nó (1938). How far, then, does such activity spread horizontally to influence the input–output activities of the adjacent radially orientated structure? There are no vertical barriers to limit the horizontal spread of excitation and inhibition across the axonal and dendritic distances that have been measured by Colonnier (1966), Szentágothai (1969) and others. The very important discovery of functionally organized radial columns in somaesthetic cortex (Mountcastle, 1957) and in visual cortex (Hubel and Wiesel, 1962) may, perhaps, have encouraged the expectation of vertical barriers, but until very recently there has been no microscopical evidence that they might exist. 'The anatomical columns are not distinct, separate morphological entities. The tangential overlap is considerable . . . The physiological column results from a focus of effective stimulation of a number of definite units by the input, coupled with the inhibition of surrounding units through the basket cell axons.' (Colonnier, 1966.) Quasi-horizontal transmission of the *integrated* output of any part of the radial organization to any other part would presumably be taken care of by those pyramidal neurones whose axons form the shorter or longer U-fibres which would interconnect closely adjacent columns as well as more widely spaced areas.

Though the neocortex is everywhere characterized by this radial input–output structure, the regional variations in its cyto- and myeloarchitectonics are well known, and these make it important to look at the specific features of any area in which one is interested and not to transfer data uncritically from one area to another. The discovery of functional columns was made in the somaesthetic and visual receiving areas; the concept of columnar organization is being developed in relation to the feature-extracting functions of these areas, and forms what is arguably the most exciting growth area of contemporary neurophysiology. It is the supreme illustration of what Le Gros Clark (1962b) called 'the sorting principle in sensory analysis'. In its first phases, investigation has necessarily been concentrated upon the inputs to the different columns; investigations of the nature of the integrated outputs from their pyramidal neurones, and the different destinations to which these outputs are projected (identified by antidromic stimulation) are on the way (Singer, 1975). The anatomical correlates for the functional columns have been discovered in tangential sections of lamina IV: in the zebra-striped arrangement of the ocular dominance columns in area 17 of the monkey (Le Vay et al., 1975) and in the barrel-shaped representations of individual whiskers in the somaesthetic cortex of the mouse (T. A. Woolsey and Van der Loos, 1970).

The motor cortex of area 4 differs from that of area 17 in that its neurones are more widely spaced; that is to say, they are separated by a larger bulk of neuropil, which would be expected to provide for richer and more flexible interconnexions. In the cortex of man's brain, the density of neuronal packing is highest in the striate area and lowest in the precentral gyrus (Sholl, 1956). Area 4 contains the largest pyramidal neurones in the whole of the neocortex. These can be identified antidromically by stimulation of the various targets to which they project (Chapters 3 and 4). They are the collectors, integrators and dischargers of corticofugal output. An important task for research is to specify the inputs that are brought to bear on the dendrites of PT neurones and parapyramidal neurones which project to identified targets, by the radially organized thalamocortical and association fibres and the stellate interneurones which are directly related to them. Some of the inputs would be those from 'sources of command' in touch with environmental events though far removed from any direct connexions with peripheral receptors (Mountcastle et al., 1975). Others would be more directly related to peripheral receptors and would come within the category of external feedback.

Nothing has yet been reported in tangential sections of area 4 to correspond with the structures that have been seen in lamina IV of monkey's visual cortex and of mouse's somaesthetic cortex. In area 4 in monkeys, the largest pyramidal neurones of lamina V tend to occur in clusters, and in tangential sections, Sloper (1973) and others have noted the grouping of their apical dendrites into obvious bundles, separated by relatively wide masses of neuropil. After ventrolateral thalamic lesions, the degenerating synapses seem to be concentrated in the neighbourhood of these bundles (Sloper, 1973). It is tempting to associate these appearances with the 'hot spots' that can be detected by microstimulation, which would mark zones of high input–output density within the 'total projection areas' of Jankowska et al (1975b; see Chapter 5).

A major cytoarchitectonic character which differentiates area 4 from the visual and somaesthetic receiving areas is that it is agranular, and has virtually no lamina IV. It is thicker than the adjacent somatosensory areas 3a, 3b, 1 and 2. Myeloarchitectonically, the inner and outer bands of Baillarger are greatly expanded and completely fused, extending outwards from the subcortical white matter as far as the outer zone of lamina III

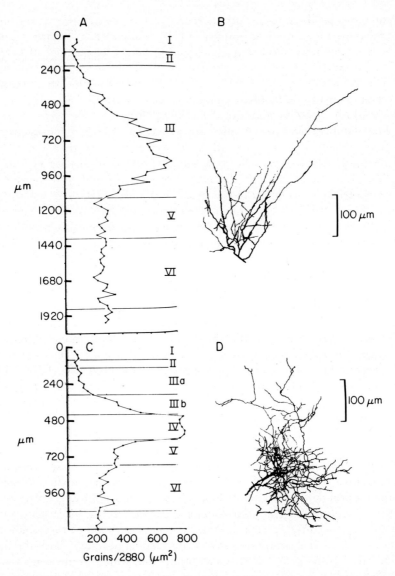

FIG. 6.2. The contrast between the thalamocortical projection from VL to the agranular cortex of area 4, and from VPL to the granular cortex of area 3 in the squirrel monkey (Jones 1975).

A. Distribution of silver grains across the cortical laminae in autoradiographs of area 4 five days after injection of H^3-proline into thalamic ventral nuclear complex. Control of background levels of activity, estimated by counts across the entorhinal cortex, is shown by vertical stippling along edge of ordinates. Densest distribution is in lamina IIIb.

B. Camera lucida drawing of Golgi-impregnated thalamocortical arborization in area 4. In this agranular cortex, the obliquely-lying parent axon is at the junction between laminae III and V.

(Jones, 1975). The main distribution of thalamocortical afferents from the ventrolateral thalamic nucleus is in lamina III, but some of their terminal ramifications reach lamina I. The contrast between these structural features of area 4 and area 3 in the squirrel monkey is illustrated in Fig. 6.2 (Jones, 1975).

As in other cortical areas, there is ample provision for horizontal spread of excitation and inhibition between neighbouring parts of the radially arranged input–output structure. Gatter and Powell (personal communication) find that the spread of degenerating intrinsic connexions in area 4 of monkeys may be as great as 2 or 3 mm in any direction from a minute intracortical lesion produced with a microelectrode. Their experiments do not show any evidence of intra-areal linkages by short U-fibres dipping into the subcortical white matter.

The input–output arrangements in area 4 are indisputably *radial*. The proposition (Asanuma, 1975) that they are organized into *columns*, which is fully justified by its evident fertility as a generator of fresh experiments, goes somewhat further and there is need for clear thinking about precisely what is entailed. Comparing the motor and association areas with the sensory receiving areas of the neocortex, Colonnier (1966) commented: 'What the significance and modality of the columns would be in an association or motor area of cortex is more difficult to imagine, but the anatomical similarity of all parts of the neocortex suggests that a functional counterpart is present in all areas. The structural design of the whole neocortex is such that it should be conceived as a mosaic of overlapping columns each possessing its own functional specificity on the basis of its tangential articulation with incoming fibres and each processing this information up and down within the column for a significant output.' This passage admirably defines the microanatomist's challenge to the electroanatomist. Whereas, in a cortical receiving area, it is logical to start at the input end and work towards the output, in a 'motor area' it is not only logical, but also technically inviting, to start at the output end and work backwards towards the input. In area 4, where more than one modality of input would presumably be involved in adjusting the flow of output, one should not necessarily expect to find the same type of columnar organization that one finds in a cortical receiving area, whose function is the primary processing of sensory data.

Before coming to consider actual or possible experiments, it will be useful to define some possible structural arrangements of input and output

C. As in A, but in area 3 after injection in VPL. In this granular cortex the densest distribution of silver grains is in lamina IV.

D. Camera lucida drawing of Golgi-impregnated thalamocortical arborization in area 3. Obliquely lying parent axon in lamina IV. In B and D the deeper-lying parts of the parent axons are not impregnated; in lamina V and VI they are 'heavily myelinated'.

(Jones, 1975.)

whose existence we might be able to affirm or deny as the result of an experimental search. The discovery of any particular arrangement need not exclude the coexistence of other arrangements, and should not be regarded as a reason for calling off the search.

The elemental unit of output is the neocortical pyramidal neurone. Situated within its synaptic cladding of radially organized thalamocortical axons and cartridge synapses (Fig. 6.1), it forms the *minimal input–output module* of area 4. Such modules may project to local or remote targets in the cortex, to subcortical structures and to the spinal cord. Some are centred on lamina III (e.g. corticorubral: Chapter 4). Our first interest, however, is in those modules which are centred on lamina V and which project to the spinal cord. We have already discussed, in Chapter 5 and in the opening paragraphs of this chapter, the possible horizontal distances across which such modules could interact by spread of excitation and inhibition.

The inputs to the minimal modules would cover a spectrum from commands at one end to external feedbacks at the other. Some might be focused on the core, others connected more diffusely at the fringes. Experiments have to begin with antidromic labelling of the output neurone, followed by specification of its inputs. Command inputs can be investigated by electrical stimulation of nucleus VL of the thalamus, feedback inputs by stimulation of muscular and cutaneous afferents. Especially in chloralose anaesthesia, the convergence of inputs from a synchronous volley of impulses in an afferent nerve or tract will give an indication of maximum input connectivity. Not all of these inputs would necessarily be expected to be 'open' in all functional contexts, and considerable advances in knowledge of what inputs are usually open have been made by recording from antidromically labelled neurones in monkeys which have been trained to make active movements, and to accept natural stimulation, for reward. Labelled neurones whose discharges are related to a specific movement are presumably obeying a command. We shall see that neurones are also responsive to specific peripheral stimuli. Closely adjacent neurones which do not respond to antidromic stimulation might be presumed to be stellate interneurones which form part of the input structure of the minimal module: their inputs might be compared to those of the output neurone, and might be found to contribute a limited fraction only of what will emerge as the final integrated output of the module.

The next question is whether the minimal input–output modules are aggregated systematically into larger assemblies or *columns*, and if so, whether these aggregations are to be specified in terms of a common input or combination of inputs, of a common target, or of some specific combination of input with output. Such a combination might be local, of input from a small peripheral field with motor output to the same periphery, or multiple, of functionally associated inputs and targets which would generally be coactivated in a specific, more or less stereotyped pattern of movement.

Aggregations of modules with common inputs would be discoverable by collecting as many antidromically labelled PTN or CSTN as possible from closely adjacent microelectrode tracks and specifying their inputs as completely as possible, to see if they did, or did not, share common commands and common peripheral fields and modalities of input. The tracks would need to be examined histologically to relate the positions of the neurones to the radial structure. The inputs to the interspersed stellate neurones would also need to be added to the description.

Aggregations of modules with common targets have been discovered by orthodromic experiments which we have already considered in detail in Chapter 5. In those experiments, we concentrated on the simplest case, that of the corticomotoneuronal projection of primates, as a possible model of the structure of projections to less easily identifiable targets. We cited evidence which rules out the possibility that every CST neurone which projects to the motoneurone pool of a particular muscle is confined within a single cylindrical column whose radius is determined by the span of tangential arborization of thalamocortical axons—say 0.5 mm—and which makes it highly unlikely that any such column would contain no modules which projected to any other target.

The modules which project to a particular motoneurone pool are collected within larger territories which we have called 'projection areas' (Jankowska *et al.*, 1975b). These areas may contain one or more foci of high output density. They overlap the projection areas which contain the modules projecting to other pools. The areas probably also contain 'parapyramidal' modules whose integrated outputs are projected to subcortical loci, as well as 'pyramidal' modules which project to brain stem and spinal loci, mediating disynaptic and polysynaptic excitation and inhibition to ascending systems as well as to spinal motoneurones. As we have seen (Chapter 4), pyramidal axons may branch to supply more than one target. We have to over-simplify in order to experiment at all, but must never allow ourselves to forget the very real complexity of our living material.

Aggregations of modules with common input–output combinations could be sought by two methods. Intracortical microstimulation (Asanuma, 1975) is capable of addressing a specific target from a specific hot spot, though it cannot easily be proved that no outputs have been discharged to other targets, nor has it been established that the entire corticofugal output has been projected from within the 'spot' (Chapter 5). Having found a 'hot spot', one can try to define its inputs by recording from single PTN, CSTN and stellate neurones within it, in order to discover whether they have some demonstrable relationship to the target. The second method, and the latest to be introduced, relies on recording from single PTN and adjacent stellate neurones in monkeys which have been trained to perform stereotyped movements. The inputs to PTN whose discharges are commanded in relation to a specific movement or component of a movement can then be defined by natural stimulation of afferent input zones (Lemon and Porter, 1976). Systematic probing, combined with histological verification of loci, is capable of showing whether minimal modules with specific input–output combinations are grouped together into columns. This method has the great advantage over microstimulation that the investigation is not necessarily restricted to hot spots.

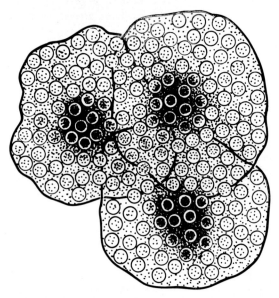

FIG. 6.3. Three overlapping *projection areas* (more can be imagined within the same cortical territory), built up of *minimal input–output modules* (dots), each centred on a PTN which forms its core and discharges its integrated output. The modules which project to the specific target of each projection area are most densely packed at the centre of the area and most loosely packed at its edges. The circles (= cylinders) suggest that the modules might be aggregated into *columns* which are smaller than the projection areas. These columns might be differentiated in terms of their thalamocortical inputs. They need not be cylindrical. Much painstaking experimental work will be needed to establish whether such a columnar organization really exists within the overlapping projection areas of area 4.

Figure 6.3 illustrates the conception of overlapping projection areas which are built up of minimal input–output modules, each of which is represented by a dot. The density of distribution of modules in area 4 is assumed to be uniform; but the diagram shows only those modules which project to one of the three common targets—one target for each of the three projection areas. The modules which belong to each projection area are concentrated at its hot spot and become less densely distributed toward its boundaries. The question whether the minimal modules are the 'minimal input–output building blocks' of the motor cortex (Brooks and Stoney, 1971), or whether these 'blocks' are assemblies of minimal modules which are aggregated into columns, is begged by the circles in the diagram. These circles (representing cylinders) should overlap if they are to correspond with Colonnier's conception (1966) of a 'mosaic of overlapping columns'. They need not be cylindrical. It seems likely that the diagram is too stark and simple to correspond with the more subtle neurological reality.

As in previous chapters, we shall deal with cat and monkey separately; in view of our own interests, we shall devote more attention to the latter. We shall be concerned with the inputs to areas adjacent to area 4, especially area 3a, as well as with inputs to area 4 itself; and with the detection of inputs by the recording of evoked potentials, as well as by recording from single neurones with microelectrodes. An important question will be how far the inputs to area 4 are transmitted directly from the thalamus and how far they are transmitted corticocortically from adjacent areas.

6.3   Electroanatomy of inputs to PT neurones in the cat

6.3.1   INPUTS FROM STRIATUM, THALAMUS AND CEREBELLUM

The main anatomical connexions between the association areas of the neocortex and the basal ganglia, cerebellum, thalamus and motor cortex have already been outlined in Fig. 1.2 (p. 8), which is based on the synthesis of Kemp and Powell (1971). To go into details of these interconnexions would take us too far afield. Their complexity will be appreciated by anyone who cares to consult some relevant reviews (Purpura and Yahr, 1966; Eccles et al., 1967; Evarts and Thach, 1969; Wiesendanger, 1969; Brooks and Stoney, 1971; Evarts et al., 1971; Massion, 1973; Massion and Paillard, 1974; Allen and Tsukahara, 1974). Electroanatomical research has been able to specify that some of the connexions which are indicated in Fig. 1.2 are excitatory and others are inhibitory, without, of course, being able to imitate or discover anything about the complex spatial and temporal patternings of neural activity which are the basis of learned performance.

Of experimental evidence for these connexions, a few examples only must suffice. Stimulation of the caudate nucleus suppresses responses to stimulation of the motor cortex (Mettler et al., 1939). Intracellular recording from antidromically identified PTN reveals that caudate stimulation evokes massive postsynaptic inhibition (Klee and Lux, 1962). Stimulation of the midline ('unspecific') thalamic nuclei also inhibits PTN (Lux and Klee, 1962).

Stimulation of the ventrolateral nucleus (VL), which is an important convergence point for signals from the neocortex, the midline thalamic nuclei, the globus pallidus and the cerebellum (Kemp and Powell, 1971), as well as of a limited range of wide-field inputs from the periphery (Asanuma *et al.*, 1974; Nyquist, 1975), exerts a powerful excitatory action on PTN. Branch and Martin (1958) found that antidromically identified PTN were commonly excited at a latency of 2.0 to 3.0 ms (range 1.0 to 20.0 ms), but that some cells received postsynaptic inhibition only. Stimulation at 30 Hz caused a build-up to a continuous high-frequency discharge of PTN. Purpura *et al* (1964) found that the EPSPs evoked by stimulation of VL generated high-frequency bursts of impulses and were sometimes large enough to inactivate, by excessive depolarization, the impulse-generating membrane of an impaled PTN.

Golgi pictures of the thalamocortical axons and of their sometimes multiple terminal arborizations, and collateral experiments in which these arborizations were stimulated antidromically from the cortex, showed that VL neurones project diffusely, as well as more narrowly, to the pre- and postcruciate cortex (Asanuma *et al.*, 1974); but Strick (1973), who made small lesions in VL and followed degenerating axons into the cortex with the Fink–Heimer and Eager methods, found only diffuse projections. In the experiments of Rispal-Padel *et al.* (1973), 8/29 anti-dromically identified thalamocortical neurones branched to project to 2, 3 or even 4 well-separated cortical loci. Possibly a rather small proportion of the neuronal population of VL projects to the cortex: about 1 in 40, though this result may merely mean that the safety factor for propagation of an antidromic impulse into the soma is low in these particular neurones. The thalamocortical axons make monosynaptic connexions with fast PTN, but excite the slow PTN indirectly via cortical interneurones (Yoshida *et al.*, 1966).

If individual VL neurones in the cat are concerned in relaying aspects of a central command to PTNs, these particular aspects will be delivered to neurones distributed over a wide zone of motor cortex. The same features of the command would possibly be available to a very large number of output neurones and the effects produced (as judged from the power of the synaptic influences recorded by Purpura *et al.*, 1964) could be large and significant. But no appropriate information exists about the coding of these features by neurones in VL of the cat.

In 1912 Rossi discovered that stimulation of cerebellar cortex lowers the electrical threshold of the motor area, and Moruzzi (1950) has since found that it can also inhibit the motor area. In the cat, much attention has been devoted to the role of nucleus interpositus which is associated with the intermediate zone of the cerebellar cortex and which projects to the small-celled part of the red nucleus and to VL. The neurones of this nucleus are tonically active, and are believed to maintain an excitatory pressure on the neurones of VL and thence on those of the motor cortex (Eccles *et al.*, 1967). The action of the cerebellar cortical Purkinje cells is to inhibit the neurones of the cerebellar nuclei. Thus stimulation of the cortex of the intermediate zone would be expected to depress, and not to enhance, the excitability of the motor cortex: inhibition of the nuclear cells should disfacilitate the neurones of VL and thence those of the motor cortex. This matter deserves further study. A possible explanation of Rossi's classical result might be found in the prolonged *silence* of the Purkinje cells which follows repetitive stimulation (Granit and Phillips, 1957).

The results of single-pulse stimulation of the cerebellar nuclei by Rispal-Padel and Latreille (1974) are that all three deep nuclei give rise to a surface-positive evoked potential in the contralateral motor cortex, at a latency of <3.0 ms. When recorded with a penetrating electrode the polarity of the wave reversed so that at a depth of 500 μm a large negative wave was recorded. The dentate nucleus projected at short latency (<3.0 ms) to the medial precruciate part of area 4 and to area 6, and at longer latency (3 to 7 ms) to the lateral precruciate and, more weakly, to the postcruciate part of area 4. The fastigio-thalamo-cortical projection was roughly similar. The posterior part of the nucleus interpositus projected only to the lateral part of area 4, without much sign of a late component; its anterior part projected diffusely to the whole of areas 4 and 6, with both early and late components.

The implications of the connexions between the cerebellum and the cerebral cortex and their possible significance for movement control have been reviewed by Allen and Tsukahara (1974). They point out that the application of the newer anatomical techniques at the cellular level and the use of single neurone recording at strategic sites on pathways for communication of signals about movement will need to be extended to reveal the details of the operation of the system.

6.3.2   INPUTS FROM THE PERIPHERY

Interest in possible inputs from the periphery to the cat's PT was aroused by the discovery by Adrian and Moruzzi (1939) that, in cats under chloralose anaesthesia, a well-synchronized volley can be set up in the PT by a peripheral stimulus. These 'relayed pyramidal discharges' have been studied in particular detail by Buser (1966) and his colleagues. The afferent pathways are evidently polysynaptic, for the mean latency for the PT discharge in response to a flash of light is 25 ms; to a bang, 15 ms; to a shock to the forelimb, 10 ms, and to the hindlimb, 20 ms. The discharge is associated with an evoked potential at the motor cortex. The mixing of the different modalities has already taken place at subcortical levels. Stations on the 'sensory-motor ascending pathway' include midline thalamus and mesencephalic reticular formation. Stimulation at these loci results in an evoked potential at the motor cortex and an associated pyramidal volley; lesions in or focal cooling of them result in blocking of the response that would otherwise be evoked from the periphery. Transmission can also be depressed by stimulation of the caudate nucleus and medial thalamic nuclei (centre median etc.). For the response to a flash of light, the primary visual receiving area of the cortex is not essential (Wall et al., 1953). A pyramidal volley can also be discharged in response to an afferent volley in the vestibular nerve (Megirian and Troth, 1964).

Buser and Imbert (1961) recorded extracellularly from single neurones in the cat's motor cortex, located at a depth appropriate for PTN but not identified as such by the antidromic method. Of these neurones 92 per cent were 'polysensory', discharging impulses in response to electrical stimulation of the skin of the limbs (latency 12 to 29 ms), to clicks (latency 25 to 45 ms), and to flashes (latency 45 to 90 ms). Such 'polysensory' behaviour is in contrast with the exquisitely circumscribed, shorter-latency responsiveness of neurones in the adjacent somatosensory cortex to localized stimulation of the skin (Mountcastle, 1957). Batuev et al. (1974) have since recorded intracellularly from 27 antidromically labelled PTN, and have found that stimuli such as those given by Buser and Imbert (1961) evoked EPSPs; to shocks to skin of forepaw at 9 to 20 ms latency, to clicks at 14 to 32 ms, and to flashes at 18 to 30 ms. The EPSPs were followed by IPSPs.

The interest of investigators turned next to the possibility of better-circumscribed inputs from the skin, and away from the use of chloralose as the usual anaesthetic. Brooks et al. (1961a, b) applied natural stimuli to the limbs and trunks of locally anaesthetised, paralysed cats. They found that the skin fields from which fifty-one PTN could be discharged were of three kinds. Seventeen were 'fixed local fields': these were confined to part of a contralateral limb, and responded to movement of hairs, light touch, pressure or movement of a joint. The edges of these fields were sharpened by 'surround inhibition'; the specific stimulus suppressed the discharge from the centre of the field when applied to a surrounding area. Neurones responding in this way were classified as 's' neurones by Towe et al. (1964). PTN which respond thus are generally fast PTN (Wettstein and Handwerker, 1970). Of the remainder of the collection of Brooks et al. (1961a,b), 15 PTN had 'fixed wide fields', which were usually bilateral and showed discontinuities (the 'm' neurones of Towe et al., 1964); only half were stimulus-specific. The fields of the remaining 19 PTN were 'labile': they enlarged when stimulation was prolonged, and they then responded to additional modalities of stimulation. Responses could sometimes be suppressed by simultaneous stimulation of another modality; for example, the response to touching the skin might be suppressed by moving a joint. Another type of suppression ('inhibition') was seen when a remote field (sometimes on another limb) was stimulated. In two freely moving cats wearing an implanted microelectrode introducer, Baker *et al.* (1971) found that a higher proportion of unidentified pericruciate neurones had wide fields after a small dose of chloralose than when the same animals were awake, when small fields predominated.

Electrical stimulation is a useful adjunct to natural stimulation if one wishes to compare the length and synaptic complexity of central afferent pathways to the PTN by measuring latency of response. Patton *et al.* (1962) used it for a comparison of the responses of 66 identified PTN to afferent volleys evoked by shocks to the central toe-pads of the contralateral and ipsilateral forepaws of lightly chloralosed cats. Some PTN also responded to sounds and flashes. The responses to stimulation to the contralateral toe-pad were evidently transmitted by a more direct pathway than those from the ipsilateral pad. Contralateral volleys evoked a large number of impulses per burst from the PTN, and at a shorter latency (mean difference 14 ms). Repetitive contralateral volleys were transmitted more reliably. The latency of the relayed pyramidal volley (cf. Patton and Amassian, 1960) was 10–12 ms in response to the contralateral input and 15–20 ms in response to the ipsilateral input. Cutting the corpus callosum abolished the first component of the massed pyramidal response to the ipsilateral volley without affecting the response to the contralateral volley.

Because PT axons may be distributed to targets in the brain stem and not in the spinal cord (Chapter 4), it is necessary, if one wishes to categorize the inputs to corticospinal neurones from receptive fields of the limbs, to label these neurones by antidromic stimulation of the LCST and not the PT. This has been done for CST neurones of area 4 in the primate (Wiesendanger, 1973), and now needs to be done for area 4 in the cat. In the second somatosensory area (SII; Fig. 2.9, p. 47), Atkinson *et al.* (1974) collected 34 CST neurones from cats anaesthetized with 50 per cent nitrous oxide supplemented by minimal doses of short-acting barbiturate. Of these neurones, 12 per cent had small fields, 44 per cent medium fields and 35 per cent large fields (e.g. head, both forelimbs and shoulders and left hindlimb), and 9 per cent were unresponsive to peripheral stimulation. The targets of CST neurones need not, of course, be related only to motor output; they may also be related to afferent input (Chapter 4), as Atkinson *et al.* (1974) have suggested for this projection from SII.

The notion that the inputs to the cat's motor cortex might be organized in a columnar arrangement of 'minimal input–output building blocks' was introduced by Welt *et al.* (1967), whose experiments were a development of those of Brooks *et al.* (1961a,b) using natural stimulation of the skin. They collected 215 neurones in 25 penetrations of 'pericruciate motorsensory cortex' and found no differences between the properties of PTN and of unidentified cells. Of the total, 75 per cent had fixed fields, but these were 'not stimulus-pure'. Histological reconstruction of the electrode-tracks in relation to the radially orientated structure of the cortex found that the greatest cross-column distance for particular fields was 0.37 mm and the mean cross-column traverse was 0.14 mm; but 'sufficiently detailed evidence was not available to determine whether an *anatomically* defined single column of cells exhibits homogeneity with respect to peripheral location of activating receptive fields'. Thus it was not possible to prove that the input from a particular area of skin was confined to an anatomically defined column. The remaining 25 per cent of the neuronal sample showed no trace of columnar organization: their wide and sometimes bilateral fields were found to 'project to neurones within these somatotopically organized columns' of the fixed fields 'in a heterogeneous, convergent manner'. Any 'radial array' of neurones would include some which received multimodal inputs from wide areas and some from narrow; this was true of the cortical interneurones as well as of the pyramidal neurones which would constitute the integrated outputs of the radial arrays.

6.3.3   TOPOGRAPHICAL RELATIONS BETWEEN CUTANEOUS INPUT ZONES AND TARGETS OF MOTOR OUTPUT

These experiments have all been primarily concerned with the inputs. Although plenty of records have been collected from antidromically identified PTN, the ultimate destinations of their axons have remained unknown, and it has been possible to view them simply as integrators of their inputs and nothing more. Credit for the first attempt to link known input to known output in the radially orientated structure of the cortex is due to Asanuma *et al.* (1968), who combined the recording of afferent inputs to single cortical neurones with the mapping of 'efferent zones' by microstimulation through the same microelectrode. Their sample of 288 neurones, which was collected from cats which were sedated with small doses of barbiturate and were free to move, resembled in general those of Brooks *et al.* (1961a,b) and Welt *et al.* (1967) in the preponderance of inputs from the skin. The neurones received multimodal inputs, but only one-third responded to deep pressure or to passive movement of joints. There was no relation between the direction of joint movement and the direction of the response to microstimulation.

We have already discussed the micromapping of efferent zones at some length in Chapter 5, and must now consider how the polymodal inputs to the radial arrays may be associated with the possible types of target we have outlined in Fig. 6.3. In these experiments the targets were the motoneurone pools of some muscles of the forelimb, or, more strictly, the interneurones which are interposed between the CST neurones and the motoneurones of the cat (Chapter 4). We have considered the difficulties which stand in the way of accepting the existence of single narrow columns which circumscribe the entire cortical projection to single motoneurone pools and which do not project to any other pools. Thus, in discussing their 'multiple-effect zones', Asanuma et al. (1968) considered two possibilities: they 'may simply represent the overlapping fringes of neighboring single-effect zones' or may 'represent functionally organized, more complex, cortical efferent colonies'. Let us look again at the hypothesis of Fig. 6.3, that there are overlapping projection areas in the cat (as there are in the primate), and that each is built up of many 'minimal input–output building blocks'. Asanuma (1975) writes: 'A likely interpretation seems to be that several of these afferent columns' (i.e. those of Welt et al., 1967; diameter about 0.1 to 0.4 mm) constitute a given efferent column that has an average diameter of 1.0 mm'. We can provisionally conclude from the results of Welt et al. (1967) and Asanuma et al. (1968) that each minimal input–output building block receives multimodal inputs. We can now ask if the output of each such 'block' is projected to a single target or to multiple targets. The *minimal input–output module* would have a single CST neurone as its output. The axons of some CST neurones supply branches to the lumbar as well as the cervical enlargement (Asanuma et al., 1976b). Thus the output of a single neurone and, hence, of a minimal module could be multiple.

A larger block would contain more than one CST neurone (Fig. 6.3, circles). Would these few cells project to one or to more than one target? This question is possibly unanswerable by microstimulation, since, as we have seen, the originally reasonable assumptions of Asanuma et al. (1968), (1) that repetitive stimulation with 2.0 µA is capable of exciting 'repetitive activity of one or two cortical neurones within an efferent colony', and (2) that their discharges 'can lead to muscle contraction', have been weakened by more recent evidence about horizontal intracortical spread of excitation and now stand in need of fresh experimental support. Microstimulation, however, is readily capable of revealing differences in the relative density of projection from the cores and from the fringes of projection areas. Further use of it, preferably in combination with the facilitation and inhibition of monosynaptic reflexes (Asanuma and Sakata, 1967) rather than with electromyography, should succeed in showing whether the 'high-threshold regions' of Asanuma et al. (1968) do, or do not, contain thin-textured excitatory outputs as well as some of the dense inhibitory outputs found by Asanuma and Sakata (1967). Thompson and Fernandez (1975) attempted to examine this point for cortical projections to hindlimb motor pools in the cat's spinal cord and concluded that 'microstimulation produced effects on a given spinal reflex independently of systematic reciprocal effects on the reflex of the antagonist'. They argued for overlapping fringes of the areas for producing different effects but for separation of their centres without mingling of excitatory and inhibitory influences. On the input side, there is already some evidence of local variations in input density; for although neurones associated with every type of receptive field were found to be distributed equally throughout the 'high-threshold regions' as well as the 'low-threshold regions' the regions of *overlap* of the wide fields did seem to converge upon local concentrations of output.

There was some indication (Asanuma *et al.*, 1968) that, 'while cutaneous receptive fields of neurons within any given efferent zone are scattered over large areas of the forelimb', the inputs from those skin areas in which there was maximal *overlap* of afferent fields would 'cause excitation predominantly of neurons of the particular efferent zone. In general, a given efferent zone receives cutaneous inputs predominantly from skin regions which lie in the pathway of limb movement produced by contraction of the muscle to which the zone projects.' Thus, contact with such an area of overlap would be expected to drive the forepaw towards the stimulating object, as, for example, in the contact placing reaction (Bard, 1938; Amassian *et al.*, 1972). This was obviously an attractive and reasonable theory. In the case of some of the cutaneous areas the validity of this generalization was not self-evident, and special arguments were developed which we have not space to reproduce in full and must urge every interested reader to study in detail (Asanuma *et al.*, 1968, pp. 676–677). Reviewing this work along with that of Sakata and Miyamoto (1968), who had concluded independently that the limb was moved away from the point of contact, by stimulation in cortical efferent zones which received inputs from the contacted skin, Brooks and Stoney (1971) stated: 'We have not been able to reconcile these results . . . Additional experiments are needed for clarification of input–output relations of primate motor cortex and for reconciliation of the different conclusions reached by studies of cat MsI.'

6.3.4   INPUTS FROM MUSCLE

At about the same time, researchers began to turn their attention to the inputs from receptors in muscle. Until the work of Amassian and Berlin (1958) there had been no evidence of any projection from muscle spindles to the cerebral cortex (Mountcastle *et al.*, 1952). The discovery of such a projection from the forelimb was followed up in detail by Oscarsson and Rosén (1963, 1966). In cats under barbiturate anaesthesia, they showed

that an electrically evoked afferent volley in the group Ia axons of a forelimb nerve, or a rapid stretch which lengthened the muscle by 60 μm and
excited the primary endings of the muscle spindles, resulted in the delivery
of a thalamocortical volley to the rostro-lateral part of the primary somatosensory receiving area at a latency of about 5 ms; this volley then evoked a
localized surface-negative potential wave. Transmission through the
cuneate and thalamic relays was very secure, with little need for spatial
summation. The focus of input was at the 'postcruciate dimple', which,
according to Hassler and Muhs-Clement (1964), marks the position of
area 3a, which lies immediately adjacent posteriorly to the classical motor
area, between it and the classical receiving area for the input from skin and
joints. Single neurones in this area, which were not invaded antidromically
from the PT, showed excitatory and inhibitory PSPs at a latency of about
5 ms after a group Ia volley.

Oscarsson *et al.* (1966) found that the neurones that were excited in
area 3a by group I afferent volleys received extensive convergence from
muscles working at different joints, from muscles which were antagonists
at the same joint, and also (at longer latency) from cutaneous afferents.
None of these neurones could be antidromically excited from the PT.
Of 17 PTN, 8 gave no response, and 9 gave longer-latency responses
from the skin. No PTN were ever discharged by muscle afferent volleys,
but subliminal excitatory actions or weak inhibitory actions were excluded
in only 4 cells. Exceptionally, a PT neurone was found which responded
directly to the input from the muscle spindles (Swett and Bourassa, 1967).

It was at first supposed that the muscle input was exclusively from the
forelimb, which, in contrast to the hindlimb which is mainly a postural
and locomotor organ, is used in a wide variety of exploratory and manipulative behaviour. The region of the 'postcruciate dimple' is cytoarchitectonic-
ally transitional between the motor cortex of area 4 and that of the somaesthetic areas 3b, 1 and 2 (Hassler and Muhs-Clement, 1964). Jones and
Powell (1968) found that this area, 3a, was also represented on the medial
aspect of the hemisphere and predicted that the muscle input from the
hindlimb would be found there. Their prediction was quite independently
verified by Landgren and Silfvenius (1968, 1969). The signals are not
transmitted through nucleus gracilis (as the signals from the forelimb are
transmitted through nucleus cuneatus), but through a separate nucleus Z
(Landgren and Silfvenius, 1971).

A degree of differentiation of muscle receptors into 'low threshold' and
'high threshold' was achieved by Murphy *et al.* (1975), who isolated m.
palmaris longus and m. extensor digitorum communis in the cat's forelimb,
denervated other structures, and stretched the muscles by 80 μm at 8 mm s^{-1}
('low-threshold': presumed to stimulate the primary endings of the
muscle spindles) or by 250 *u*m at 25 mm s-^{1} ('high-threshold': presumed to

stimulate secondary endings and possibly Golgi tendon organs). Of 129 neurones collected from area 4 y, 73 were in receipt of low-threshold inputs and 56 received high-threshold. Three neurones were suppressed by low threshold and 4 by high-threshold stimuli. In one of the 14 experiments 10 neurones were antidromically stimulated from the pyramid; they were in layers III or V and were all affected by high-threshold stimuli.

The high-threshold responses were unaffected by injection of succinyl-choline, but the low-threshold responses were increased by it, which supports their characterization as due to inputs from primary endings. Histology confirmed that all tracks were in area 4 γ. In experiments in which multiple tracks were made, all low-threshold cells were 'restricted to columns of cortex oriented orthogonally to the cortical layers. The input columns were approximately 0.5 to 2.0 mm in diameter.' The high-threshold cells were scattered diffusely; 'the density of such cells, located presumably in the low-threshold columns for other muscles, was far less than that found in the muscle's own low-threshold response column'. The rest of the limb was denervated, so it is not known whether any or all of these neurones also received a cutaneous input.

The relation of these inputs to the outputs to the muscles was tested by microstimulation in 4/14 cats (3–300 pulses at 300 Hz, <30 µA; light halothane anaesthesia). With 30 pulses at 16 µA, EDC gave more than 40 g tension, latency 20–25 ms, and PL relaxed minimally during the stimulation. Threshold and tension varied with depth of anaesthesia and with EEG arousal; local desynchronization was associated with higher tension. 'Despite this extreme sensitivity to fluctuations in experimental conditions, stimulation was selective for one muscle or the other, with a zone of overlap whence both muscles responded (one more than the other).' The localization was different in different animals but 'output column coincided with input column' in every case. Here again we are dealing with coaxial condensations of one class of input with one class of output, without any certainty that the output is restricted to the stimulated site and does not contain corticofugal cells belonging to other outputs. The approximate coincidence refers to the low-threshold input only: the high-threshold input from each muscle was diffuse and widespread.

6.3.5   CORTICOCORTICAL AND THALAMOCORTICAL TRANSMISSION OF INPUTS TO AREA 4

The pathways by which the inputs from skin and muscle reach the motor cortex and the PTN are not fully known. The immediate proximity of somaesthetic cortex (SI; Fig. 2.9, p. 47) suggests that they might be transmitted corticocortically. The existence of plentiful short association fibres which interlink these areas (Jones and Powell, 1968; Grant et al., 1975) reinforces the suggestion that the inputs arriving in SI from the ventro-basal (VB) nucleus of the thalamus could be relayed to area 4. The direct route from thalamus to area 4, that from nucleus VL, is the other main candidate; but the peripheral inputs to its neurones are few and ill characterized (Asanuma et al., 1974; Nyquist, 1975; Asanuma and Hunsperger, 1975). The possibility of transmission of inputs from VB to area 4 requires more investigation.

W. D. Thompson et al. (1970) recorded from neurones at the lateral end of the cruciate sulcus, including some antidromically identified PTN, and stimulated the surface of SI with surface-anodal pulses, 0.2 to 0.9 mA. 'Although SmI cortex near the caudal end of the coronal sulcus was explored, low threshold regions for exciting MsI cells were found, in all instances, to be near the lateral end of the post-cruciate dimple.' As we have seen, this dimple generally marks the position of area 3a, but in these experiments on locally anaesthetized and paralysed cats, the receptive fields of the cells near the dimple were cutaneous. There was a strong tendency towards contiguity of receptive fields of neurones in corresponding 'regions of SmI and MsI'. The time for transmission from the dimple to MsI neurones (a distance of about 5 mm) ranged from about 1.0 to 9.0 ms with a peak at about 3.0 ms. The possibility of cortico-subcortico-cortical transmission could not be excluded. The results of cooling the dimple in an attempt to block transmission to MsI were equivocal.

Coming next to the possibility of corticocortical transmission of the inputs from muscle from area 3a to area 4, F. J. Thompson et al. (1973) stimulated the deep (motor) radial nerve in lightly nembutalized cats and recorded the evoked potential in area 3a. They then probed this area with a stimulating microcathode (10 μA) and recorded intracellularly from neurones in that part of the motor area which gave responses of radial muscles at lowest threshold. Of 120 neurones, only two were made to discharge impulses by microstimulation within 3a; 17 responded with EPSPs and 14 with IPSPs. The control of motor output by corticocortical transmission of feedback from muscle could therefore be more subtle than would be provided for by a simple excitatory drive.

Murphy et al (1975) recorded responses to low threshold stretching of EDC in area 3a as well as in area 4. 'Discrete EDC columns were found both in the dimple region (area 3a) and in motor cortex (area 4 γ).' The interrelations were not tested with microstimulation. No responses were obtained from 4 tracks in the intervening cortex. When the 'dimple' was cooled to 16°C at a locus medial to the responsive cells, the responses in area 4 were hardly reduced. Latencies were 11 ms (measured from the mechanical stimulus to the muscle). This evidence all strengthens the possibility that there are parallel lemnisco-thalamo-cortical projections from primary afferents of muscle spindles to neurones in area 3a and to non-PT neurones in area 4. Most of these low-threshold neurones were found in lamina III of area 4.

The corticipetal transmission of the high-threshold input (spindle secondaries, tendon organs) is considerably slower, the earliest activity reaching its peak at 17 ms. The neurones responding to it are found in all laminae of area 4. The response of 51/56 neurones was decreased by cooling nucleus interpositus of the cerebellum to 15°C, and Murphy et al. (1975) have drawn a diagram which shows the pathway as passing through this nucleus on its way to the cortex.

If it could be proved that nucleus interpositus is, in fact, a *relay* nucleus, this would have great theoretical interest which cannot be allowed to pass without comment. The deep cerebellar nuclei are analogous to the vestibular nuclei in that they receive excitatory inputs from outside the cerebellum, and are subject to inhibition by the cerebellar Purkinje cells. Thus transmission through nucleus interpositus would be inhibited by the cortex of the intermediate region, as transmission through the vestibular nuclei is inhibited by the cortex of the flocculonodular lobe. One of the vestibular nuclei contains the second-order neurones of the vestibulo-ocular reflex and the cortex of the flocculo-nodular lobe receives a parallel afferent input of mossy fibres from the vestibular apparatus. When the normal relationship between the directions of rotation of the head and of the visual field is artificially reversed, the vestibulo-ocular reflex undergoes an appropriate 'plastic' change (Gonshor and Melvill Jones, 1976); and there is evidence that this change depends on a modification of the inhibitory action of the cortex on the nucleus (Ghelarducci et al., 1975).

The cortex of the intermediate region receives information of length, rate of change of length, and tension of the muscles (Fig. 4.8, p. 118). So if nucleus interpositus is actually responsible for transmission of signals of muscle length (from spindle secondaries) and tension (from Golgi tendon organs) to the motor cortex, there would be interesting possibilities of cerebellar modification of their actions on its output, whether by short-term 'switching' or by long-term 'plastic' change (cf. Chapter 8, section 8.3.6).

6.3.6.   CALLOSAL AFFERENTS

Finally, we come to electroanatomical evidence that the two motor areas are interconnected by the corpus callosum. Corticocallosal neurones were identified antidromically by stimulation of the opposite motor area by Asanuma and Okamoto (1959). Asanuma and Okuda (1962) found that orthodromic excitation of a PTN can be evoked from a circumscribed part of the opposite cortex, apparently the homologue of the region containing the PTN. In intracellular records the discharge was seen to arise from an EPSP. The excitatory point was surrounded by a zone whose stimulation suppressed the discharge that was evoked from the centre.

6.4 Afferent input to the motor cortex in the monkey

6.4.1 THALAMIC PROJECTIONS TO AREA 4

The multitude of connexions made with the surfaces of PTNs provides the anatomical basis for influences of many brain structures to be exerted on the motor cortex. This region receives connexions from other cortical zones, from the opposite hemisphere and from the thalamus. Projections from the thalamus have been studied using a number of anatomical techniques. In area 4 of the squirrel monkey, terminals of thalamic afferents, traced by staining them with the Nauta method during degeneration and also revealed by autoradiography fill much of layer III (see Fig. 6.2). A small proportion of thalamic afferents also end in layer I. In Golgi preparations, the terminal unmyelinated portions of presumed thalamic afferents to area 4 enter layer III obliquely and divide

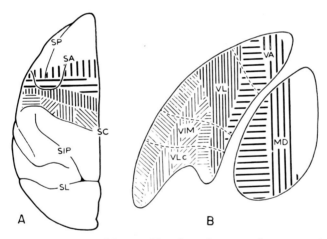

FIG. 6.4. Injection of horseradish peroxidase into the areas of cortex marked on the diagram of a monkey's left hemisphere (A) resulted in retrograde marking of neurones in those thalamic nuclei which are outlined on a diagram of a horizontal plane of the thalamus (B). These are the nuclei which receive most of the projections from the dentate and interpositus nuclei of the cerebellum. In A, note, from medial to lateral: face area (horizontal hatching); hand area (ascending oblique hatching); area intermediate between hand and foot areas (vertical hatching); and foot area (descending oblique hatching). Note the corresponding hatchings in the thalamic nuclei in B. After injections into the precentral gyrus, labelled neurones were also found in nucleus centralis lateralis and in the most caudal part of centrum medianum.

SC, central sulcus; VA, nucleus ventralis anterior; VL, nucleus ventralis lateralis; VIM, nucleus ventralis intermedius (or ventralis 'posterior lateralis pars oralis); VLc, nucleus ventralis pars caudalis; MD, nucleus medialis dorsalis.

(Kievit and Kuypers, 1975.)

to produce beaded secondary and tertiary branches which ascend more or less vertically through the deeper half to two-thirds of this layer (Jones, 1975). Each set of branches could extend for several hundred microns.

Kievit and Kuypers (1975) examined the cells of origin of thalamic afferents to the motor cortex of the monkey by injecting horseradish peroxidase into the arm area of the precentral gyrus. They studied the distribution of the thalamic cells to which this label had been transported in a retrograde direction from their axon terminals in the cortex. The results of their thalamocortical mapping are summarized in Fig. 6.4. Strick (1975) also concluded that area 4 received thalamic input from multiple sources. The arm area projections were from both ventrolateral (VL_o) and adjacent ventro-posterolateral (VPL_o) nuclei. The cells of origin occupied a distinct continuous zone through these two nuclei midway between the internal and external laminae. A large injection in the arm area caused all the cells in this zone to be labelled. Strick (1975) also confirmed that a distinct part of the intralaminar nuclear group was labelled—the centrolateral (CL) nucleus and the immediately adjacent region of the centromedian (CM) nucleus contained cells whose axons projected to the arm area. Large injections of horseradish peroxidase in the arm area caused labelling of all the cells in a crescent of CL. These experiments do not demonstrate whether the separate thalamic nuclei project to different layers of area 4.

6.4.2   ELECTROANATOMICAL INVESTIGATION OF PERIPHERAL INPUTS TO
         AREA 4

Thalamocortical projections to the motor cortex of the monkey provide one set of pathways by which influences originating in peripheral receptors activated by movement could be relayed to output neurones of area 4. These influences could reach area 4 relatively directly, possibly through VPL_o, or they could be routed through the cerebellum and then relayed through VL_o (Kemp and Powell, 1971). But many other pathways are also available, through the somatosensory receiving cortex (SI) (Pandya and Kuypers, 1969), or by longer routes involving the basal ganglia (and again thalamic nuclei VL and VA), the reticular formation or the intra-laminar nuclei. A detailed examination of these pathways in the monkey, concerned with the precise microanatomy of the many parallel courses along which peripheral feedback could be conveyed to the output cells of the motor cortex, has not been undertaken. But, even without this knowledge, it is possible to examine the effects of stimulation of peripheral receptors or their afferent fibres on cells in area 4 and, in particular, to attempt to describe the afferent input zones of PTNs.

It is clear that the motor cortex includes receiving (sensory) elements:

inputs, as well as transmitting (motor) elements; outputs. A study of inputs from the periphery is most conveniently conducted using electrical registration of nervous activity because the number of synapses interposed in the pathways from the periphery places severe limitations on conventional anatomical methods. Evoked potentials (Adrian, 1941) may be detected on the surface of the intact cerebral cortex when stimuli are delivered to peripheral receptors or to afferent nerve fibres. In the monkey, such evoked potentials have been recorded over precentral as well as over postcentral regions. Malis *et al.* (1953) stimulated the sciatic nerve of anaesthetized monkeys and recorded evoked potentials before and after ablation of regions which could have been concerned in the relay of nervous influences to precentral cortex. They found that the responses in the leg area of motor cortex to sciatic nerve shocks were unaltered by resection of the adjacent postcentral cortex, by removing both pre- and postcentral cortex of the other hemisphere or by resection of the cerebellum. They deduced that the precentral motor area received its own projection from peripheral afferents independent of afferent projections to these other regions.

They also analysed the possibility that, because most evoked potentials produced by natural cutaneous stimulation were limited to points on the postcentral gyrus, their precentral responses might have originated by way of 'proprioceptive' inputs from deep tissues. They found that cutaneous as well as deep stimuli were capable of causing evoked responses in precentral cortex and concluded that projections from both superficial and deep receptors must converge upon this region.

Adey *et al.* (1954) also recorded evoked potentials from the cortex of anaesthetized monkeys. The responses which were produced by stimulation of deep tissues could be recorded in both precentral and postcentral zones. The positions on the cortical surface at which these potentials had their shortest latency from a given peripheral site (fingers, toes, face, etc.) were topographically separated and each of the shortest latency fields (for the fingers) was situated close to or on the central sulcus (sometimes more clearly in front of it than behind). Measurements made within the sulcus indicated that the earliest effects of a peripheral stimulus could be detected in the depths of the sulcus, 5 ms or less after stimulation of the hand.

Like Malis *et al.* (1953), these authors concluded that some precentral projections were independent of responses in postcentral cortex. Moreover, they reported the occurrence of ipsilateral projections from deep tissues to homologous regions of cortex. These ipsilateral projections were less effective in producing evoked potentials which were usually more variable, were evident in smaller zones of the cortex and had longer latencies than the responses produced by contralateral stimulation.

The problems of interpreting the results of evoked potential studies have been referred to in later work (Phillips *et al.*, 1971). Potential changes recorded from the pia-covered surface of the cortex may have their origin in deep or distant regions. If the source of the responses is to be examined, electrodes must be inserted into the cortex and attempts must be made to activate only selected populations of receptors in identified regions.

Albe-Fessard and Liebeskind (1966) examined the responses of single neurones in regions of the motor cortex from which evoked potentials could be recorded in chloralose-anaesthetized monkeys. Both electrical stimulation of the hands and feet and natural activation of receptors in the limbs were used. The inputs to cells in area 4 were topographically separated to the extent that neurones in the arm area were influenced mainly from the arm and those in the leg area mainly from the leg. In contrast to neurones in the postcentral receiving cortex of the same animals whose discharges were almost exclusively influenced by 'tactile' stimuli, the majority of cells in the motor cortex were excited by stimulation of deep structures and particularly by movement of limbs. Convergence of influences was a feature of the responses of motor cortex cells to limb movement and this convergence was revealed particularly in cells whose discharges were promoted by movement of a particular joint and inhibited by movement of the corresponding joint on the opposite side (Fig. 6.5). When limb muscles were dissected, motor cortex cells could be shown to respond to traction on the tendons of muscles and to light pressure on denuded muscles, providing direct evidence for an input from these sources which could possibly be activated during natural movement in the intact monkey.

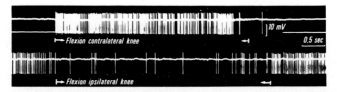

FIG. 6.5. Recordings from a neurone in the motor cortex of a monkey *(M. speciosa)* under chloralose anaesthesia. The cell is excited by flexion of the contralateral knee (top tracing). During sustained flexion of this contralateral limb (bottom tracing), flexion of the ipsilateral knee produces inhibition of the cell's discharge. (Albe-Fessard and Liebeskind, 1966.)

A clear demonstration of an afferent projection from particular muscle spindles to a few neurones in the motor cortex was provided by the experiment of Albe-Fessard *et al.* (1966). Stimulation of fusimotor fibres to the muscle spindles of the semitendinosus muscle, after critical curarization had been produced so that contractions of extrafusal muscle fibres were abolished but not those of intrafusal fibres, caused activation of four precentral neurones in the leg area of motor cortex.

Phillips *et al.* (1971) delivered electrical shocks to the deep radial nerve and to the deep palmar branch of the ulnar nerve in anaesthetized baboons. When weak shocks, capable of exciting only low threshold group I afferents in these motor nerves were delivered, evoked responses completely localized within area 3a deep in the central sulcus were the only responses obtained. The locations of the responses from the deep radial and the deep palmar branch of the ulnar nerve were topographically separated. The latencies of the evoked responses were short (3.8 to 5.2 ms after the arrival of the group I volley at the cord) and transmission through the synapses in the afferent pathway was secure because distinct, separate waves were produced when three separate shocks were delivered at high frequency (330 Hz). These responses were abolished by section of the dorsal columns. Under the anaesthetic conditions used in these experiments (nitrous oxide and pentobarbitone) and with stimuli limited to muscle afferent fibres of group I conduction velocity, no evoked responses were recorded in area 4, even though microelectrode penetrations were made through the full depth and through an appropriate region of this cortex.

Within the localized zone of cortex (area 3a) which had been shown to receive an input from group I muscle afferents, Phillips *et al.* (1971) recorded the responses of 143 single neurones. The majority of these could be caused to discharge when single shocks of intensities too weak to cause a maximal group I volley in the motor nerves were used. Only a small proportion of the cells which responded to stimulation of afferents in one motor nerve could also be discharged by stimuli applied to the other nerve; so the inputs to individual cells appeared to be topographically separated.

A small number of neurones which could be discharged by weak stimulation of group I afferent fibres in motor nerves also responded to brief stretch of innervated muscles in that nerve's territory or to vibration of a muscle. Responses were consistent with an input from the primary endings of muscle spindle receptors. Neurones in area 3a also responded to brisk movement of joints (which could have activated muscle, tendon and/or joint receptors) but these were not influenced by gentle stroking of the skin. The cells which responded to inputs were not output cells sending their axons into the corticospinal tract. Area 3a neurones whose responses have been described must therefore be thought of as 'receiving' neurones responding particularly to the afferent input from primary endings of muscle spindles in particular muscle groups.

Although the above experiments did not indicate a short-latency, well-defined input from primary endings of muscle spindles to neurones in area 4, Wiesendanger (1973) confirmed earlier work of Albe-Fessard and her colleagues in experiments on baboons and monkeys anaesthetized with nitrous oxide–oxygen mixtures and chloralose. Using electrical stimulation of the deep and superficial radial nerves and of the deep ulnar nerve, Wiesendanger demonstrated convergence of afferent inputs from different territories, both deep and superficial, on to individual PT cells. This contrasted with the topographical separation of inputs which had been found for cells in area 3a and it differed somewhat from the findings of Albe-Fessard and Liebeskind (1966) who, with natural activation of receptors, did not demonstrate convergence of inputs from cutaneous and deep afferents on cells in area 4. The shortest latency of a PTN response to electrical stimulation of a peripheral nerve occurred 12 ms after the afferent volley entered the spinal cord—some 7 ms longer than the earliest responses in area 3a.

Identified PTNs in area 4 were not excited by half maximal group I volleys in motor nerves. The threshold for a response of such a neurone was always in a range which could have allowed more slowly conducting group II afferent fibres to be implicated in the production of the response. Moreover, these effects were apparently exerted mainly on PTNs with rapidly conducting axons because even the large, complicated volleys produced by maximal stimulation of peripheral nerves had a low probability of influencing PTNs with slowly conducting axons.

Passive manipulation of joints (which again could have influenced muscle, skin and tendon receptors as well as joint afferents) could modulate the firing of PTNs and maintained 'tonic' changes in firing were reported following joint movement (see also Fig. 6.4). Succinylcholine which causes activation of the primary endings of muscle spindles to a much greater degree than any influence on secondary endings, did not influence the firing of PTNs. Taken together with the other results listed above, these findings were interpreted as indicating that the inputs from muscles to PTNs in the motor cortex must derive from secondary endings of muscle spindles. In fact, other area 4 neurones not identified as sending their axons into the corticospinal tract, also exhibited exactly similar responses to the stimuli used in these experiments.

An alternative approach to the study of muscle afferent projections to the motor cortex has been used by Hore et al. (1976) and by Lucier et al. (1975). These workers applied controlled stretches to hindlimb and forelimb muscles respectively in baboons and monkeys and studied the responses of neurones in both areas 3a and 4. Our interest must relate particularly to the responses of area 4. In the studies of Hore et al. units with the greatest sensitivity to static changes in length of the stretched muscle were found in area 4. While velocity sensitivity (measured by the dynamic index of the unit's discharges when the muscle was subjected to a ramp stretch) was highest for cells in area 3a, some area 4 units also exhibited velocity sensitivity in their firing. This was considered to be an indicator of some influence arising in velocity sensitive (primary) endings in muscle spindles as well as the more characteristic length sensitivity contributed by secondary endings (Matthews, 1972).

Lucier *et al.* (1975) came to a similar conclusion for PTNs (output cells) and non-PT cells in the forelimb area of the motor cortex of monkeys when they provided stretch of a muscle, sinusoidal changes in length and high-frequency vibration. PTNs were found to be sensitive to high-frequency (100 to 300 Hz) sinusoidal vibration of muscle tendons with low amplitudes of stretch (indicating an input from primary endings) and to respond to this stimulus with minimum latencies of the order of 20 ms. But the response was not a strong one in these anaesthetized animals and considerable variation in latency was evident (Fig. 6.6). The

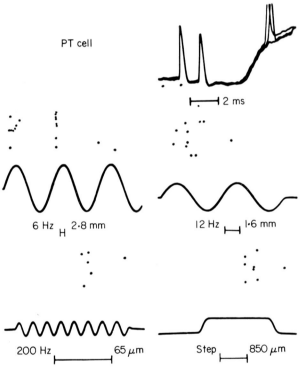

FIG. 6.6. Discharge pattern of a fast-conducting corticospinal (PT) neurone. Antidromic and late orthodromic responses (five-times superimposed) elicited by a pair of electrical stimuli at 1 ms interval (indicated by two dots) applied to the dorsolateral funiculus. Illustrated are only the responses to selected frequencies to show partial driving of the cell with 6 Hz sinusoidal stretching at high displacement amplitudes and lack of driving when the frequency was increased to 12 Hz. Note the conspicuous fall in minimal displacement amplitude as high-frequency vibration was used. The modulation of discharges with individual cycles of stretching and the short burst responses to vibration and step displacements were classified as 'dynamic' responses. Time calibrations for dot-rasters: 20 ms. (Lucier *et al.*, 1975.)

best site for detecting stretch-evoked responses in the motor cortex (from stretching extensor digitorum communis) was found to coincide with the area of lowest threshold for eliciting a twitch response of contralateral hand and finger extensors with surface anodal stimuli. But many cells, even within these limited input zones, did not respond to changes in muscle length.

This discussion has concentrated on the possible involvement of inputs from muscle receptors in producing the evoked responses which have been seen in the motor cortex when peripheral afferents have been stimulated. The conclusion must be that muscle afferents have access to the motor cortex. In addition, some convergence of cutaneous afferents on to cells in this area has been found. But technical difficulties have prevented an unequivocal answer being given by experiments of this sort to the question of contributions of inputs from tendon receptors or from joints.

6.4.3 TOPOGRAPHICAL RELATIONS BETWEEN INPUTS AND OUTPUTS

6.4.3.1 *Experiments on untrained, tranquillized monkeys*

The input regions appear to be ones which, when stimulated, produce outputs to muscles affecting the input zones. This general proposition has been examined in detail by Rosén and Asanuma (1972) for individual neurones in the forelimb area of the monkey's motor cortex. These authors used 'tranquillized' cebus monkeys, kept quiet by repeated injections of small doses of barbiturates but capable of moving and accepting food and juice as the tranquillizing effect of each dose wore off. They studied the afferent inputs to cells in the hand area of the motor cortex and classified these inputs as superficial (to S-cell neurones) if the cell responded to hair bending, light touch or light pressure. The inputs were regarded as coming from deep receptors (to D cells) if the cells responded to passive joint movements and/or pressure on deep structures. Only 45 per cent of the 192 cells studied in this work could be influenced by the peripheral stimuli used, which appeared to be confined to the hand and forearm. This was in spite of the fact that cells uninfluenced from the periphery (undriven cells) could show 'large modulations of discharge frequency' when the animal moved the forelimb spontaneously, in a manner similar to the modulations observed in adjacent cells whose afferent input could be found and classified. More of the influenced cells were affected by stimulation of deep receptors (50 cells) than by activation of superficial receptors (30 cells) and only 7 cells were affected by both. With the exception of one cell, all the influenced cells were excited.

The neurones whose afferent input zones were examined were all at or close to sites where weak intracortical microstimulation (ICMS) produced motor effects of the fingers, hand or wrist. All the afferent input zones were found to be related to these motor effects. For example, Fig. 6.7 (their Fig. 2) indicates that the afferent input zones of cells located in penetrations where either flexion, extension, adduction or abduction of the thumb were produced by stimulation, were disposed on the thumb in characteristic places. 'The receptive fields of S-cells found in the different columns illustrated the characteristic localization. Two cells found in the "thumb flexion column" were both activated from the ventral aspect of the thumb. The cells found in the columns for thumb extension, adduction and abduction were activated from the distal tip, the medial aspect, and the lateral aspect of the thumb, respectively. The D-cells found in this area were all activated by passive thumb movements or thenar pressure.'

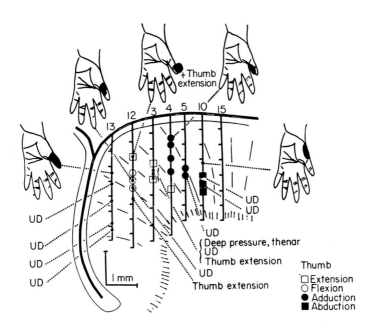

FIG. 6.7. Reconstruction of electrode tracks and cell locations. From an experiment in which several electrode penetrations (solid lines, identified by numbers) passed through efferent zones projecting to various thumb muscles (same experiment as illustrated in Figs 5.23 and 5.24).

The peripheral motor effects produced by ICMS (<5 μA) are indicated by symbols explained in the Figure. Cortical spots stimulated with 5 μA without evoking motor effects are shown by small solid lines perpendicular to the lines indicating tracks. Positions of cells encountered are indicated by dots and connected with dotted lines to descriptions of receptive fields and adequate stimuli. (Rosén and Asanuma, 1972.)

Note that the afferent input zones illustrated in this Figure are strikingly smaller than the wider receptive territories described by Brooks et al. (1961a,b), Welt et al. (1967) and Asanuma et al. (1968) in the cat. The illustration above relates principally to receptive fields on the skin from which activation of S-cells was obtained. The D cells (thoes cortical neurones influenced by deep stimuli) found in this area 'were all activated by passive thumb movements or thenar pressure'.

The nature of the superficial receptors which could influence cells in the hand area of the motor cortex in these monkeys deserves comment. Only one cell could be activated by hair bending and the majority responded with a rapidly adapting effect to touch or light pressure on glabrous skin of the hand. 'Each of the efferent zones described above received tactile input exclusively from that side of the finger or hand which was in the direction of the movement produced by ICMS.' However, this did not apply to regions which, when stimulated, produced extension of the digits. Only two S-cells were found in these zones and these responded to light touch on the tip of the thumb. 'No S-cells were found in zones projecting to the extensor muscles of the other fingers.'

The majority of the cells which responded to stimulation of deep receptors were affected by passive joint movement and most of these were driven from the joint involved in the motor effect caused by ICMS. Often, the cells influenced by joint movement could not also be driven by pressure on muscles; the conclusion then was that activation of joint receptors alone had caused the effects. Other cells were driven by pressure on muscles stretched by the joint movement which influenced the cells; these were considered to be affected by muscle afferents. A smaller proportion of cells was activated by joint movement and by pressure on muscles which would not have been stretched by the effective joint movement. Alternatively, a few cells were influenced by movement of joints in a direction opposite to that produced by ICMS. But, in general, it was concluded that the afferent input from deep receptors came from the muscle and joint activated by the movement caused by ICMS.

As a part of these same experiments, Rosén and Asanuma stimulated groups of afferent fibres in forelimb nerves and recorded evoked potentials in the depths of the cortex. They demonstrated again that the responses evoked in the motor cortex by 'cutaneous and group II deep afferents' were independent of projections to the postcentral gyrus from these peripheral nerves because cooling of the postcentral gyrus, which they reported to abolish local postcentral responses, left unchanged the latency and amplitude of precentral evoked potentials.

In these experiments it was not known whether the cells from which recordings were made were the same as the structures which were activated by the intracortical stimulus. In terms of defining local cortical territories for input–output connexions this may not have been important since both the units recorded and the structures stimulated must have been closely associated anatomically. But it could not be said that either the recordings or the stimulations were of output units (cells were not identified as corticospinal neurones); so the microstructure of the input–output organization revealed in these experiments still remains unknown. It is possible that the ICMS activated input structures (see Chapter 5) in which case the discussion of these important findings might most profitably and correctly relate to receiving (input) functions of the motor cortex alone.

6.4.3.2   *Inputs to output neurones in trained, alert monkeys*

The use of even small doses of anaesthetic agents could have modified the recordings made in these studies on tranquillized monkeys. It is clear that the results obtained in experiments of this sort depend to some degree on the use of general anaesthetic agents and on the particular agents employed. Rosén and Asanuma report that they did not find the wide-field receiving neurones in tranquillized monkeys which are often reported for chloralose anaesthetized cats (see earlier, section 6.2). But they also found a much lower proportion of motor cortex cells with responses to afferent input than had been reported by Fetz and Baker (1969). These latter authors indicated that 85 per cent of a sample of 233 single neurones recorded in the leg area of the motor cortex of unanaesthetized, free-to-move monkeys received a clear and reproducible input from passive movement of one or more joints of the contralateral leg. A smaller, additional number of cells received an input from skin receptors and very few cells were not influenced by peripheral stimuli. In a later study, Fetz *et al.* (1974) also found a high proportion of cells in the arm motor area to be in receipt of inputs from joint movement (75 per cent) or cutaneous stimulation (8 per cent).

But in asking questions about the relationships of input to output for the motor areas of the cerebral cortex, it may still be most fruitful to start with the output cells rather than with afferent projections (see above, section 6.1). Because of uncertainties in identifying output neurones by ICMS (Chapter 5), the alternative method of identifying outputs by their antidromic responses to PT stimulation and then examining their responses to afferent input would seem to offer some advantages. Moreover, if these observations can be made in conscious monkeys capable of performing natural movements, the relationship of output activity to movement performance can be examined and decisions can be taken about the particular movement with which the cell's firing is most clearly associated *before* the afferent input is studied and without the problems associated with the administration of general anaesthetics. Such an experimental procedure has been used by Lemon *et al.* (1976). It allowed responses to afferent input to be studied for neurones whose characteristic discharges occurred with active movements of proximal joints as well as for neurones whose discharges were related to active finger and hand movements. Proximal joint movements are not a prominent feature of the responses produced by ICMS and were not studied in the work of Rosén and Asanuma.

With a fully conscious monkey, testing of responses to afferent input by passive manipulation of a limb requires cooperation of the animal. These experiments were only possible after prolonged training (using food rewards) during which the animal was taught to relax while the joints of the hand and arm were moved through their full range and while natural stimuli were delivered repeatedly. That the animal was relaxed during these procedures could be assessed by the examiner; but it was also checked by continuous monitoring of EMGs from representative flexor and extensor muscles of the arm being studied.

Evaluation of the active movement with which a PTN's natural discharge is clearly associated is also a difficult and time-consuming process. But it is possible, by requiring a monkey to perform a large number of different but reproducible arm movements, to say whether the characteristic discharge is clearly locked to activity at the shoulder, elbow, wrist or fingers and then to specify the direction of the movement with which the greatest discharge is associated. More will be said in Chapter 7 of the relationships of PT cell activity to motor output. But here it is necessary to indicate the method of assessment of the 'clinical' association of some cell's activity with particular active movements at particular joints of the arm.

Monkeys were taught to reach out and pull towards themselves the small knob on the end of a horizontal lever. The lever had to be pulled into a target zone against a spring (there were no stops) and successful achievement of this displacement was indicated by an auditory cue and the presentation of a food reward. The lever movement could be used as a time reference for analysis of the relationship of neuronal discharges to the arm movements associated with lever pulling and also to the subsequent movements of the arm involved in collection of food rewards presented in different positions in space. The monkey's reach and grasp for a 'high' food reward presented immediately in front of and high above his head required protraction of the shoulder combined with roughly a right-angle flexion of the elbow, for example. Presentation of successive rewards at the same position in space allowed many repetitions of the movement of the hand to and from this place. A similar protraction of the shoulder could then be combined with almost full extension of the elbow by requiring the animal to collect food rewards from 'far' presentation in which the arm had to be stretched out to its maximum directly in front of the animal (Fig. 6.8). Discharge of cells related to the shoulder protraction should be similar for both these movements; discharges related to elbow extension should be greater for the latter than the former.

Figure 6.8 shows the range of movements of the shoulder and elbow which could be produced by presenting food rewards after they were earned by lever pulling, at four different positions: high (above the animal's head but in front of it), middle (at the position of the knob on the lever, in front of the animal), close (almost alongside the animal's chest) and far (at the maximum extent of the animal's forward reach). The measurements were made, frame by frame, from moving film of the performances of one animal. They show the very reproducible movement involved in displacing the lever and the dissociation of elbow and shoulder movements which could be achieved by food presentation in the different positions.

When these manoeuvres were combined with additional ones to require the monkey to abduct or adduct the pronated wrist to collect food placed

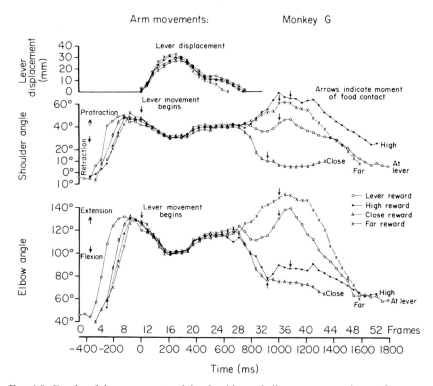

FIG. 6.8. Graphs of the movements of the shoulder and elbow accompanying performance by a monkey of the lever-pulling task and also collection of food rewards from a number of positions. All the graphs are aligned with respect to the beginning of movement of the lever (at time 0). Measurements of lever position and of shoulder and elbow angle were made using frame-by-frame analysis of movie film in many repetitions of performances of these movements. The graphs are representative examples of the performances for each of four different food collection positions: high (above the animal's head and slightly in front), lever (at the position of the knob on the lever), close (near the animal's chest and directly in front of him) and far (requiring maximum extension of the arm to reach the reward). The reproducibility of the displacements of shoulder and elbow accompanying the stereotyped displacement of the lever is indicated by the coincidence of the four lines during the whole of 600 to 700 ms beginning just before and continuing through the period of the lever pull. After this time, a series of combinations of shoulder protraction or retraction with elbow flexion or extension could be achieved about 1 s after the beginning of movement of the lever by presenting the food reward in different positions. The moment of contact of the hand with the food reward is indicated by the arrows about 1 s after the beginning of lever displacement. (Lemon et al., 1976.)

to the right or left in front of him, to collect the food from above or below with wrist pronated or supinated, from the far side or the near side of a barrier with the wrist flexed or extended, it will be seen that a given shoulder and elbow movement could be combined with a variety of wrist displacements. Finally, the need to extend a single finger (the index)

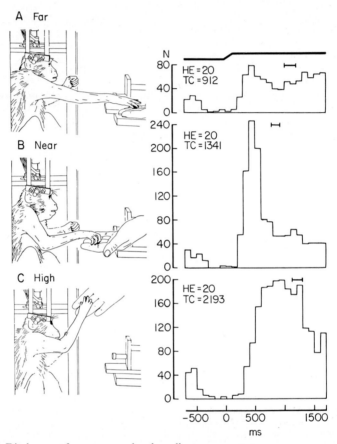

FIG. 6.9. Discharges of a neurone related to elbow movements.

The activity of this neurone is shown during movement to three different positions of the reward. When the food was presented in the far position (A) the shoulder was protracted and elbow extended. The activity associated with this movement is indicated by the upper histogram on the right; the horizontal bar above the histogram represents the variation in the time interval between the beginning of lever movement (at 0 ms) and the moment of contact with the food reward. In B, with the food in the near position, the shoulder was partially retracted and the elbow flexed. Rapid withdrawal of the arm from the lever prior to food collection was always associated with a brisk discharge of the cell. In C, the shoulder was protracted (as in A) but the elbow was still flexed (as in B), and there was a long-lasting discharge of the neurone associated with the prolonged holding of the arm in this position (note that the food was collected later in C than in B). (Lemon et al., 1976.)

while keeping all the others flexed in retrieving food from a small hole in a board allowed flexion and extension of this digit, combined with opposition of it to the thumb, to be examined separately from the flexion of all digits in concert which is used to collect food rewards from a flat surface.

The 'clinical' evaluation of the active movement with which a given PTN's discharges were associated was time-consuming and recordings had to be made from individual neurones for long periods, but it allowed a large number of cells to be classified according to the movement with which the characteristic discharge was most clearly associated. A typical example is shown in Fig. 6.9 of a unit whose discharges were clearly related to active movements of the elbow. When the food was presented in the 'far' position (A), the shoulder was protracted and the elbow extended. The activity associated with this movement is indicated by the upper histogram on the right. In B, with the food in the 'near' position, the shoulder was partially retracted and the elbow flexed. Rapid withdrawal of the arm from the lever prior to food collection in this position was always associated with a brisk discharge of the cell. In C, the shoulder was protracted (as in A) but the elbow was still flexed (as in B), and there was a long-lasting discharge of the neurone associated with the prolonged holding of the arm in this position. The food was collected much later in C than in B.

The responses of a unit discharging only during movements involving protraction of the shoulder joint are indicated in Fig. 6.10. Here the protraction needed to collect a high reward was associated with a much more intense discharge (left-hand histogram) than the retraction needed to collect a near reward (right-hand histogram) even though the elbow angle was similar in both cases. Finally, the very much more intense activity of a cell associated with individual finger movement, rather than with whole hand flexion for collection of food is indicated in Fig. 6.11.

These few examples serve to indicate how the relationship of neuronal activity to movement performance was evaluated. If the cell could be identified as a PTN, it was an output neurone and its afferent input could be analysed.

Some general comments about the afferent inputs as defined by Lemon and Porter (1976) for movement-related precentral neurones in conscious monkeys must be made because they relate to the work already described. Each cell had to be studied for a prolonged period, never for less than 10 minutes and usually for up to an hour. All joints were moved through their normal range a number of times and the effects of static position of the joint and movement in each direction were tested repeatedly. During the movements of one joint, the others were held in a stationary position. Hair bending, light touch and deep pressure were applied to the skin of both arms, trunk and face with a variety of probes and light brushes. Tapping, prodding and squeezing muscles, tendons and joints through the skin

while joints were held stationary were also tested. In a few cases the animal
allowed a small hand-held vibrator to be applied over muscle bellies, but
this test was usually resisted by animals. Noxious stimuli were not used.
All details of the responses to this variety of stimuli were mapped on to a

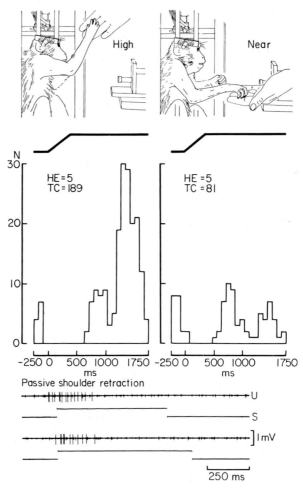

FIG. 6.10. Responses of a neurone related to active and passive shoulder movements.
   This cell discharged maximally only during movements involving protraction of the
shoulder joint, for instance, when the monkey collected high rewards, as shown in the
diagram at the top left of the Figure. The histogram for cell activity during five high
reward collections is shown on the left. On the right is the histogram for collection of
five rewards placed close to the animal (near rewards) requiring retraction of the shoulder
joint. Much less activity was associated with this movement. At the bottom of the figure
are records showing the response of this neurone (U) to passive shoulder retraction.
Approximate indication of the onset and duration of this movement is given by the step
in the signal pulse (S). (Lemon et al., 1976.)

chart of the animal's body, and recorded on a multichannel tape recorder with a voice commentary and indicators of the approximate timing of each joint movement, muscle tap, etc. Throughout the whole period, the animal was rewarded for remaining relaxed by being given food to collect with the other hand.

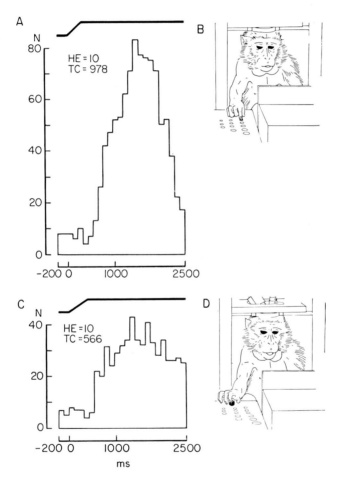

FIG. 6.11. Neuronal activity during different types of finger movement.
   The cell was strongly associated with active finger movements. When the monkey collected the reward from a small food-well (B) which task required independent movements of the thumb and particularly the index finger, with the other digits flexed out of the way, there was a very strong discharge before and during the collection of the food (histogram in A). Discharge frequency fell off rapidly once the animal had finished manipulating the food (about 2 s after the lever movement) and placed the food in his mouth. When the monkey collected the food from a flat surface (D), employing all of his digits in a more general movement of the hand, far less discharge was observed (histogram in C). (Lemon *et al.*, 1976.)

In the description of the effects of afferent inputs, the term 'receptive field' for the territory from within which these effects could be produced has been reserved for territories on the surface of the body. Here its use is in line with the common practice of physiologists who study sensation. A great deal is known about the receptor populations which are activated by stimulation of receptive fields on the skin. But many of the inputs studied by Lemon and Porter involved manipulation of joints. The domains within which the receptors could be located were deep and could be in

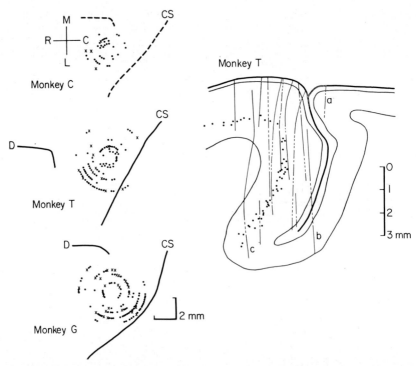

FIG. 6.12. On the left is shown the surface topography of electrode penetrations made in three monkeys (C, T and G). Successful penetrations in which cells with no apparent afferent input were encountered are marked by a cross. The positions of penetrations have been plotted in relation to the central sulcus (CS) and dimple (D). Approximate positions only (dotted lines) are shown for monkey C. (R, rostral; M, medial; C, caudal and L, lateral).

On the right is a parasagittal section through the region of the central sulcus in one monkey (T) showing some of the identified electrode tracks and all of the tracks in this 1 mm slab of cortex. The illustration is made up by superimposing 40, 25 μm thick serial sections and the solid lines show the segments of electrode tracks visualized in these sections. The dots represent the position of some of the Betz cells. Examples of tracks from penetrations directly into the postcentral gyrus (a) and penetrating the post-central gyrus in the depth of the sulcus (b) and tracks reaching the bottom of the anterior bank of the sulcus (c) are shown. The scale has been adjusted to allow for tissue shrinkage during preparation and refers to the depth during life. (Lemon and Porter, 1976.)

the joints, in muscles or their tendons or in other deep structures (e.g. fascia) disturbed by joint movement. We cannot give an accurate account of the territory affected or the receptor populations within it which are influenced. Hence we have not called the charts made of these influences maps of receptive fields. They may have nothing to do with sensation and we have preferred the term 'afferent input zone' for these inaccurately defined regions and our inadequate knowledge of their receptive properties.

At the end of the experiment, the location of the cell from which recordings has been made was charted approximately by histological reconstruction of electrode tracks and micrometer measurements made during the recording period. These locations must be subject to more error than those mapped in acute experiments because only electrical indicators of initial contact of the electrode with the surface of the cortex exist. Even so, estimates of depth of the cortical grey matter made in each electrode track during the experiment correlated well with the thickness of the cortex at these sites measured histologically. Both confirmed that many electrode tracks had penetrated the full depth of the anterior bank of the central sulcus and that cells in this zone, possibly those involved in the output to most accessible muscles (Chapters 2, 4 and 5) had been sampled (Fig. 6.12).

Of 359 cells studied in the precentral 'arm area' of three monkeys, only 257 were fully investigated with regard both to their afferent input and their activity during voluntary movements. (Often cells were 'lost' before the prolonged study of them had been completed.) Only 51 of the fully studied cells were identified PTNs. We shall describe some of the general features of the examination of the whole population of cells and then focus on the special characteristics of the PTNs.

Lemon and Porter (1976) emphasized that many cells would respond at first to an 'arousal' stimulus such as brushing hairs anywhere on the contralateral arm. But this was not a reproducible response and frequently it was accompanied by general movement and EMG activity or restlessness (alerting) of the animal. This arousal response could well have been due to the active movement of the animal, since all the neurones being studied were ones whose discharges were modulated during voluntary movement.

In contrast, the responses obtained by natural stimuli within afferent input zones were highly reproducible, were obtained during periods of complete EMG quiescence, were quite specific to particular stimuli delivered at particular places and showed a close temporal relationship between stimulus and response.

Afferent input zones for individual neurones were found in all parts of the arm, as indicated in Table 6.1. The numbers in brackets refer to the number of PT neurones recorded in two animals expressed as a fraction of the total number of cells with these input zones sampled in the same cortical area of the same two animals. These figures indicate that PT cells could have afferent territories in either proximal or distal parts of the contralateral limb.

TABLE 6.1

Distribution of afferent input zones for movement-related precentral neurones

Principal location of input zone	Number of neurones	PT
Shoulder	19	(5/14)
Elbow	71	(19/48)
Wrist	61	(7/29)
Hand	14	(1/12)
Fingers	37	(10/29)
Thumb	12	(1/4)
No apparent input	43	(8/31)
TOTAL	257	(51/167)

The 43 cells which had no apparent input were tested over a long period. They could have been in receipt of subthreshold influences from the natural stimuli used or they could have been weakly inhibited and this influence could have gone undetected. Alternatively, their afferent input zone might have been outside the region tested. With these qualifications, they have been regarded as having no *apparent* afferent input.

The most common adequate stimulus was joint movement and 190 cells (74 per cent of the sample) responded to joint movement, either alone or in combination with other procedures. The input zone could be very small, limited to a single joint on a digit. Figure 6.13 shows the reproducible responses of a precentral neurone to five successive applications of flexion to a single joint, the metacarpo-phalangeal joint of the middle finger. No response was obtained to movement of adjacent joints on the same finger or to other directions of movement at this joint. Ninety-eight cells responded to a single movement at a single joint, a further 12 to more than one movement at the same joint (for instance, shoulder retraction and abduction) and 42 cells responded to movement at two or more joints. The afferent input zone for this last category could still be small, since some of these cells responded to movement of two joints on the same finger.

Neurones responding to joint movement usually responded to movement only in one direction: movement in the opposite direction either had no effect or, in some tonically active cells, produced inhibition. Only three cells responded to movement of one joint in both directions; for other cells apparently showing bidirectional effects, the response in one direction was often associated with EMG activity and this response disappeared when the animal was relaxed. The responses were usually to joint *movement* rather than to joint position and the cells ceased firing when the joint came to rest in its new position (167 of 190 cells responded in this way). Joints were moved at speeds varying from 10° to 50° per second and these were well within the range of speeds observed during voluntary movement (see Fig. 6.8). There were, however, 23 cells which all received inputs from the wrist, elbow or shoulder, and showed a maintained change in firing rate for a maintained joint position—usually at the extreme end of the range of movement of that joint (Fig. 6.13C).

For cells responding only to joint movement, 135 of 152 responded to movement through a wide angle (greater than 50°) like that illustrated in Fig. 6.14A–C. The remaining 17 cells responded to movement through relatively small angles. These cells all received inputs from the shoulder or elbow and the smallest range of movement to which a cell would respond

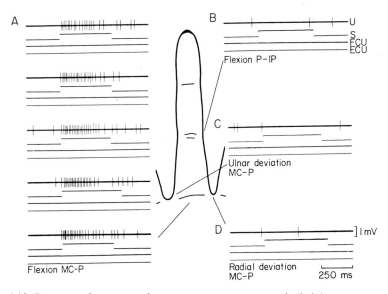

FIG. 6.13. Response of a precentral neurone to movement at a single joint.
    This neurone responded only to flexion of the metacarpo-phalangeal joint (MC-P) of the middle finger. For each set of recordings the signal marker (S) gives an *approximate* indication of the onset (upward) and end (downward deflection) of natural stimulation after which time the joint was held in its flexed position. Records from this cell (U) shows a reproducible discharge pattern for each of the five successive flexions shown in A. The EMG traces (bottom two lines of each set) show no activity and indicate the relaxed state of the animal. B, flexion of the proximal interphalangeal joint (P-IP), C, ulnar, and D, radial deviation of MC-P joint, were all ineffective stimuli for this neurone. In this Figure ECU and FCU are EMG recordings from extensor carpi ulnaris and flexor carpi ulnaris. (Lemon and Porter, 1976.)

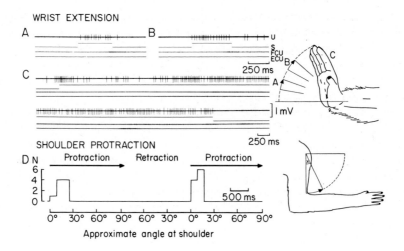

FIG. 6.14. Responses of precentral neurones to joint movement.

A, B. Records showing a neurone responding to extension of the wrist joint through a wide angle. The cell discharged when the joint was moved anywhere in the range from a flat position of the wrist to full extension. Responses are illustrated to movement through the two segments (A and B) illustrated in the diagram on the right. Cell discharge fell off rapidly once movement ceased. When the wrist was maintained at full extension tonic discharge of the cell was observed. The two sets of recordings at C are continuous. The elevations of the signal marker (S) in A and B indicate the approximate duration of the movements indicated in the diagram to the right of the records. During the elevation of the signal marker in the two parts of the continuous record, C, the joint was held in the extended position. The fact that the discharge apparently begins before movement to C is an artefact caused by the fact that the experimenter operated the signal marker and the joint movement separately. Note difference in time scales and quiescence of the EMG recordings. D. Response of another neurone to protraction of the shoulder joint, as illustrated on the right. The cell only fired when the joint was moved through a small angle (x) of approximately 30°. The number (N) of discharges recorded during a cycle of protraction, retraction and then protraction again are shown plotted against the angular movement of the shoulder. Note the lack of response during the retraction phase. (Lemon and Porter, 1976.)

was about 20°. The cell illustrated in Fig. 6.14D, responded to passive protraction of the shoulder through 15° to 30°. No response was obtained when the joint was moved in the opposite direction (retraction).

The responsiveness of any one neurone to joint movement could be affected by the position of other joints, movements of which did not themselves affect the neurone. The majority of cells responding to joint movement could not also be influenced by prodding, tapping or squeezing related or adjacent muscles or by tapping tendons. They were also unaffected by cutaneous inputs. Tapping the appropriate joint caused responses in some cells but the effect was less marked than for joint movement.

Joint movement is, of course, an effective stimulus for muscle receptors. But, if muscle receptors were the source of the clear definite effects recorded in response to joint movement, the finding that a single movement at one joint (particularly of the fingers) caused this response, must indicate a projection from receptors localized in a small group of muscles affected by that movement at that joint.

That joint receptors may also be involved requires to be examined critically because of the fact that the responses were usually to movement in one direction and that the most powerful effects occurred at the extremes of joint movement. We do not know how joint receptors in the monkey's forelimb behave during movement. But studies by Burgess and Clark (1969) and Skoglund (1956) on knee joint receptors in the cat indicate that these are very active at the extremes of joint movement, with little activity in response to intermediate angles. Moreover, the responses of knee joint afferents in the cat are strongly influenced by the attitude of other joints in the limb: a common finding also for the responses of precentral neurones in the monkey to joint movement.

Joint receptors themselves could help to explain the input, for a majority of cells, from only a single joint. But, again from the observations on cat knee joint receptors (Burgess and Clark, 1969) joint receptors would not account for the directional sensitivity of the influenced neurones or for the responses of some of them to movement through small angles.

Continuing the examination of the work of Lemon and Porter (1976) we can turn to the second most common form of response in precentral neurones: 35 cells (13.6 per cent of the responding population) were influenced by muscle palpation, including 26 which were also driven by joint movement. None of these cells was recorded at a depth sufficient for it to be located in area 3a. The best stimulus for each of the 25 cells was a brief tap to a local region of a muscle belly which usually evoked a small burst of discharges. The area over which such a stimulus was effective was small (less than 2 cm²) and usually arranged in an elliptiform shape with its long axis along the length of the muscle belly. Squeezing the muscle belly with maintained pressure was only effective for four cells. Nine cells responded to muscle palpation but failed to respond to any movements of related joints.

The most common finding (for 21 of 26 neurones which responded to muscle palpation and joint movement) is indicated in Fig. 6.15. Tapping a localized site over the surface of flexor carpi ulnaris (Fig. 6.15A) caused a brief burst of discharges of the cell. Rapid extension of the wrist, stretching this muscle, produced an increase in the firing of the cell which then adapted rapidly (Fig. 6.15B). When the wrist was rapidly extended at (1), and then rapidly flexed at (2), to stretch and then shorten the muscle, shortening was followed by a distinct pause in the discharge (Fig. 6.15C).

It was usually the case that a neurone responding to tapping and stretching of a muscle in this way was most active during voluntary movements when that muscle was actively contracted. Figure 6.15D shows that the cell illustrated here discharged most intensely when the animal flexed the ulnar-deviated wrist to obtain a food reward (after pulling the lever). The intense discharge during food collection in this case was associated with pronounced EMG activity in flexor carpi ulnaris. The remaining 5 of 26 neurones responding to muscle tap and to joint movement discharged with joint movement in a direction which would have *shortened* the muscle to which tapping was an effective stimulus.

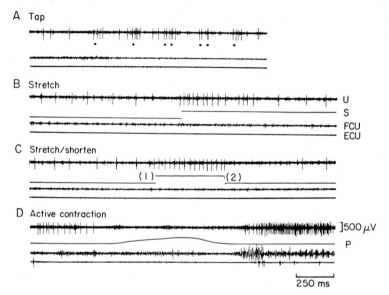

FIG. 6.15. Responses of a precentral neurone to muscle palpation and joint movement.

A shows the neurone responding to brief taps applied to the belly of FCU. The dots on the record represent the *approximate* times at which the taps were applied. B. FCU was stretched by extension of the wrist joint (as indicated by the upward deflection in S). This produced a burst of discharges which rapidly adapted when the wrist was kept in the same position. C. The wrist was rapidly extended at (1) and extension maintained until (2) when the wrist was rapidly flexed. This flexion produced a pause in the cell's discharge. D. When the monkey actively flexed the wrist (as indicated by the burst of activity in the EMG recording of FCU) after pulling the lever (lever position indicated by trace P) there was an intense discharge of this cell. (Lemon and Porter, 1976.)

For six cells responding to muscle palpation, the head of a small vibrator was pressed into the muscle belly at the point where tapping had proved effective and vibration at 100 and 300 Hz was then tested. Vibration at 100 Hz (with undamped displacements of the probe through 0.5 to 1 mm) was effective in increasing the discharge of all six cells, but 300 Hz affected only two. There was a general increase in discharge frequency of the units, particularly at the onset of vibration, but no evidence of entrainment to the vibrator frequency.

In the experiments of Lemon and Porter (1976) only 27 cells (10.5 per cent of the population) responded to cutaneous stimulation. Light touch was the optimal stimulus for 15 cells, deep pressure for 4 and hair movement for 8 cells. The responses were always very transient. All the cutaneous fields with the exception of one were confined to the hand; the exception was a cell with a 'stocking' field for hair movement over the entire surface of the arm. But most cutaneous receptive fields were small; 22 cells had fields of less than 5 cm² in area.

Only 15 of the cells had a purely cutaneous field, the remaining 12 had fields associated with joint movement and there was usually a close relationship between the two inputs. The cell illustrated in Fig. 6.16A–D, for example, had a small skin field on the ventral surface of the tip of the thumb; it also responded to flexion of the interphalangeal and metacarpo-phalangeal joints of the thumb.

6.4.3.3 *Oligosynaptic nature of inputs*

The nature of the stimuli which were effective in influencing precentral neurones made it very difficult to calculate latencies for the responses of most of them. But for 14 cells responding to light touch and for 11 cells responding to muscle taps it was possible to carry out the stimulation with a light probe carrying a small piezoelectric device. Fifty to 100 stimuli were delivered and the responses measured by hand from filmed records of the unit's discharges and the simultaneous output from the probe which indicated first contact with the tissue. The responses of a PTN to brief light taps applied in a localized spot over the belly of biceps brachii are illustrated in Fig. 6.17A–C. The peristimulus time histogram for this cell, made up of the responses to 50 such muscle taps, is shown in Fig. 6.17E. The latency at the $p < 0.001$ level was 6.0 ms for this PTN's responses to muscle taps, and was the shortest latency found in this sample. The latency distributions for skin inputs and muscle inputs to the other neurones which could be studied in this way are indicated in Fig. 6.17F, G. Nineteen of 25 cells responded with latencies of less than 20 ms and 8 cells responded in less than 10 ms, including three identified PTNs. This short latency is consistent with the findings of Devanandan and Heath (1975) for some precentral neurones responding to shocks in forelimb nerves.

This general survey of afferent input zones may be compared with observations made by others and continues to emphasize the predominant projections from deep receptors to precentral neurones. But it further stresses that the inputs for particular cells arise from very limited peripheral territories, whether in joints, muscle or skin and that the inputs from muscle and skin are capable of affecting precentral neurones, including PTNs, after a very brief latency.

No precise information exists about the pathways over which these inputs from peripheral receptors reach precentral neurones in monkeys. The localized peripheral territories, the short latencies and the clearly characterized responses would appear to suggest a direct spino-thalamo-cortical projection similar to the ones which direct precise responses from

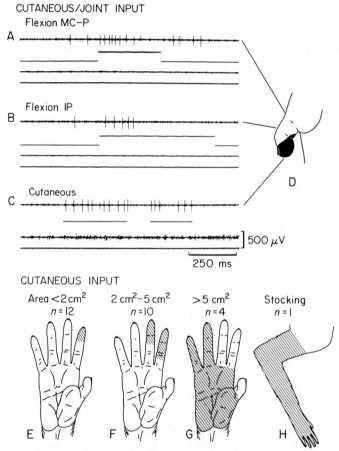

FIG. 6.16. Cutaneous inputs to precentral neurones.

A–D illustrate a neurone with an afferent input zone on the thumb. Adequate stimuli for this neurone included flexion of the metacarpo-phalangeal (MC-P) and interphalangeal (IP) joints of the thumb, and light touch over the black area shown in D. Responses to these three stimuli are shown in A, B and C respectively.

E–H show the distribution of cutaneous fields for 27 precentral neurones responding to tactile cutaneous stimulation. Receptive fields were classed according to area, and an example of a field in each category is shown by the hatched area. The stocking field in H included the entire hairy surface of the right arm and was exceptional. (Lemon and Porter, 1976.)

receptors to the sensory receiving cortex (Mountcastle and Powell, 1959). Indeed, the somatic sensory cortex (S1) sends axons into area 4 and could be a source of the inputs we have described. Against this is the apparent preservation of precentral evoked potentials from stimulation of deep and

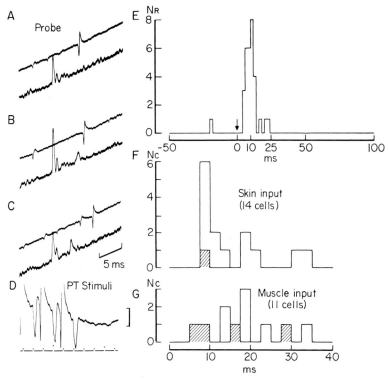

FIG. 6.17. Latency of neuronal responses to peripheral stimuli.

A, B and C are from filmed records of a PT neurone (the largest deflection in the upper trace of each pair) that responded to light taps applied to the belly of the biceps muscle with a blunt probe. The records have been filmed with R-C coupling and the waveform of the action potentials has been differentiated. The moment of application of the tap to the muscle belly is indicated by the sharp upward deflection in the rectified output signal from a piezoelectric device mounted at the tip of the probe (the peak of this signal represents an indentation of the order of 0.25 mm). D illustrates the responses of the same cell to high-frequency stimulation (500 Hz) of the medullary pyramid with three shocks of 420 μA each. The shape of the action potentials is more monophasic because this record is undifferentiated and made with direct coupling to the amplifier. The stimulus artefacts are large and complex and the sweep is triggered by the first of three stimulus artefacts. Time scale 1 and 5 ms. Voltage calibration 500 μV for A to C, 300 μV for D. E shows the peristimulus time histogram for this same cell for 50 taps applied to biceps muscle. Cell discharges occurring 50 ms before and 100 ms after the tap stimulus have been placed in 2 ms bins. F and G show the distribution of latencies at the $p < 0.001$ confidence limit for cells responding to light touch applied to a cutaneous field (F) and taps to muscle bellies (G). Latencies of PT cells are shown in hatched shading. (Lemon and Porter, 1976.)

superficial peripheral afferents after removal of postcentral cortex (Malis et al., 1953). But the proposition deserves thorough study of responses of individual precentral neurones and the examination of their afferent inputs in the absence of postcentral cortex.

Responses in area 3a have been reported to be abolished upon section of the dorsal columns (Phillips et al., 1971). But the afferent input to neurones in area 4 has not been studied under these conditions. Moreover, it is clear from recent work that, in the monkey at least, spinothalamic tract neurones with their axons in the ventral white matter of the spinal cord are capable of transmitting precise information from localized tactile receptive fields and from receptors in deep tissues including muscle (Willis et al., 1974; Applebaum et al., 1975). A proportion of these spinothalamic units responded to joint movement and a few had receptive fields in skin and were additionally influenced by deep receptors. The further projection of these ventral spinothalamic influences has not been investigated, but it could conceivably be through thalamocortical influences on area 4.

The sensory relay nucleus of the thalamus, VPL, has been regarded as projecting almost exclusively to somatic receiving cortex and the existence of a separate projection of part of it into area 4 did not at first attract attention (Strick, 1975). To our knowledge this zone has not been studied with microelectrode techniques to examine its possible role in the relay of afferent information to output structures in the motor cortex. But parts of the ventrolateral nucleus have been examined. This structure receives a very complicated series of inputs, partly from the cerebellum and partly from the basal ganglia, but also from the cerebral cortex itself, including area 4. Different cells or different regions of VL may have quite different connexions and functional significance. Kievit and Kuypers (1975: Fig. 6.4) and Strick (1975) have indicated that there is some topographical organization of the VL cells which provide their outputs to the arm or the leg motor area in the monkey.

Different workers may have studied different elements of VL. Evarts (1970) studied the discharges of VL neurones in relation to movement performance but made no comment on their responses to peripheral stimuli. The receptive fields of individual neurones in the ventrolateral nucleus of the cat were studied by Asanuma and Fernandez (1974, 1975) but no localized inputs from circumscribed limb territories were found in this species. Albe-Fessard and Bowsher (1960) had also indicated a lack of specific, topographically organized inputs to VL in the monkey anaesthetized with chloralose. Joffroy and Lamarre (1974) recorded the influences of peripheral stimuli on VL cells in the awake monkey. They noted that about half the cells located in the ventral part of the complex could be activated by sharp pressure on deep tissues or by taps on tendons or muscles in one or several limbs 'either contralateral or homolateral'.

Cells in the dorsal part of the nucleus did not respond to peripheral stimuli. The latency of some of the responses to sharp taps on muscle was found to be 15 to 20 ms and these cells also discharged naturally in advance of movement performance.

It is not clear how the zones from which recordings have been made in the ventrolateral nucleus of the monkey's thalamus relate to the areas of origin of thalamocortical projections to area 4 defined by Strick (1975). But the evidence so far does not make VL a prime candidate for transmitting the specific peripheral afferent influences referred to earlier in this section to neurones in area 4.

Single cell recordings have been made in the thalamus of patients undergoing stereotaxic surgery for Parkinson's disease. Jasper and Bertrand (1966) found that cells which they believed to be located in and around VL were not responsive to peripheral somatic stimulation or to passive movement of limbs. Albe-Fessard *et al.* (1967) also noted that the bursts of discharge of cells which accompanied tremor, and which were also believed to be located in VL, were not responses to peripheral stimuli. Donaldson (1973), however, has exposed the weakness of the topographical foundations on which all putative localizations of microelectrode placements in the human thalamus have had to be based.

It could be that other thalamic sites deserve attention as candidates for the transmission of specific, localized afferent inputs to neurones in area 4. As has been indicated already, VPL could deserve study, as could the intralaminar nucleus, CL, which has long been known to project upon area 4 in the monkey (confirmed by Kievit and Kuypers, 1975, and Strick, 1975). But this does not exclude VL from further consideration as a major contributor of input to the motor cortex. The task must be to examine precisely what functional contribution the cells in this complex region make.

Finally, it is necessary to examine appropriate cells in the cerebellum and its output nuclei to study how their inputs relate to the inputs of the motor cortex. It is not enough to remark that cerebellar ablation leaves intact the projections to the motor cortex which can be revealed by study of evoked potentials. The cerebellum may, perhaps, select or modulate specific input characteristics or direct them to particular and appropriate cells. Any such influences will be detected only by careful analysis and rigorous timing of the responses of cerebellar units to just those stimuli which are now known to influence neurones in area 4. To our knowledge no such careful studies, directed to particular regions of the topographically organized zones of the monkey's cerebellum, have been published. But some information relating to an involvement of projections through the cerebellum in modifying the responses of cortical cells to disturbances of movement performance will be mentioned in Chapter 7.

It must, of course, be self-evident that feedback about the performance of a movement can come from receptors other than those in the moving part. A prime influence in many motor tasks must be the input from vision. But it has been shown by Evarts and Tanji (1974) that the inputs from visual stimuli influence PTNs with much longer delays than the inputs from kinaesthetic stimuli which have commanded so much of our attention.

6.4.3.4 *Comparison of inputs to PTN and neighbouring intracortical neurones*

But we began this section by asking specifically about the afferent input zones of identified output neurones. As is the case in all studies of this sort (see Chapter 7) a disappointingly small proportion of the cells from which recordings are made can be so identified, but this may in part reflect the small proportion of cortical neurones which send their axons into the PT. Only 51 of the 257 cells fully investigated by Lemon and Porter (1976) were proven PTNs. These had axonal conduction velocities ranging from 30 to 70 ms^{-1}. These 51 PTNs can be compared with the 116 other neurones recorded in the same vicinities in the same animals. In general, the afferent input to the two populations was similar. But a number of differences, which could be important if they are confirmed to be representative of the inputs to PTNs in general, were revealed.

A greater proportion (20 per cent) of PTNs received their input from distal joints and the muscles acting about distal joints than did unidentified cells (12 per cent). There was more evidence of convergent inputs to PTNs than to other cells: more PTNs with cutaneous inputs had larger fields (>4 cm^2) than unidentified cells, and a greater proportion of PTNs (31 per cent) received inputs from two or more joints than did unidentified cells (12 per cent). This difference was also reflected in the fact that a smaller proportion of PTNs (33 per cent) received inputs from only one joint than did unidentified cells (48 per cent). The proportion of PTNs with no apparent afferent input was 16 per cent (8 of 51), while 20 per cent (23 of 116) of unidentified cells in the same regions were in this class.

6.4.4 CONCLUSIONS ON INPUT–OUTPUT ARRANGEMENTS

From studies of this sort it is possible to ask how the afferent input to the precentral gyrus is organized. Are projections from particular peripheral territories segregated and distributed exclusively to output neurones with particular destinations? Precise histological reconstruction of the position of each recording site is not feasible in experiments during which very large numbers of tracks are made over a period of several weeks and very large numbers of units are studied. But some general observations can be made with confidence.

Most cells in Lemon and Porter's study which responded to natural stimulation of the extremities (hand and digits) lay within the bank of the central sulcus and all cells with cutaneous receptive fields were found in this region. In general, the further away from the central sulcus a penetration was made, even though still within area 4 and still examining the convexity of the precentral gyrus, the higher was the proportion of cells with no detectable afferent input. For example, in one monkey 21 of 58 cells (36 per cent) recorded in tracks which entered the convexity of the gyrus had no apparent input, while only 8 per cent (6 of 71 cells) recorded in tracks which traversed the anterior bank of the sulcus were undriven.

If the afferent inputs of closely adjacent neurones, either those recorded simultaneously with a single electrode in a given track (which are presumed to be situated close together) or those recorded within 500 μm of one another in the same track and, therefore, capable of being well within the same or an immediately adjacent cortical efferent zone 1 mm in diameter (Asanuma and Rosén, 1972) were examined, some evidence about the anatomical organization of afferent inputs could be obtained. Of 18 pairs of neurones recorded at the same point or located close together (within 500 μm) in the same track, 11 pairs had closely related afferent input zones. Examples for pairs of simultaneously recorded neurones are shown in Fig. 6.18. For the pair of units recorded at B, one received a cutaneous input from the index finger and one from both index and middle fingers. The pair recorded at A had widely separated afferent input zones, flexion of the terminal joint of the index finger and protraction of the shoulder respectively.

Groups of three cells, all within 500 μm of one another and located in the same electrode track, were encountered on four occasions. Two of the groups contained cells all of which had the same afferent input zone (on the digits for one group, at the wrist for the other). In the other two groups, two of the cells had the same afferent input with the third receiving its afferent influences from an unrelated zone. One of the most interesting observations was made in one electrode track in which four responsive cells, each with a separate input, were encountered: the inputs to each of these cells came from the hand, fingers, wrist and elbow respectively. Therefore, although there is a general tendency for cells in a local region of cortex to receive inputs from a particular peripheral territory, these local regions of cortex also contain cells with quite distinct and separate afferent input zones. The very precise topographical segregation of inputs to separate cellular regions reported for the precentral cortex of tranquillized monkeys by Rosén and Asanuma (1972) was not seen in this later work on conscious monkeys where many more units responded to peripheral stimuli and where units with quite widely separated afferent inputs were found close together in the same restricted region of cortex.

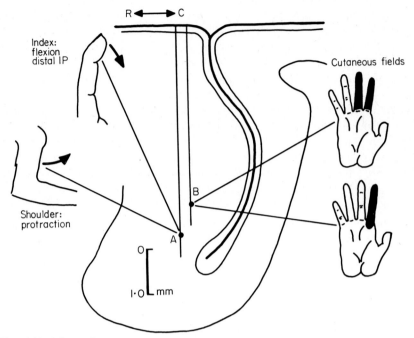

FIG. 6.18. Afferent input to simultaneously recorded precentral neurones

 Pairs of cells were recorded by the same electrode. Two tracks that yielded simultaneous records from cells pairs are shown diagrammatically. Of the pair recorded at A, one cell responded to passive flexion of the distal interphalangeal (IP) joint of the index finger, while the other responded to protraction of the shoulder joint. The pair of cells recorded at B had similar cutaneous fields (black areas) on the ventral surface of the right hand. (Lemon and Porter, 1976.)

 But it is still possible to investigate whether each input is precisely related to the apparent output function of the cell from which recordings are being made. In addition to the definition of the output pathway of the cell's axon (into the pyramidal tract), the relationship of the cell's discharge to particular directions of movement at particular joints has been studied (Lemon *et al.*, 1976). For most of the neurones examined, the relationships could not be said to specify anything about the output of the motor cortex because the cells from which the recordings were made were not identified as output neurones. For this large population, all of which could conceivably be the neurones which receive and process afferent information, comparison of the discharges during active movement with those defined by passive manipulation of the limb could reflect changes in the afferent *input pattern* caused by active versus passive production of the same displacement (see Fig. 6.19,1). But for some of the PT cells, the same comparison could reflect the anatomical organization of the input and output properties of those particular cells in relation to the production of particular movements (see Fig. 6.19,2). The method, therefore, deserves attention because of its potential ability to answer this fundamental question of input–output relationships at the level of individual cells. As yet the number of observations collected is very small and the conclusions must be tentative. But they indicate a point of departure for future work on this very challenging topic.

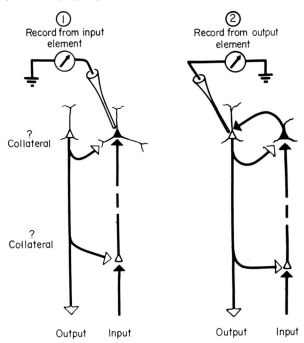

FIG. 6.19. Elements in the precentral cortex from which recordings could be made. 1. For an input receiving element collaterals of an output cell could determine the discharge during movement or could influence transmission from receptors during movement. In the second case, comparison between 'passive' and 'active' responses reveals the differences in transmission through the input pathway under the two conditions. 2. Discharges of output elements may be compared during active movement and during passive movement to detect the input–output organization of this cellular element.

The majority of neurones studied, whether PTNs or unidentified neurones, showed a strong relationship between their afferent input zone and the particular active movement with which their natural discharge was specifically associated. This strong relationship was considered to exist if the afferent input zone was completely confined within the area involved in the particular active movement with which that cell's discharges were associated. Of the proven output neurones (PTNs), 79 per cent exhibited such closely associated active–passive behaviour and this particular relationship was most clearly revealed for cells whose output and input were related to movements of the distal parts of the limb. (70 per cent of unidentified cells also had a strong active–passive relationship.) An example of a neurone with this strong relationship is shown in Fig. 6.20. Active and passive movements in the same direction at the one joint (in this case the wrist) were associated with discharges of the cell.

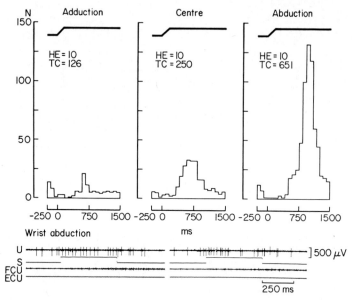

FIG. 6.20. Active and passive responses of a neurone related to wrist movements.
This Figure shows peri-response time histograms obtained for a neurone when the food reward was collected from three different positions. The monkey was required to place his arm through a perspex guide tube, which prevented large displacements of the arm from side to side. Food was placed to one side of the tube so that with the wrist in the pronated position, either *adduction* (radial deviation) or *abduction* (ulnar deviation) of the wrist was required to collect the reward. Rewards were also placed in the *centre* of the tube, and this required the pronated wrist to be held straight. The histograms show that this cell increased its activity when the wrist was progressively abducted for the reward. The records below the histograms show the response of the cell to two passive abductions of the wrist. The *approximate* timing of the beginning and end of the passive abduction movement is indicated by the elevation of the signal pulse (S). EMG records are from flexor carpi ulnaris (FCU) and extensor carpi ulnaris (ECU). (Lemon *et al.*, 1976.)

A very small number of cells exhibited discharge during active movements of either hand. These cells were exceptional because the vast majority of precentral units were related only to contralateral movements. But it is of some interest that these cells with a bilateral relationship to movement could also have bilateral afferent input zones confined within the regions moved during the characteristic active responses (usually in the hand and fingers). A similar finding in man was reported by Goldring and Ratcheson (1972).

For other neurones, the afferent input zone included the joint moved during the characteristic active discharge of the cell, but the zone was not confined to this limited region. The input and apparent output associations of these cells were regarded as being related—but not so strongly as the majority referred to above. Such cells could have an afferent input zone from both shoulder and elbow but active discharges associated only with movements of the elbow. Alternatively, they could exhibit active discharges in association with the movements of only a single digit (in retrieving food with the index finger from a small hole in a board) but have an afferent input zone involving the whole hand. This class of related but not so strongly related active–passive behaviour accounted for another 15 per cent of the associations (and 17 per cent of the PTNs exhibited this form of behaviour). Only 13 per cent of the cells studied had an active–passive behaviour in which the input and apparent output discharges were not related to the same region of the limb and it was very uncommon for PTNs to show unrelated behaviour.

The adequate stimulus which influenced about half of the neurones with a strongly related active–passive response was movement of a single joint. The proportion of these for which the effective passive movement at this joint was in the same direction as the active movement with which the natural discharges were associated was 75 per cent. An example is indicated in Fig. 6.20 where active and passive wrist abduction caused the cell to discharge. For the other 25 per cent of cells with input limited to a single joint, movement in opposite directions under active and passive conditions was effective. The cell in Fig. 6.10 is an example (active shoulder protraction and passive shoulder retraction were associated with discharge of the cell). Again it was more common for movements in the same direction to be effective when the active and passive associations were with movements about the distal joints of the limb.

For cells which responded to muscle palpation as well as to passive movement at a single joint, it was more common for the muscle containing the receptive elements to be stretched during the passive movement and contracted during the active movement with which discharges were associated. About half the cells with a demonstrated muscle afferent input behaved in this way. But other associations, e.g. that the muscle would be stretched during the effective passive movement and relaxed during the associated active movement, also existed (see Table 6.2).

Although cutaneous fields were found for only a small proportion of the neurones, the cells which received this input most often discharged with active movements which advanced the receptive field towards an object. As has already been noted, most of these fields were on the glabrous skin of the ventral surface of the fingers and hand and the neurones influenced by these fields discharged during active flexion of the digits or wrist. The discharge during active movement preceded contact of the receptive field with any surface or object. These findings tend to confirm the generalizations provided by Rosén and Asanuma (1972) for the S-cells in their studies. But exceptions exist. A few cells with cutaneous receptive fields discharged during active movements which withdrew the receptive field from any contact.

TABLE 6.2

Precentral neurones responding to passive joint movement and muscle palpation. Comparison of muscle state under active and passive conditions

		Condition		Number of neurones
		(a) Passive	(b) Active	
A.	Muscle	Stretched	Contracted	9
B.	Muscle	Stretched	Relaxed	5
C.	Muscle	Shortened	Contracted	3
			TOTAL	17

For neurones responding to both palpation of a muscle and movement of a joint at which the muscle acted, a comparison has been made of the state of the muscle providing afferent input to a neurone under (a) passive conditions—the direction of passive joint movement which activated the cell could either stretch or shorten the muscle; and (b) active conditions—by either direct observation or, where possible, examination of EMG records, the state of the muscle (contracted or relaxed) during the active movements with which the cell's discharge was associated could be determined.

It remains to examine the anatomical disposition in the cortex of the neurones whose active and passive discharge characteristics have been studied to see what can be learned about the arrangement of the input–output modules. Again the behaviour of adjacent or neighbouring cells and a comparison of the responses of groups of cells situated close together in the same track should provide some indications of the microanatomical organization. The first general point concerns output associations. While neighbouring cells were frequently concerned with movements about the same joint, it was quite common for adjacent cells to be associated with active movements in different directions or with quite different movements at separate joints (see also Chapter 7).

Figure 6.21 shows histograms of two pairs of cells recorded in separate tracks. Each pair was recorded simultaneously with the same electrode. The neurones of one pair (Fig. 6.21A,B) had a very similar relationship to the motor task and both responded during active and passive extension of the wrist. The other pair is represented in Fig. 6.21E. One cell was strongly related to finger movements. It discharged briefly during the lever grip phase and again later when the monkey collected the food reward (Fig. 6.21D). This cell was completely quiescent during the pull phase and had an afferent input zone confined to the index and middle fingers. The other cell, recorded with the smaller deflection spikes in Fig. 6.21E, was strongly related to flexion of the elbow; it was quiescent when the monkey extended his arm to the lever and discharged strongly during the pull phase (Fig. 6.21C). This cell responded to passive elbow flexion.

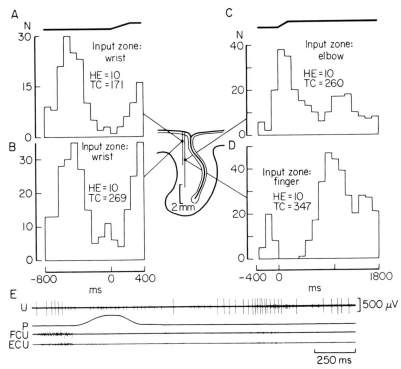

FIG. 6.21. Behaviour of simultaneously recorded precental neurones.

The diagram in the centre of the Figure shows two electrode tracks and the approximate position in each track at which a pair of neurones were recorded simultaneously by the same electrode. For the pair A and B, both cells were associated with active extension of the wrist prior to grip of the lever knob and had similar peri-response time histograms. Both cells also responded to passive extension of the wrist joint. For the pair of cells C and D located in the other track, one (C) was strongly related to flexion of the elbow and discharged just before and during pull of the lever and later (1 s after lever movement) when the monkey flexed his arm to bring the food reward to his mouth. This cell is recorded with the smaller of the two deflections in the original records shown below in E. It responded to passive flexion of the elbow joint. The other cell in the pair (D), which is recorded with the larger deflections in E, discharged during finger movements, including lever grip, and later during collection and manipulation of the food (note that this phase of discharge begins at about 500 ms and reaches its peak at about 900 ms before withdrawal of the hand with the food began). This neurone was silent during the pull phase. It had a cutaneous field on the index and middle fingers and also responded to flexion of several joints of these two fingers. This Figure hence indicates that neighbouring cells could show very similar relationships to input and output (A and B) or quite different relationships (C and D). (Lemon et al., 1976.)

While some adjacent cells could be related to active movements at the same joint, these movements could be in the same or opposite directions. Other adjacent cells could be related to active movements at different joints. Many groups of cells situated close together (within 500 μm) included neurones whose activity was related to movement involving the same part of the arm, but all of these groups contained at least one cell that was related to movements at a different joint. The afferent input zones were usually, but not always, related to part of the limb with whose active movements the cell's natural discharge was associated.

Relevant to this question of the anatomical situation of neurones whose activity was related to voluntary movement of a particular joint was the observation that cells discharging in association with the same active movement at the same joint could be recorded at cortical locations which were quite distant from each other (up to 5 mm apart). Thus, in one monkey, although most cells whose active discharge was related to finger movements were found in tracks which penetrated the cortex near the central sulcus, several cells related to finger movement were found in the convexity of the gyrus. Conversely, many cells related to shoulder movement were found on the convexity, but it was not uncommon to find such cells in the anterior bank of the sulcus.

6.5 Summary

Each of the corticospinal projection areas whose overlapping architecture we surveyed in Chapter 5 is built up of PTN which project to a common motoneuronal target, though their branching axons (Chapter 4) must also connect them to other targets, possibly in functionally significant combinations. Each PTN forms the axis of a radially oriented minimal input–output module of cortex. The horizontal dendritic branches which spring from its radially oriented apical dendrite spread horizontally as far as 1.0 mm, and receive synaptic contacts from the widely ramifying terminal arborizations of thalamocortical axons which may have entered the cortex a further 0.5 mm distant horizontally from the apical dendritic shaft. The axon of the PTN gives off intracortical collaterals which spread mono-synaptic excitation and disynaptic inhibition across similar horizontal distances. There are different types of stellate interneurones: some form 'climbing' or 'cartridge' synapses along the apical dendritic shafts of PTN; others, with horizontally running axons, form baskets of synapses on the perikarya of PTN which may be more than 0.5 mm away. The suggestion that the cartridge synapses are excitatory and the basket synapses are inhibitory is plausible but unproven. Richly though the minimal modules thus interdigitate with their neighbours, the pre-dominantly radial orientation of the incoming thalamocortical axons, and of the apical dendrites and axons of the PTN, strongly suggest that the input–output connexions of a single PTN are preponderantly coaxial. But the distance across which a radially activated minimal module could excite and inhibit its neighbours may be as great as 2 to 3 mm in any direction.

Detailed knowledge of the thalamic loci which project to different parts of area 4 is incomplete. Thalamic neurones send to the PTN 'commands' from other parts of the cortex, presumably derived from internal programmes which are related to environmental events though far removed from any direct connexions with peripheral receptors. Thalamic neurones also transmit signals generated by 'internal feedbacks' (e.g. cortico-cerebello-thalamo-cortical), and signals generated by 'external' feedbacks arising in peripheral receptors in the moving parts. Research is trying to find out whether single cortical interneurones and single PTN receive inputs from single or multiple sources. It is obvious that the responses of antidromically labelled PTN, which are the dischargers of the integrated output of the minimal input–output modules, are of special interest and importance.

In cats, the minimal modules receive multimodal inputs, some from narrow and some from wide peripheral fields. Their output targets have been investigated by microcathodal stimulation, which is subject to all the difficult technical and interpretative problems which we have discussed at length in Chapter 5, and which has been limited to the 'hot spots' of the projection areas. It is in general true that inputs from the distal parts of the limbs are related to outputs to the muscles of the same parts. Though the intracortical connectivity is essentially *radial*, the multimodal inputs and the uncertainty about the specificity of the outputs gave us leave to doubt the possibility of proving that there exist *columns* made up of aggregations of minimal modules with similar combinations of input and output.

Experiments on the much larger brains of monkeys have sometimes used chloralose as the anaesthetic and synchronous volleys in skin and muscle nerves as the inputs: under these conditions the inputs to the PTN are multimodal. As in the cat, there is a general topographical relationship between the peripheral origin of the inputs to unidentified cortical neurones, which in the monkey can usually be elicited by natural stimulation from more restricted areas of the forelimb digits, and the distal muscles which are activated by microcathodal stimulation at the same electrode site (whenever this happens to lie in a hot spot).

A complementary method of investigation, which avoids the difficulties inherent in microstimulation, entails recording from antidromically labelled PTN, and from adjacent cortical neurones, in monkeys which have been trained not only to perform a stereotyped motor task but also to remain relaxed while their limbs are probed and manipulated by the experimenter. Discharge of a PTN in regular association with, and in advance of, a particular component of the motor performance (Chapter 7) implies that the PTN is under command. Such PTN need not be confined to hot spots. Their inputs (feedbacks) can also be stimulated by imposing movements on different joints and by deep and superficial probing of the appropriate limb. About 90 per cent of the neuronal responses are to deep probing and to movement of joints. There is apt to be wider convergence on PTN than on unidentified neurones (which may be collectors of part only of the inputs which converge on the PTN as the 'final common path' which leads out of the module). The latency of response of some neurones in area 4 to probing the limb is so brief that the signals must be transmitted by a direct spino-thalamo-cortical pathway. Recording from two or more closely adjacent neurones provides a powerful analytical tool for establishing whether all those input–output modules with similar inputs and outputs are aggregated into specific columns, or whether such modules are more widely dispersed within the cortex.

The results of these experiments support a cortical organization made up of input–output modules in which the peripheral territories with which both input and output are associated are the same or very closely related. While the modules tend to be aggregated in such a way that those dealing with a particular territory are close neighbours, they can be concerned with that territory in opposite senses (e.g. for flexion or extension) and they will have interspersed among them modules concerned with remote territories in the same limb. Finally, the modules are not confined within very limited zones having sharp boundaries because outlying members of the group of modules related to a given territory have been found in cortex several mm removed from the major aggregation.

7
Electrophysiology of neurones of cortical projection areas in relation to conditioned and voluntary movement

7.1 Pyramidal tract discharge and movement

We have indicated already much of the evidence on which conclusions about the connexions of the pyramidal tract are based. We have examined the organization in the cerebral cortex of the neurones which give rise to the pyramidal tract and we have seen how this organization has been studied. PTN have been found to be receivers of nerve signals. Their activities are determined by the inputs to them, and in the previous chapter we reviewed the relationship of one of the inputs (feedback from peripheral receptors) to apparent output function. It remains to ask what aspects of the movement performance output are related to natural function of PTNs and to study how these output functions have been investigated.

It will become clear that PTNs become active before the movements with which their discharges are associated begin. This activity cannot therefore be determined solely by the feedback influences studied in Chapter 6. Discharges of some PTNs have been shown to change according to the force which needs to be developed in prime mover muscles in order to execute movement. But the force required may also, apparently, be signalled by the number of PTNs which become active immediately in advance of the contraction of those muscles. There is commanding evidence for a relationship of the discharges of many PTNs to the timing of particular muscle contractions in the production of movement. As yet, the determinants of these particular relations in commands from a programme up-stream from the PTN themselves remain matters for conjecture and for further study.

An important technological advance in the study of pyramidal tract function was the development of a method for the examination of impulse activity in identified PTN of conscious, free-to-move monkeys. This allowed the signals transmitted along efferent fibres from the motor cortex to be analysed in relation to normal behavioural responses of the animal. It was demonstrated by Evarts (1964, 1965a, b) that stimulating electrodes could be implanted in the PT of a monkey and that microelectrodes could subsequently be inserted into the motor area of the cerebral cortex through a previously prepared defect in the bony cranium. The operations for preparation of the animal were carried out under general anaesthesia and with full aseptic precautions. Then, when the animal awakened, and on separate occasions for some weeks subsequently, fine metal microelectrodes could be driven slowly through the dura and into the cortex. These electrodes caused the animal no discomfort. Indeed, the monkeys appeared to be completely unaware of the probing. Once the electrode came close enough to a cell in the cerebral cortex to record its discharges selectively (without interference from the impulse activity of neighbouring neurones), the cell could be tested to discover whether or not its axon travelled in the PT. Antidromic responses with short, constant latency and the ability to follow brief trains of high-frequency stimuli delivered to the PT were observed in a proportion of the cells from which recordings were made.

Evarts found that all of the antidromic responses occurred with short latencies (usually less than 5 ms, corresponding to an axonal conduction velocity of greater than 10 ms^{-1}). Hence the method sampled only the activities of those PTN which have relatively rapidly conducting axons. An example of this sampling is shown in Fig. 7.1 which plots the estimated axonal conduction velocities of 172 PTN examined in another study (Lewis, 1974). The bias towards recordings from cells with rapidly conducting axons is clear.

In this study, all but 20 of the 172 neurones had axonal conduction velocities above 25 ms^{-1} and the most common conduction velocity was of the order of 60 ms^{-1}. The errors in estimating the conduction velocity of PT axons in these experiments are large. Stimulation is carried out with implanted electrodes and can be delivered only at one site. The action potential does not necessarily arise precisely at the cathode of the stimulating pair and the length of the conduction path to the cell body in the motor cortex can be measured only approximately. There may, in fact, be no PT axons with conduction velocities above 80 ms^{-1} in these monkeys and the presence of this group in the sample of Fig. 7.1 may arise from overestimates of the length of the conduction path. In the species of monkey used for these studies, *Maca fascicularis*,[1] the majority (85 per cent) of fibres in the medullary PT are said to be less than 1 μm in diameter and only 2–3 per cent of the fibres measure above 6 μm in diameter (Verhaart 1948).

[1]Earlier called *M.irus* or Java Monkey and also referred to as crab–eating macaque cynomolgus monkey (Napier and Napier, 1967).

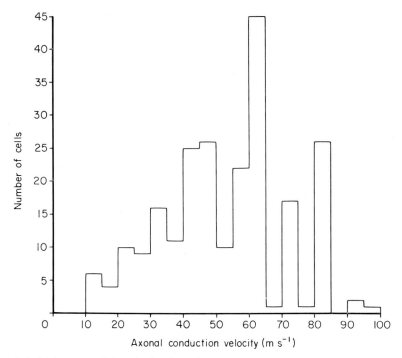

FIG. 7.1. A histogram of the calculated conduction velocities of 172 PT axons sampled in studies of a number of conscious monkeys. Recordings were made of the discharge of individual cells in area 4 whose axons could be stimulated by shocks delivered to a pair of electrodes implanted in the ipsilateral pyramidal tract. Conduction velocities of the axons were calculated from measurements of the latency of the antidromic action potential and of the approximate conduction distance from the stimulating to the recording electrode. (Lewis, 1974.)

Evarts (1965b) noted that, within his sample of PTN, two populations could be identified. The cells with antidromic response latencies of less than 1 ms (and axonal conduction velocities probably around 45 to 50 m s^{-1} or greater) had very low frequencies of impulse discharge while the monkey sat quietly at rest. Twenty-two of 28 such units had discharge frequencies below 4 spikes per second and some were silent for many seconds at a time. On the other hand, PTN with antidromic response latencies of 1 ms or greater tended to be firing even when the animal sat still. These differences are illustrated in Fig. 7.2, which summarizes the observations on 62 PTN studied by Evarts (1965b, Table I). It is not clear whether the two groups of PTN are related to the fast and slow PT fibres of Brookhart (1952) (see Chapter 3).

When the monkey moved its contralateral arm, the activity of the PTN changed. Those cells which had been almost silent at rest discharged bursts of nerve impulses during movement. Discharges of an individual neurone sometimes reached frequencies of 80 to 100 impulses per second with certain arm movements. But, when discharges were averaged over several minutes, during which a series of movements of the hand were occurring, interspersed with periods without movement, the average frequencies were much lower. Figure 7.2 compares the average frequency during periods of more or less constant use of the hand for scratching, grooming, food-handling, etc. (moving) with the average frequency of the same units during periods when the monkey was still. Cells with antidromic latencies less than 1 ms are plotted in black and these had the most marked overall change in frequency associated with movement. Some units with longer antidromic response latencies showed a decrease in impulse activity during movement.

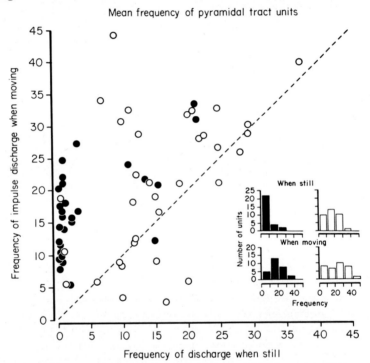

Fig. 7.2. Each dot on the graph plots the mean frequency of discharge of a PTN, recorded while a monkey sat still, against the mean frequency of discharge of the same PTN during periods when the animal was moving. Units with antidromic response latencies of less than 1 ms (and hence high axonal conduction velocities) are shown in black while units with antidromic response latencies of greater than 1 ms are shown in white. The inset histograms show the mean frequencies of these two groups of PTNs both when the animal was still and when it was moving. (Evarts, 1965.)

The characteristic average frequencies of PT unit discharge associated with movement were not high. Evarts' results for discharge during

movement performance, which are summarized in Fig. 7.2, suggest an
almost complete overlap of the average firing frequencies for PTN with more
slowly conducting and more rapidly conducting axons. These observations
were made in monkeys which were completely free to move their limbs in
any way, and the movements performed may have varied widely from one
set of observations to another. It was, therefore, of some interest to examine
the characteristic frequencies of discharge associated with a stereotyped
lever-pulling task. Figure 7.3 illustrates the results for a similar sample of
43 PT units whose discharges were studied in relation to the repetitive
performance of a natural flexion movement of the right arm to pull a lever.
Although the observations are scattered, the PTN with rapidly conducting
axons tended to show higher characteristic frequencies of discharge with
this movement performance than did the PTN with more slowly conducting axons. Although the mean frequencies of firing of PTN tended to be
below 100 Hz, instantaneous frequencies of discharge much higher than
this were common during phasic bursts of activity. Intervals between
successive impulses could be as brief as 1.5 ms and were commonly less

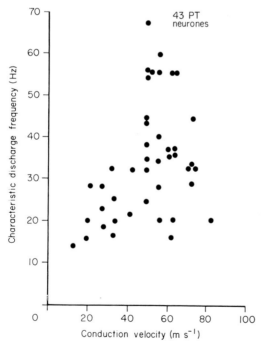

FIG. 7.3. The characteristic frequencies of discharge of 43 PTNs studied during periods
of stereotyped movement performance (pulling a horizontal lever) have been plotted
against the estimated axonal conduction velocity of each PTN. Units with higher axonal
conduction velocities tended to have higher rates of discharge in relation to this movement
task. (Lewis, 1974.)

than 5 ms, placing these intervals in the range for which temporal facilitation at corticomotoneuronal synapses has been found to be significant
(Chapter 3).

It has been demonstrated that intracortical inhibition of small PTN in
the cat occurred via recurrent axon collaterals when large PT axons were
stimulated electrically (Armstrong, 1965; Takahashi *et al.*, 1967). If the
same effects occur in monkey PTNs, this inhibition could serve to keep the
firing of the small PTN low when adjacent large cells were highly active
in association with movement. In addition the lower frequency but more
tonic firing of the neurones with more slowly conducting axons could be
related to their concern with postural adjustments in the movement
rather than with the active movement itself (see Chapter 3 and Brookhart,
1952). Tonic firing of some cells did seem to be related to posture of the
contralateral arm. PTN which were tonically active in relation to one
posture of the arm have been shown to change their firing when the limb
was held in another posture. Sometimes the previously tonically firing
unit became silent with the arm in the new posture and then the cell could
behave phasically with movement away from this second posture (Porter
and Lewis, personal observation).

The relationship of the most intense discharge of particular PTN to
characteristic movements of a limb has been demonstrated by requiring an
animal to collect food rewards with the right hand in various postures
(see Chapter 6). Some cells could be shown to be strongly related to
movement at one particular joint and independent of movements at
adjacent or related joints. Thus a cell could be shown to discharge every
time the wrist was flexed, although the shoulder, elbow and digits were in a
variety of different positions. Similarly, some cells could be shown always
to discharge most in relation to the movement of ulnar or radial deviation
of the wrist by presenting food to be collected by the right hand but
placed to the right or the left of the animal. An example is shown in Fig.
6.20 (p. 260). Many units associated specifically with movements of the
digits in the 'precision grip' (discussed by Phillips, 1971) would show most
discharge if the animal had to collect small morsels of food using individual
finger movements whether the arm was projected to the food in a high, low,
left or right position. If the food reward was large and could be collected
in a fist made by closure of the whole hand such 'finger movement related'
PTN showed much less intense activity.

A semi-quantitative demonstration of the different intensities of cellular
discharge which accompanied different active movements could be obtained
by requiring the animal to perform a task (pulling a lever) in order to gain a
food reward. Different food rewards could then be presented in different
positions for collection as discussed in Chapter 6. The discharges of the
neurone which accompanied the lever-pulling task and the food collection

could be summed to make a peri-response time histogram (Fig. 7.4) using the performance of the lever-pulling task as the response. Histograms created for food collection using the hand in different attitudes clearly revealed the association of most active cell firing in relation to a characteristic movement or attitude of the hand or arm (Lemon *et al.*, 1976). This same close relationship between cellular activity in the precentral gyrus and the contractions of a particular muscle group has also been demonstrated elegantly by operant conditioning (Fetz and Finocchio, 1975).

Evarts (1965b) reported that cells which were close together in the cortex usually changed their firing rate in relation to movements about the same joint. They could show discharge patterns which were in phase with one another or which altered in a reciprocal manner during movement. Also the correlation between the discharges of a pair of adjacent PTN being studied simultaneously could vary depending on the movements which the monkey was making. This observation achieves significance in considerations of the localization of cells concerned with movement performance and of the organization of this localization, and it has been discussed in Chapter 6.

Changes in discharge of PT units were also noted during sleep (Evarts, 1964, 1965a). In general, those units which had short antidromic response latencies and which were relatively silent when the animal was awake but still, increased their firing during slow-wave sleep. The units with longer antidromic response latencies, which exhibited tonic, maintained discharge during wakefulness without movement, tended to fire less with slow-wave sleep. The same unit could change its firing pattern with different phases of sleep. Some of the highest-frequency bursts of activity were recorded during sleep accompanied by low-voltage fast EEG records (REM sleep). But these bursts were not associated with movement. Hence movement must have been correlated with factors additional to the high-frequency discharge of single PTN. In-phase activity of large numbers of pyramidal cells may have been required and it may have been necessary for the excitability at subcortical and spinal levels to be appropriate for this more or less synchronous discharge of many PT cells to become effective.

7.2   The timing of pyramidal tract discharge in relation to movement

In order to examine the temporal relationship between PT activity in the awake monkey and movement performance it was necessary to train monkeys to perform a well-defined, repeatable movement and investigate the relationship between change in neuronal discharge and the onset of

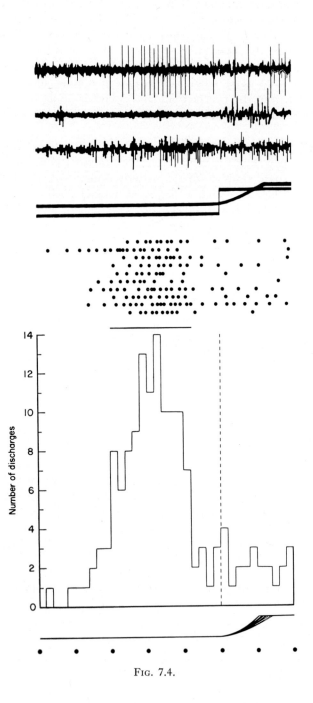

Fig. 7.4.

this movement. In initial experiments, a conditioned extension of the wrist, carried out briskly in response to a light flash, was used as the movement task. If the monkey performed the wrist extension to release a telegraph key in a response time of less than 350 ms, it was rewarded with delivery of juice into its mouth. Electromyographic responses in flexor and extensor muscles acting on the wrist were recorded through the skin using electrodes taped to the monkey's forearm and, during the performance of the conditioned response, recordings were made of the activities of PT cells in the arm area of the motor cortex.

A large proportion of the PT units showed changes in their discharge in association with the performance of the conditioned movement task. These cells did not respond to the signal to move and only changed their activity when this signal resulted in performance of the movement task. Many of these units altered their firing before the onset of EMG activity in the extensor muscles of the wrist (Fig. 7.5). In many neurones with short antidromic response latencies, this change was a burst of discharge beginning about 50 to 80 ms before the onset of the extensor EMG response. For some individual cells it could be shown that, as the latency of onset of the cell's firing varied following the conditioning light stimulus, so did the reaction time. There was a clear, positive correlation between unit response latency and reaction time. It was the nerve cell's discharges and the movement response which were temporally correlated.

Responses which occurred prior to the onset of muscle activity could not have been caused by alteration in afferent discharge from the moving hand. Also, some of the units which discharged after the onset of extension

FIG. 7.4. The upper part of the Figure shows a sample of filmed recording of the discharges of a precentral neurone (top trace) in relation to the electrical activity in two representative arm muscles, *biceps brachii* (second trace) and *flexor carpi ulnaris* (third trace), when the lever was pulled forwards through 15 mm in generating a force from 200 g (when movement started and the step occurred in the fifth trace) to 600 g (fourth trace). During ten repetitions of such a movement performance, all aligned with respect to the beginning of forward movement of the lever, the discharges of this neurone were indicated by dots in successive rows of the raster which occupies the middle section of the Figure. A histogram (event correlogram) has been compiled by adding the occurrences of neuronal discharges in successive 20 ms time periods before and after the beginning of forward movement of the lever (dashed vertical line) in a number of repetitions of the movement task. These movement performances have been superimposed at the bottom of the histogram so that an indication of the average performance and its variability has been obtained. The histogram clearly shows the average 'burst' of activity in this neurone which uniformly preceded the movement task. The average duration of this representative burst of firing, time locked to the movement performance, has been defined as the period during which the columns of the histogram exceeded the level which would have resulted from a uniform distribution of discharges across the total time period (700 ms). This average duration of the characteristic burst of neuronal discharge for the cell is indicated by the horizontal line above the histogram. Time scale at the bottom of the Figure is common to all parts of the Figure and dots are separated by 100 ms. (Porter and Lewis, 1975.)

could have been related to the contraction of flexor muscles at the end of the task. These particular experiments involving stereotyped conditioned responses could not clearly distinguish this from a response to the effect of extension on peripheral detectors of movement.

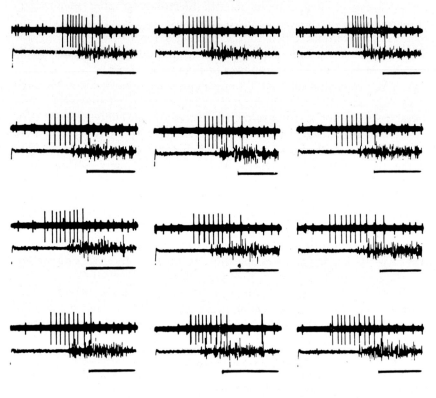

FIG. 7.5. In a series of 12 trials a light came on as a signal for a monkey to make a brief extension movement of the wrist. Each of the twelve trials is illustrated by means of a record of the discharges of a PTN (upper trace in each case) which was silent during flexion and which discharged prior to extension of the contralateral wrist on each occasion. All traces begin at the onset of the light stimulus. The minimum response latency for the PTN discharge was about 120 ms. This was associated with an EMG response latency in the extensor muscles (second trace in each case) of 170 ms and a reaction time (to lift the hand off a telegraph key and break contact) of 220 ms. In general, the shortest latency PTN responses were associated with the shortest latency EMG responses. The bottom line in each case appeared when the contact opened. Time marks are 50 ms apart. (Evarts, 1966.)

The majority of PT units responded only when the conditioned movement was performed with the contralateral hand, but a few units were found to respond when the ipsilateral hand was used. Discharges of the same cell accompanying either ipsilateral or contralateral hand movements have also been reported by Lemon *et al.* (1976) for a small proportion of PTN. A similar small proportion of neurones in the precentral gyrus of man has been shown to discharge with ipsilateral hand movements (Goldring and Ratcheson, 1972).

The temporal relationship to movement performance of the responses of a large number of precentral and postcentral neurones has recently been examined by Evarts (1972a, b). Figure 7.6 shows that, in association with the performance of an abrupt flexion or extension movement of the wrist, precentral neurones could begin to discharge as early as 140 ms before the movement response and commonly changed their activity 60 ms before the movement. In contrast, most neurones in the postcentral gyrus of the same monkey showed responses beginning after the movement as though influenced by it. As Evarts pointed out, it was not possible to do better than time these discharges with reference to the movement itself, because different muscles became active at different times before, during and after the movement. It was not possible to discover in these experiments which particular muscle response was most closely associated with the discharges of any particular unit.

In a more complicated but completely natural movement, monkeys have been trained to reach out, extend the fingers, grasp a small knob firmly with the right hand and pull the knob briskly and horizontally

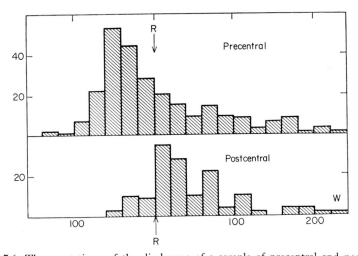

FIG. 7.6. The onset times of the discharges of a sample of precentral and postcentral neurones in relation to flexion and extension movements of the contralateral wrist have been measured. The two distributions of peri-response latencies (to onset of discharge in relation to the movement response, R) have been plotted. The abscissa indicates the time in ms before or after R at which each individual cell began to discharge. The ordinate is the number of cells in each population exhibiting that peri-response latency. (Evarts, 1972a.)

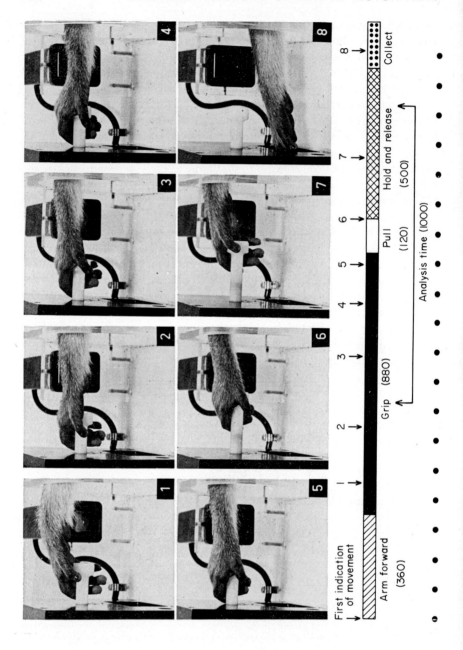

towards them through a short distance of 15 to 20 mm (Fig. 7.7). Precentral neurones changed their discharge at different times in relation to this movement. Some cells became active during reaching and finger extension, others during the grip of the hand on the knob and yet others during the pull phase of the movement task. The discharges of these groups of cells overlapped one another in time so that the population of active cells could be considered to be changing continuously with time during the total movement performance. Yet this population could be divided artificially into separate groups whose activity closely preceded reaching, grasping or pulling. In Fig. 7.8 this has been done for a sample population of precentral PTN. Of these pyramidal tract units, 60 were active well before the pull was performed, while 24 became active immediately before and during the pull phase. It is likely that this activity in functionally different groups of PTN preceded the contractions of different groups of muscles. The progressive temporal changes in the population of cells which were active were associated with the progressive sequence of muscle contractions involved in the smooth execution of the movement. The graphs show the number of cells in each group which were discharging at particular times in relation to the pull phase of the movement performance. Those cells which were discharging well before the pull phase progressively dropped out (ceased firing) as the second group (associated with flexion of the arm and movement of the knob) began to be recruited. These latter cells tended still to be firing at the completion of the task when most of the cells whose discharges had been initiated earlier had completed their bursts of activity.

When one considers the orderly sequence and continuously changing activity in the limb musculature which accompanies any task performance together with the association of each individual PTN's activity with a clearly defined aspect of movement performance (e.g. wrist pronation) whenever it was carried out, the aggregate of the PT activity (even though

FIG. 7.7. A series of photographs of characteristic attitudes of a monkey's hand during a lever-pulling task performance. At the bottom of the Figure is indicated the average period occupied by the grip, pull and hold phases of the task and the approximate times during these periods at which the hand was in the attitudes represented by the numbered photographs. A relatively long period was occupied in adjusting the grip and pronating the wrist (photographs 1–5) prior to the brief pull phase of the task (6). But this long period was not necessarily characteristic of all animals' performances and it may have been that extension of the arm through a perspex tube and the visual distortions introduced by this and the animal's view of his hand through a perspex 'window' caused this long period of grip adjustment. In other experiments, without the perspex tube, and with no front on the recording cage, the grip phase often occupies a very brief period and the animals tend to go straight from reaching out to pulling (see Fig. 6.8, p. 239). At the end of the pull phase, the animal released the grip (7), the lever was returned to its rest position by a spring, and the hand was extended into a food compartment to collect the reward (8). Time scale: dots separated by 100 ms. (Porter and Lewis, 1975.)

sampled from many animals) suggests that each PTN may have been related to the modulation of contraction in a particular muscle or muscles. As aggregations of PTNs become involved in characteristic temporal association with the movement performance, their particular motor units in an associated muscle or muscles would be recruited to the peripheral sequence.

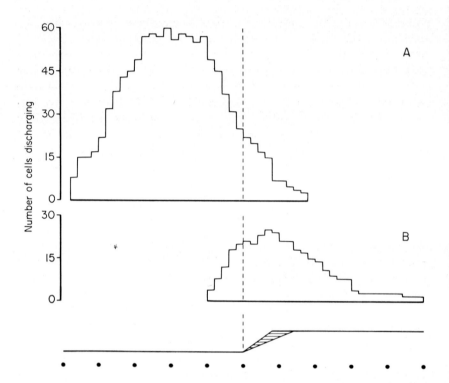

FIG. 7.8. The population of PTN firing bursts of impulses in relation to repetitions of the movement performance has been artificially divided into those beginning their burst within 100 ms of the start of movement (B, 24 cells) and those beginning their discharge earlier than this (A, 60 cells). In both histograms the number of cells discharging in each 20 ms time period has been plotted. Histogram A reveals that, in the early firing group of PTN, more and more cells were becoming active in the period from 500 ms to 200 ms before the pull started (in a period when the grip was being perfected (see Fig. 7.7)). Thereafter there was a relatively constant number of these cells in action up to about 100 ms before the onset of pull movement when the number of cells discharging fell off continuously. Histogram B reveals that the number of cells which began to fire bursts of impulses in close temporal relationship to the pull phase of the task increased in a 'ramp' which preceded the movement and its force ramp by 100 ms. Some additional cells were recruited to this population during the development of the force ramp. But the number of these cells which were active decreased after the end of the 'pull' phase and during the 'hold' period. The bottom trace represents the movement of the lever. The shaded area indicates the scatter of ramp durations in different repetitions of the pull task. Time scale: 100 ms. (Porter and Lewis, 1975.)

7.3   Relationship of pyramidal tract discharge to force of muscular contraction

A better understanding of the relationship between PT neuronal discharge and movement performance resulted from the experimental manipulation of some aspect of the movement and a study of the influence of this manipulation on the activity of identified cells. Evarts (1968) succeeded in dissociating the position achieved by the wrist in a repetitive flexion-extension task from the force required to be produced in flexor and extensor muscles in order to achieve and maintain a given position. As illustrated in Fig. 7.9, monkeys were trained to carry out this task in order to obtain a juice reward. Once a PTN had been found whose discharges were related to some aspect of the movement performance, the task could be modified by the addition of loads to the lever. By means of pulleys, these loads could be applied to oppose or to aid a given direction of movement. The same position of the wrist (e.g. flexion) could thereby be associated with more or less activity in flexor muscles producing the movement to that position.

Figure 7.10 illustrates the discharges of a PTN associated with the repetitive performance of the wrist flexion-extension task under three load conditions. When the load opposed flexion (upper trace) much more discharge occurred for the same movement excursion than was exhibited by this cell when the lever alone was being moved (no-load condition, second trace). Moreover, the discharge of the unit continued into the extension phase of the repetitive movement, presumably in association with the continuing contraction of flexor muscles to control the 'paying out' of the load. But when the load was so placed as to aid the flexion movement, which could thus be accomplished without contraction of flexor muscles, the cell was almost silent during the performance of the same movement to the same position (third trace).

Not all PTN showed such a clear relationship to the force exerted by the muscle groups with which discharge was associated. But a general tendency for the mean frequency of discharges in the associated bursts of activity to be related more to force than to position was demonstrated. Some units showed very phasic responses which could be more readily related to rate of change of force in the movement task. But rate of change of force in a given direction usually had to be superimposed on some threshold level of force development before changes in neuronal firing were evident. These observations led Evarts to suggest that the PTN were related both to force and to the rate at which force was changing in a given muscle group.

Out of a sample of more than 100 PTN studied in relation to this task, 26 showed a relationship of their discharge frequency to force development and these were not coding the position to be taken up by the wrist. Five other units showed discharges associated regularly with one direction of movement but were not clearly related to the force needed to produce the movement. The discharges of these units were also not related to the position achieved or to the speed of the movement accomplished. But the conclusion from these experiments and the selected sample of cells which

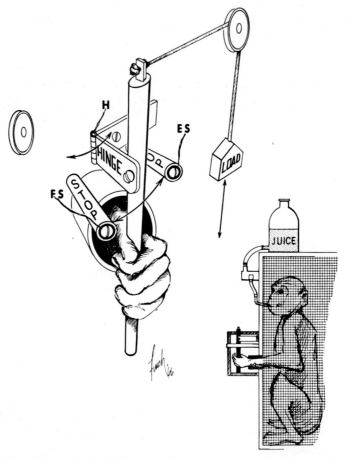

FIG. 7.9. In order to gain a fruit juice reward, a monkey was required to grasp the vertical rod attached to a hinge and to move it back and forth from one stop to the other. The stops are labelled FS (flexor stop) and ES (extensor stop). If the period between breaking contact with the flexor stop and making contact with the extensor stop was between 400–700 ms, and if the previous movement in the opposite direction also fell within these time limits, the solenoid valve was automatically operated and a reward was delivered. The forearm was held in a slot so that movements could be produced only by alternate flexion and extension movements of the wrist. Attachment of a load to the rod and allowing it to exert force opposing either flexion or extension could be achieved by placing the cord over one or other pulley. The same position could be combined with no load, a load opposing movement to that position or a load aiding movement in that direction. (Evarts, 1968.)

was studied in detail was 'that variations of force were very strongly represented in PTN (pyramidal tract neurone) output' (Evarts 1968, p. 25).

A summary of the results obtained in the 31 cells studied in detail by Evarts is included in Fig. 7.11. It is clear that some units were more active with loads opposing extension than with loads opposing flexion (graphs grouped at bottom right of Fig. 7.11) and others were more active with flexor loads (graphs grouped at bottom left of Fig. 7.11). It is also clear that

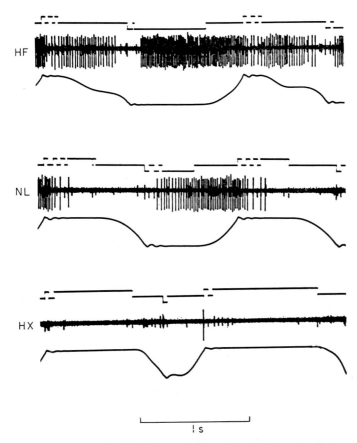

FIG. 7.10. The discharges of a PTN in association with repetitions of a flexion-extension movement at the wrist. Wrist displacement is indicated by the third trace. Contact with the extensor stop is represented by the lowest level of this trace, and the flexor stop is contacted when the trace reaches its upper position. With no load attached to the rod (NL) the unit discharged before and during the movement to flexion, but was silent during the movement to extension. When a load of 400 g opposed the movement to flexion (HF), increased flexor force was required to move the rod and the cell was much more active. Conversely, when the load of 400 g aided flexion (HX) and little or no flexor muscle force was required to produce the movement, the unit was almost totally silent. (Evarts, 1968.)

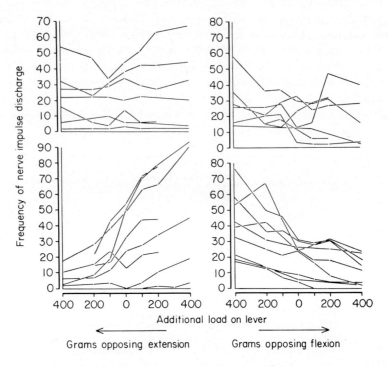

Fig. 7.11. Each of the 31 PTNs analysed in detail by Evarts (1968) has been represented by a line which plots the relationship between that neurone's discharge in the movement to the flexion stop against the load added to the lever to aid or oppose the flexion movement. Some PTNs increased their discharge with additional loads opposing flexion, others decreased their discharge and a more complicated relationship was found for some.

the discharge frequencies with maximum responsiveness usually did not exceed 100 per second. (For one of these units the discharge reached 147 per second in the extensor position with a maximum load opposing extension. This unit is illustrated in Fig. 7.12.) Some units showed peak frequencies of discharge at loads intermediate between the largest opposing flexion and opposing extension and five units showed no consistent variation in discharge frequency in relation to load. The summarizing diagram (Fig. 7.11) refers only to the discharges accompanying the movement to flexor displacement, but it was usual for similar variation in behaviour to be exhibited by these same units when their discharges during the movement to extension of the wrist were studied, but then the changes tended to be in the opposite direction for given load conditions. This variation for 6 of the same 31 PTN is indicated in Fig. 7.12. Some units increased their firing with increase in the load opposing extension, some reduced their discharge, some showed maximum discharge at an intermediate level of force requirement and some were relatively unaffected by changing loads (this last category tended to fire at low rates anyway).

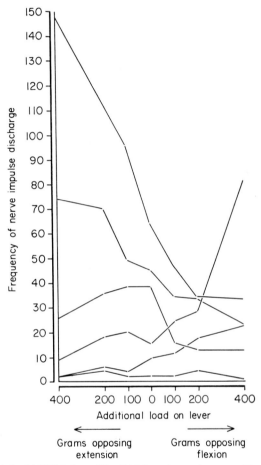

FIG. 7.12. Six of the 31 PTNs from Fig. 7.11 have been chosen to illustrate the range of responsiveness to added loads seen in the experiments of Evarts (1968). In this case each line plots the discharge frequency of the neurone during movements to the extensor stop against the load opposing (to the left) or aiding (to the right) the extension movement.

It is important to consider the significance of this variation in behaviour. The most important finding was the one emphasized by Evarts, viz. that a small proportion of the PT units (perhaps only 10 per cent of the total sample studied) showed a clear monotonic relationship to the force required in order to accomplish the movement. These units, if they made appropriate connexions in the spinal cord, could have been specifying the output of motoneurones to the force developing prime movers of the wrist joint. The other units, while undoubtedly related to the task, could have been influencing the spinal output to other muscles whose contractions had a different function in the movement, for example, as fixators of a more proximal joint rather than developers of the force required to move the lever or lift the load. In such a case, the appropriate output for their function need not be expected to be proportional to load. It is further possible that only some of the cells whose output was changing in relation to movement performance were related to force development in the muscles whose motoneurones they influenced. Others may have been concerned in other aspects of the movement, e.g. displacement velocity, or they may have been influencing transmission in afferent pathways whose activities would be modified by the movement.

In studying a different movement task, involving development of force between the fingers and thumb of the monkey's hand in gripping a small force-measuring disc, Smith *et al.* (1975) also found that a proportion of neurones in the area of motor cortex which contained a low threshold zone for eliciting hand movements with intracortical stimulation showed responses which preceded force development. These cells had discharges which could be related to the rate of change of force with time, or to a combination of force and the rate of change of force.

Lewis and Porter (1974) have confirmed, for a different movement task, that some PTN changed their firing rate with changes in the load to be moved. Usually, these changes were not so great as the examples having the steepest slopes in Figs 7.11 and 7.12. Indeed, an increase in load of 200 g usually resulted in an average change in frequency of less than 15 per cent of the frequency during the same task without the load. A few cells increased their average discharge by 30 per cent with an added load of 200 g and one cell, which was firing at 35 impulses per second during movement of the unloaded lever, ceased firing altogether when a load of 400 g was added to the lever. PTN which were discharging earliest in relation to the lever pulling task (such as those in the upper graph of Fig. 7.8) showed a reduction of their firing rate in relation to the task when the load opposed the pull phase. Those discharging in the second group of Fig. 7.8, in temporal association with the pull action, increased their discharge when an additional load was added to the lever. It was clear that the beginning of the change in discharge, appropriate for the change in load, frequently occurred before the movement to lift the load and could not, therefore, have been produced by afferent feedback about the resistance to performance of the movement task. These animals and those studied by Evarts had been trained to carry out the movement against a variety of loads. So some learned programme for force development could have been influencing the PTN even if loads were changed without warning and in an apparently random manner. Peripheral feedback from receptors capable of detecting the 'feel' of the loaded lever could also have modified the later discharges (after the first impulse or two) in the bursts produced by the PTN, if it reached the cerebral cortex early enough.

In a subsequent study, Evarts (1969) examined the behaviour of PTN in a monkey trained to maintain a given wrist position even when loads were applied to the manipulandum in a direction to displace the wrist from this position. Maintenance of wrist position could again be achieved by contraction predominantly of flexor muscles (if the load opposed flexion) or by contraction of extensor muscles (if the load condition were reversed). Of 102 PTN studied in relation to this motor performance, 33 discharged with the associated movements but were not active during the fixation task, and 48 were related to contractions of muscles acting about the wrist during the fixation task but were much better related in their discharge patterns to non-task movements of the fingers, wrist, arm or shoulder. Only 12 of the 102 PTN were more clearly related to the fixation task than to other movements. Six of these units became more active with loads opposing flexion (requiring flexor muscle contraction to be increased) and the remainder were most active with loads opposing extension. These units showed a monotonic relationship between the load and their average discharge frequency during the maintenance of position. But much higher frequencies of firing than the average occurred with the small fluctuations in force during postural fixation: the discharge rate was by no means steady. Evarts concluded that these experiments further demonstrated that PTN activity varied in relation to the pattern of muscular contraction acting about a joint and not in relation to the position of the joint (which in these instances was held more or less fixed).

The experiments on discharge during postural fixation again demonstrated that a given PTN could be active during many different movements, discharging more in relation to some and less in relation to others. This could reflect the innervation by these PTN of motor pools concerned in the supply of muscles whose involvement was different in these different movements.

Humphrey (1972) attempted a quantitative summary of the relationship of firing rates of cells in the motor cortex to the output variables of movement performance. The movement studied was rotation of a joystick using the contralateral forelimb. The torque applied to the joystick gives a measure of the force generated by the muscles. He assumed that the firing rate of a population of cortical cells could be considered as the input to a linear control system consisting of the motoneurones together with the musculo-skeletal apparatus which generated changes in net muscular torque or joint position and whose performance could be characterized mathematically. In order to match the theoretical predictions of a linear

system receiving this input and experimental observations on the relationship between firing rate of individual cells and the measured torque and
position of the joystick, an optimum response of the linear system could
be defined. The first requirement was a delay between impulse activity
and torque development. This delay had to be set at a value of the order
of 50 to 100 ms. The response of the system could then be described by
one of three similar functions which was optimal for relating impulse
activity in a given cell to torque development. Six of 31 units (which
included both PT and non-identified neurones) showed variation in firing
rate over approximately the same time-course as the changes in torque,
17 showed more transient or 'phasic' changes which seemed to be related
to the first derivative of torque with the time, and 8 were intermediate in
their responsiveness. Each of the optimal functions used to relate these
three groups of cellular activity to torque output had the characteristics
of a simple second-order control system and the impulse response of each
system was said to strongly resemble the twitch-tension output time-
course of whole skeletal muscle.

The discharges of some cells which fired phasically with movement did
not appear to be proportional to torque or muscular force, and Humphrey
suggested that their discharge might be related to the rate of change of
torque rather than to force development in other contracting muscles.
Generalizing from the results of the experiments mentioned above, he
suggested that the control signal from the motor cortex, $F_{(t)}$, might be
related to the net muscular tension or torque, $T_{(t)}$ by an equation of the
form:

$$F_{(t)} = a \frac{d^2t}{dt^2} + \beta \frac{dT}{dt} + \mu T$$

where α, β and μ are constants. He further suggested that the matching of
experimentally recorded cellular discharges to torque output by an optimal
linear control system, which gave a much better correlation than a more
simple model of proportionality, indicated that different components of the
cortical signal could be transmitted with different emphasis by different
neuronal subgroups, 'some related to more proportional and some to more
derivative aspects of the force output'.

Humphrey et al. (1970), with a number of microelectrodes in the motor
cortex, succeeded in recording simultaneous activity in groups of 3 to 8
separate neurones discharging in relation to a given movement. One third
to one half of these neurones were identified as sending their axons into
the PT and these had short antidromic response latencies usually of less
than 3 ms. However, these authors reported that non-identified cortical
units in the arm area of the motor cortex showed discharges which were
quite as highly correlated with movement as were the activities of the PTN.

Weighted means of the rates of discharge within successive 50 ms time periods of these simultaneously recorded sets of cells were considered as the input signal to a control system whose impulse response was character-ized as a smooth curve which reached its peak within 100 ms and decayed to zero again in another 150 ms (Fig. 7.13). After this transformation, the firing of the sets of cortical neurones could be matched closely to the force output with time of the contralateral arm if the real force trace were shifted backwards by an average of 100 ms.

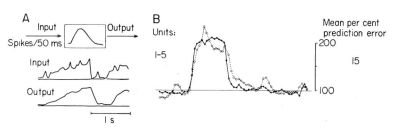

Fig. 7.13. A. The technique used in obtaining smoothed output is indicated. The output of a digital filter in response to a single neuronal spike is shown as a continuous curve in the upper part of the Figure: it reached a peak within 100 ms and decayed to zero in another 150 ms. The second trace (input) shows a segment of the weighted mean discharge of a PT cell constructed by summing spikes in each 50 ms. The output produced by this is illustrated in the third trace.

B. An example of the accuracy in predicting the time-course of the force trace when a number of simultaneously observed spike trains are used in the prediction equation. The dots represent the observed force values and the open circles those predicted. The numbers to the left indicate the units used in the prediction equation. The numbers to the right indicate the average prediction error (percentage). 100 g opposed flexion.

(Re-drawn from Humphrey, Schmidt and Thompson, 1970.)

The inclusion of the activities of groups of neurones in the input to the system gave a smoother output than that seen from the responses of single cells, and the results were in better agreement with the experimentally observed torque trace. Not only did this transformation give a reliable prediction of the force development in the movements with which the discharges were associated, but it gave an almost equally accurate prediction of the displacement achieved, the velocity of the movement and the rate of change of force with time. These authors, therefore, concluded that, if consideration were given to the slow dynamic responsiveness of muscles and the associated loads involved in limb movement, cortical neuronal discharges were theoretically capable of specifying not only force of muscular contraction acting about a joint but the time-course of this force development and hence the resultant displacement. However, in the movement task these animals performed, force output and displacement were related. So an association of neuronal responses with one of these would automatically lead to correlations with the other.

7.4 Pattern of pyramidal tract discharge and the time of onset of muscular contraction

The behavioural effects of PT section in monkeys suggest a function for pyramidal tract neurones in conferring skill and precision on movement performance and in permitting independent movement of individual digits (Lawrence and Kuypers, 1968; Woolsey *et al.*, 1972). Precision of movement performance could be achieved by the accurate control of time-courses of sequences of muscle contractions. It was therefore of interest to examine the relationship between discharge of PTN and the time of onset of the muscle contractions with which those discharges appeared to be invariably associated. As had been found by Evarts (1968), the mean frequency of firing of individual PTN was not closely correlated with the time of onset of muscle contraction after the first impulse in a burst of activity. The temporal pattern of impulses within the bursts often showed a peak of instantaneous frequency (represented by the shortest interval within the burst) which was much higher than the mean frequency of impulse discharge for the burst. These brief intervals, as a result of temporal summation in the postsynaptic neurone, could be expected to contribute most strongly in bringing motoneurones rapidly towards threshold depolarization for impulse initiation. In corticomotoneuronal fibres, temporal facilitation of synaptic effectiveness would confer an even greater significance on the briefest intervals in a burst (Chapter 3). Accordingly, it was possible that the time of occurrence of the shortest interval in a burst of impulses might be related to the time of initiation of a motor response.

An examination of the repetitive bursts of activity in representative PTN during repetitive 'grasp and pull' movements of a lever has indeed revealed a high degree of correlation between the time of occurrence of the least interval (highest instantaneous frequency) in each burst and the time of onset of electromyographic evidence of muscle contraction in the movement associated with that burst (Porter, 1972). An example of such a relationship for the successive bursts of activity of a PTN with an axonal conduction velocity of 56 m s^{-1} is shown in Fig. 7.14 which plots the latency of the shortest interval in each burst (measured from the first spike of the burst) against the time between the first spike and the onset of electromyographic evidence of muscle contraction in the lever-pulling movements. The two variables were highly correlated (correlation coefficient, $r = 0.88$) and it was possible that the cells of which this example was representative were capable of influencing the time of onset of muscle contraction in some muscle groups and hence of modifying the precision of movement performance.

In this study the least interval between the discharges of a neurone was used as a single indicator of temporal factors in the neuronal burst.

Facilitation of corticomotoneuronal excitatory effects (for example) is influenced not only by the length of the interval between nerve impulses, but also by the temporal pattern of impulses which preceded this interval (Chapter 3). If the entire temporal profile of the impulses in the burst had been considered, even higher correlations might be expected between the activity of the cell and the time of onset of muscle contraction associated with that activity.

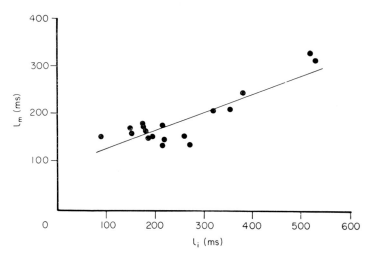

FIG. 7.14. For each natural burst of impulses in a PTN accompanying repetitive flexion movements to pull a lever, the latency after the first impulse in the burst of the shortest impulse interval (l_i) in the burst (highest instantaneous frequency) was measured. For each burst, the latency of the onset of muscle contraction (l_m) after the first impulse in the burst was also measured and, for a series of similar movement performances, the latency of each shortest interval has been plotted aaginst the latency of the muscle contraction with which its burst was associated. The line is the calculated regression line. It is very likely that the relationship between these variables is much more complicated than that implied by the line and the correlation coefficient ($r = 0.88$). Not all the shortest intervals whose latency was measured were equal intervals. The effect of the shortest interval could have been modified by the activity in the cell which preceded it: hence when the shortest interval occurred late in the burst more activity could have preceded it than when the shortest interval occurred early. A complete evaluation of these influences has not been made.

It is of great interest that the PT unit illustrated in Fig. 7.14, and a number of others whose behaviour was similar, not only showed a high degree of correlation between the time of occurrence of the least intervals in their bursts and the time of onset of muscle contraction in a sample muscle, but they also showed a weak relationship between mean frequency of discharge in these bursts and the load to be moved in the lever-pulling task. For the unit illustrated in Fig. 7.14, for example, the mean frequency of impulse discharge during bursts of activity in relation to movements of the unloaded lever was 37.2 impulses per second. When the manipulandum was loaded with an additional 200 g weight to be lifted during the pull phase, the mean frequency in the bursts increased to 46.6 impulses per second. There was no change in the time taken to perform the movement task and the least interval was still highly correlated with the time of onset of muscle contraction. These observations strengthen the suggestion that PT output may be concerned with more than one parameter of movement performance, and the results would be consistent with the proposal that even individual PTN may be able to influence both force and timing of muscle contraction. In general, however, many more individual PTN were found to show a strong correlation of the highest instantaneous frequency of their discharges with timing of muscle contraction than with the force developed.

7.5 Flexibility of the relationship between pyramidal tract discharge and muscular contraction

The demonstration of a high degree of correlation between the discharges of single PTN and the occurrence of contraction in a particular muscle does not preclude the existence of equally significant correlations with contraction of other coactivated muscles and does not necessarily indicate a causative role for the PT discharge in initiating the muscle contraction. To obtain more evidence about the meaning of the relationship between neuronal discharge and muscle contraction, Fetz and Finocchio (1971, 1972) trained a monkey to produce isometric contractions of particular forelimb muscles while the arm was held in a cast which prevented movement. They used the electromyographic records obtained from each of four muscles as reinforcement criteria in the training and were able to teach the monkey to produce isometric contraction of one of these muscles while suppressing, more or less completely, the EMG responses of the other three. It was possible for the monkey to learn to produce repeated bursts of EMG activity in one of the four sampled muscles with negligible coactivation of the other three and, after a period of about six weeks of training, the monkey could produce relatively isolated contractions of each of the four muscles in turn.

It was now possible to study the relationship between precentral cortical neuronal firing and the isometric muscle contractions. Some of the precentral cells studied were identified as PTN. It was found that some cortical cells whose discharge was strongly related to contraction of one of the muscles (e.g. *biceps brachii*) produced bursts which started about 70 ms before the EMG response and reached peak frequencies at the time of maximal muscle activity. These cells were inactive when relatively isolated contractions of other muscles (e.g. triceps) were produced. Such results indicate that, although in normal free movements of the arm contractions of many muscles, including both biceps and triceps, were occurring in association with the cortical cellular activity, the particular cortical cell's discharge was related to contraction in only one of these muscles—a fact which could be demonstrated by the operant conditioning technique.

An attempt was then made to test the stability of the relationship between cortical cellular activity and the muscular contraction with which the cell's discharge was closely related. The animal was given food reinforcement for producing bursts of cellular discharge while simultaneously suppressing all muscle contraction, including that of the closely related muscle (in the case being cited, biceps). After many repetitions, involving about 100 reinforced responses and as many unreinforced, the monkey could produce bursts of cortical cellular activity without any measurable EMG response in the sample muscles. So the relationship between neuronal discharge and contraction of the biceps muscle was flexible. This phenomenon could be dependent on other connections with the spinal final common path being so modified in their activity that they prevented a motor output in response to the corticospinal discharges. It has been mentioned already that, in sleep, bursts of high-frequency discharge may occur in PTN without motor responses (Evarts, 1964). It is also relevant that repetitive, very high frequency discharge of PTN in the vicinity of epileptic foci may occur without overt movement. The monkey, learning to produce bursts of cortical neuronal discharge without movement responses in a 'closely coupled' muscle, may have been learning to suppress the effects of these bursts of activity at a lower level in the motor system.

Although the reverse dissociation was attempted, and the monkey was rewarded for producing muscular contractions in the biceps muscle without concomitant cellular discharge in the sample cortical neurone, this dissociation was not fully achieved. Contraction with less than normal cellular discharge was seen. A possible interpretation of the difficulty of producing muscle contraction without cortical discharge is that, in order to initiate contraction of the biceps muscle fibres, some cortical discharge in cells related to the innervation of this muscle was necessary. Production of EMG responses in the biceps muscle without activity in a previously related PTN could be meaningful only if it could be shown that the muscle could be *maximally* active without concurrent discharge in the appropriate cells.

These experiments have been important in demonstrating a conditioning test for the stability of relationships between neuronal discharge in the cortex and movement performance. A very stable relationship could be a causal one and Fetz and Finocchio suggested that resistance of the relationship to dissociation might indicate a causal connection. But demonstrated flexibility of the association does not preclude a causal relationship. It could mean that, under certain circumstances, effective connexions may have their influences cancelled or suppressed by the operation of other systems. It would also be of great importance to test the stability of the relationships between PTN discharge and the contractions of muscles acting about the most distal joints of the forelimb, because other evidence points to a more significant role for PT activity in the control of these muscles than in the contractions of proximal muscles such as biceps.

Schmidt *et al.* (1974) examined the discharges of a number of cortical neurones (not identified as PTN) during repetitive flexion–extension movements of the wrist against a simulated spring load. The load was controlled electronically and could be varied without influencing the monkey or its posture. About one-third of 35 task-related cortical neurones showed a changing pattern of cellular activity in response to repetitions of identical load changes. Schmidt *et al.* argued for a plastic relationship between cellular function in the cerebral cortex and the load to be moved in a wrist flexion–extension task. They suggested that, because this plasticity exists, it is impossible to define the relationship between a cell and a specific task unless the cycle of changes in the task is repeated frequently and the relationship is shown to be independent of the previous experience of load changes. But many of the cells these authors examined appeared to be only weakly related to the particular task. A more valid test for plasticity requires that a relationship between cellular activity and muscle contraction which is very strong be shown to change with time. In fact, many PTN whose firing is so tightly related to the contractions of a particular muscle can be shown to preserve that precise relationship, particularly to the timing of contraction of the muscle, even through very large numbers of repetitions of a movement task. Plasticity of their relationship to the task seems to be minimal when stereotyped, similar tasks are performed repetitively. But flexibility of involvement is obvious when different movement tasks are studied.

Re-examining the relations of cortical cell activity to the force developed during wrist movements, Schmidt *et al.* (1975) were led to conclude that very few cells showed a clear change in discharge with change in static force development or with the rate of change of force in this task. But the cells whose discharges they studied were related in their activity to the movement task in a way that suggested involvement of the cortical cell in specifying which muscles were to be activated for the particular movement performance (see earlier, Chapter 6, and Porter and Lewis, 1975).

Demonstration of a causal involvement of the discharges of a PTN (through its corticomotoneuronal connexions) in the firing of motor units of a particular muscle could be obtained by the demonstration, in simultaneous recordings from the PTN and the muscle, of an increase in probability of motor unit activity occurring with an appropriate latency and time-course after the discharge of an impulse by the PTN. Analysis by cross-correlation of the relationships between many pairs of simultaneous recordings from PT or other precentral neurones and limb muscles has been carried out by a number of workers. Some of these studies have used electromyographic registration of muscle contraction with surface electrodes over particular muscles. Other studies have sampled the electrical activity of parts of representative muscles or of motor units in those muscles using implanted electrodes (Muir, 1975). Although several hundred cortical cell-muscle pairs have been examined during prolonged periods of time and through many tens of thousands of discharges of the cortical cell, very little evidence for a direct, short latency effect of cortical cell firing on muscular response has been produced. The probability of muscle activity increases or decreases in many muscles after the individual discharges of a sample PTN, but these changes begin late, occur slowly and are prolonged so that they provide no evidence for a direct effect of the cortical cell on muscle action.

But in a few examples (8 out of 70), particularly when the muscles studied have been those acting distally, Fetz *et al.* (1975) have demonstrated a clear-cut increase in muscle activity which begins in forearm muscles as early as 6 ms after the impulse is recorded in the cortical cell. This increase in activity has a time-course with a rising and decaying phase said to be like that of a monosynaptic corticomotoneuronal EPSP and occurs only in some of a group of muscle responses sampled simultaneously with the cortical cell. This is a most important finding. The experiment deserves to be extended and other attempts made to confirm this report. It demonstrates that, at a statistical level, when the correct pair (cortical cell and muscle) are studied together, even the tiny influence which might result from the discharge of a single corticomotoneuronal fibre impinging on the membrane of a motoneurone is capable of influencing the firing of that motoneurone and so changing the probability of occurrence of muscle action.

In another study, Fetz *et al.* (1976) examined the activities of 200 precentral neurones whose discharges covaried with movement. Of these, the discharges of 54 were followed by transient increases in EMG activity with latencies between 4.3 and 11.5 ms. Only 4 of 35 identified PT neurones showed such transient increases (post-spike facilitation) in EMG responses following their discharges. In order to demonstrate these 'post-spike facilitation' changes it was necessary to select conditions in which the cell's firing and the multi-unit EMG were in a steady-state relationship, with the animal holding a particular position. Cell firing and concomitant EMG activity which accompanied changes in position were neglected. When cortical cell activity was examined simultaneously with the EMGs of a number of muscles (more than 5 in each case), post-spike facilitation of the EMG could occur only in a single muscle or in a group of synergistic muscles acting at a single joint. Fetz *et al.* deduced that a corticomotoneuronal cell could influence motoneurones of only one muscle and hence have a very limited 'muscle field' or could branch to engage motoneurones of a number of related muscles. It is of interest that post-spike depression of EMG activity was not reported in this study, even in muscles acting antagonistically to those which were facilitated.

The conclusion that must be drawn from the infrequent observation of this possibly monosynaptic effect in cross-correlation studies is that individual PTN make limited effective connexions with spinal motoneurones. The general correlation of muscle activity with cortical cell firing which is seen in a large number of muscles could reflect changes in excitability of subcortical nuclei or spinal interneurones which follow the cortical cell's action potentials. But specific evidence for a causal role of corticomotoneuronal synapses in promoting muscle action is seen only rarely and when an appropriate combination of neurone and muscle are, by chance, sampled together. That the effect is a small one could relate to the small size of the excitatory influences produced by individual corticomotoneuronal synapses. A specific function of corticonotoneuronal connexions with particular motoneurones is suggested, however. These specific connexions could be concerned in the precise timing of the contractions of particular motor units which is so essential for the performance of skilled movement.

7.6 The influence of peripheral receptors on pyramidal tract discharge during movement performance

There is ample evidence that, in both the cat and the monkey, a large variety of peripheral afferents is capable of influencing PT neurones. This is discussed more fully in Chapter 6. The function of this influence during natural movement cannot be deduced from acute experiments or from observations made by stimulating receptors in a passive limb. As Brooks and Stoney (1971) have pointed out, the dynamic effects during movement may differ significantly from the static effects observable during an acute experiment in a non-moving animal. There is also ample evidence that movement performance may be influenced by disturbances of input from receptors in the moving limb (Mott and Sherrington, 1895). It has been possible to examine the effects of modifications of receptor function on PT activity during movement performance.

A simple, initial experiment demonstrated that, in the conscious, free-to-move monkey, impairment of afferent feedback from the receptors of the moving hand could modify the relationship between cellular activity in PTN and movement performance. Recordings were made of the discharges of PTN associated with the repetitive performance of the lever-pulling task referred to previously. Once the behaviour of the neurone had been examined quantitatively, a small dose of local anaesthetic was injected subcutaneously on the flexor aspect of the wrist of the moving hand. This anaesthetic diffused in the tissue at the wrist and caused a partial anaesthesia of the palm and the fingers which reduced the responsiveness of the animal to stimuli delivered to these skin areas. In addition, some impairment of conduction in afferent fibres from joints of the fingers and some loss of function in the small muscles of the hand probably occurred. But the animal was still capable of carrying out the lever-pulling task at the same rate as previously and with the same force development as before the interference with afferent signals from the hand. Hence it was possible to re-examine the discharges of the same pyramidal tract neurone in relation to repetitions of this very similar movement performance but in the absence of some of the afferent signals normally produced during the movement.

Figure 7.15 shows the activity of a PTN with an axonal conduction velocity of 50 m s^{-1} which produced a burst of discharge correlated with the movement of the lever. The upper histogram shows the summed activity associated with 50 repetitions of the pull phase of the lever-moving task. (The lever movement is shown at the bottom of the Figure and the average duration of the associated burst of nerve impulses is indicated by the white bar above the histogram.) After partial local anaesthesia of the moving hand, 50 repetitions of the same movement performance were accompanied by more discharge in this cell (lower histogram) and the associated burst of activity lasted longer.

However, the muscle contractions were not significantly altered. Thus there was a change in the relationship between PTN activity and muscle activity (although perhaps not individual motoneurone activity). This could have been due to the increased PT discharge replacing, in some sense, the lost effect of the normal afferent input on spinal mechanisms. Alternatively, the afferents anaesthetized could have been insignificant except in modifying the animal's knowledge of his limb. The result might then have been one of relearning, producing a change in the relationship between cellular activity and muscle activity similar to that described by Fetz and Finocchio (1972).

Local anaesthesia of the hand did not destroy the relationship between neuronal activity and the load to be moved in the lever-pulling task, nor did it alter significantly the relationship between the pattern of neuronal discharge in the bursts and the time of onset of associated muscle contractions. The PT unit illustrated in Fig. 7.14 is a representative example. With a normally sentient hand, the mean frequency of discharge of this unit increased from 37.2 to 46.6 impulses per second when the lever was loaded with an additional 200 g weight. After partial anaesthesia of the hand being used to move the lever, the discharges of the same unit changed from 42.8 to 55.1 impulses per second for the same increase in load, a strikingly similar proportional increase. Moreover, a consistent relationship between the latency of the shortest interval after the first spike in the

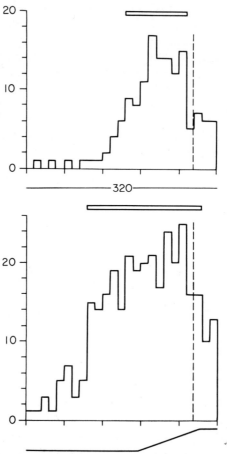

FIG. 7.15. Peri-response time histograms have been plotted of the discharges of an individual pyramidal tract neurone discharging bursts of nerve impulses in association with 50 repetitions of a lever-pulling task. The occurrences of nerve impulses have been plotted in time bins before and after the end of forward movement of the lever (indicated by interrupted vertical line), and the average movement of the lever is schematically indicated by the black line at the bottom of the Figure. The upper correlogram shows the bursts of impulses discharged in relation to movement before administration of a dose of local anaesthetic to the right wrist, while the lower correlogram shows the bursts associated with 50 repetitions of a similar movement after partial anaesthesia of the hand. In each case, the abscissa has a duration of 320 ms about the movement performance and the ordinate indicates number of occurrences of nerve impulses. The axonal conduction velocity for this pyramidal tract neurone was 50 m s⁻¹. When the load on the lever was increased by 200 g weight, it increased its firing both before and after local anaesthesia of the hand (from 32.2 to 36.0 impulses per second before and from 39.5 to 40.5 impulses per second after local anaesthesia of the hand). (Lewis and Porter, 1974.)

burst and the time of onset of associated muscle contraction could still be observed. Although there was a tendency for the onset of muscle contraction to occur slightly later, many of the observations for individual performances of the motor task were consistent with those which had been made before local anaesthetic was administered. The discharges of the unit were still clearly related both to the load to be moved and to the time of onset of muscle contraction associated with the movement. Impaired afferent feedback from the hand had not caused a gross disturbance in these relationships which must have been governed by a learned central nervous system programme or by other afferent systems (Lewis and Porter, 1974).

It might be expected that, because of the partial paralysis of the intrinsic muscles of the hand which must have resulted from the injection of local anaesthetic, 'extra' activity in other muscles (presumably the long flexors of the fingers) would be necessary to allow the animal to grasp the lever sufficiently firmly to pull it. However, any extra PTN activity necessary to drive this should occur immediately before the grasp phase of the movement and might well be seen in PTN corresponding to those of Fig. 7.8A (whose natural firing increased ahead of the grasp). The increased activity following local anaesthesia of the hand was more reliably observed in the PTN which fired their bursts immediately before the pull phase (Fig. 7.8B). This extra firing must presumably have been associated with an increased cortical drive to the motoneurones supplying the muscles which actually pull the lever.

If the injection of local anaesthetic were made subcutaneously in a region of skin not directly involved in the movement task (the skin over the lumbar region in the midline of the back or the skin on the volar aspect of the ipsilateral wrist) the influence of the injection on PT and non-identified neurones firing with the movement task was not consistent. Impairment of afferent conduction from the ipsilateral hand could influence cortical neuronal firing in relation to movement of the contra-lateral hand, but the direction of this influence was not systematic and its magnitude was small.

The influence of local anaesthesia of the moving hand was dependent on the degree of impairment of afferent conduction and larger effects on PT discharge were produced by larger doses of anaesthetic. However, the effects studied in detail were those caused by small injections because, with more anaesthesia of the hand than these produced, and spread of the drug to influence wider regions of skin and to paralyse more muscles, movement performance was impaired. Following a single injection of 0.3 to 0.5 ml of 1 per cent xylocaine with adrenaline at the right wrist, sample PTN discharging with the grasp and pull phases of movement increased their frequency of discharge by about 20 per cent without detectable alteration in the movement performance. These increases were statistically significant. For example, three PTN with similar mean frequencies of firing during bursts of activity before local anaesthesia of the right wrist (discharging at 30.3, 37.2 and 32.2 impulses per second, respectively) increased their mean firing to 44.8, 42.8 and 39.5 impulses per second in association with similar stereotyped movements carried out after the injection of local anaesthetic (Lewis and Porter, 1974).

The changes in response of PTN during movement could not have been due entirely to a different strategy of movement performance and a different sequence of muscle contractions with the partly anaesthetic and possibly partly paralysed hand, because the activity of some PTN increased after local anaesthesia of the hand even in time periods when the animal was still and not using the contralateral forelimb. The suggestion must be that afferent discharge from the hand was capable of influencing PTN continuously. For some neurones, whose discharges were related to the contraction of muscles used in grasping and pulling, this effect could be revealed as an increased overall firing of the cells when the function of afferents from the hand was impaired. Moreover, when these cells were caused to discharge in association with the contraction of their target muscles, their increased excitability (possibly due to removal of a tonic inhibitory influence resulting from input from the hand receptors) was revealed as a higher frequency of discharge and a longer duration of the associated burst.

Another approach to the relationship between activation of peripheral receptors and PT discharge during movement performance has been to introduce an external disturbance of the movement during the study of pyramidal tract activity. Monkeys were trained to position a handle, which they grasped continuously, within a target zone. Correct positioning of the handle was indicated by a light signal. After the handle had been held in the correct position for some seconds it was unexpectedly displaced by an external force which abruptly moved it out of the target zone either towards or away from the animal. The monkey was then rewarded for promptly returning the handle to the correct position. Once the animal was proficient in the performance of the task, recordings were made from pre- and postcentral neurones discharging in relation to the task. Of 500 neurones examined, 75 were identified as PTN (Evarts, 1973).

The shortest latency from perturbation of the handle to discharge of postcentral neurones was 10 ms, but a wide range of response latencies was found for the 200 postcentral cells examined. The minimum latency for response of a precentral neurone was 14 ms, but the earliest response in an identified PTN occurred 20 ms after the disturbance of position. (This cell decreased its activity in response to the movement of the handle.) The earliest increase in firing of a PTN occurred 24 ms after the perturbation of the handle. The latencies for the responses of PTN were commonly between 20 and 40 ms, early enough for receptors detecting change in position to alter the firing of PTN during movement performance if the same effects occurred also during active movement.

In response to the activation of peripheral receptors by the disturbance of position, and presumably in response to changes in muscle spindle discharge by the elongation of muscles, reflex changes in electromyographic records were seen with a latency of about 12 ms. A second and third phase of muscle response then followed with latencies respectively of 30 to 40 and about 80 ms. The short-latency (30–40 ms) response occurred only after monkeys had been trained and had learned to correct the disturbance in position by making an opposing movement. Evarts (1973) concluded that this short-latency EMG response could have occurred via a cortical loop from receptors in muscle capable of influencing PTN related to the initiation and control of muscle contraction. The process of learning could have allowed this loop to produce an effective output to muscles.

In a different experiment (Porter and Rack, 1976), a very similar latency was measured for the responses of PTN to imposed disturbances of nearly isometric muscle contraction. Monkeys were trained to generate force with the tips of their fingers against a rigid force-measuring lever. Electromyographic responses were recorded in *flexor digitorum profundus* muscle which was a prime mover in the test and was contracting almost isometrically. The activities of PTN whose discharges increased with force (and often more clearly and phasically with the small dynamic fluctuations in the force trace) were sampled. The force-measuring lever, which was held against an electromagnet, could then suddenly and unexpectedly be released, producing an abrupt unloading of the isometrically contracting flexor muscles and a brief flexion movement of the finger joints.

The monkey was not required to make any response to this sudden disturbance and was rewarded only for the maintenance of force (during periods of many seconds). The unloading disturbance was not provided during the preliminary training of the animal and was used for the first time only when recordings were being made of the activities of the first PTN to be tested. During testing, unloading was carried out in some trials and not others at a variable time after the beginning of the force development task and with no visual or auditory cue.

Electromyographic responses to the disturbance were variable. A period of reduced EMG activity sometimes followed the unloading with very short latency, but, after this, no consistent EMG changes occurred. Yet the peripheral disturbance produced a clear, definite, short-latency effect on PTN discharge. Cells which increased their discharge with increase in force of contraction sometimes showed a peak of firing 20 to 40 ms after the sudden release of the lever and unloading of the muscle

(Fig. 7.16). This peak of firing would appear to be in an appropriate direction for initiating a return to the previous force condition (to which the animal had been trained), but it did not automatically produce a muscular response in these cases. The production of a muscle response may depend on other factors, presumably related to training, in addition to PT response.

Conrad *et al.* (1974) examined the responses of 98 precentral cortical neurones to sudden and unexpected load changes during a learned elbow movement in *Cebus* monkeys. In all but two of 94 cortical cells tested, the sudden introduction of a torque pulse during the execution of the elbow movement caused a clear-cut effect on the cellular discharge. Torque pulses in opposite directions frequently produced opposite effects. The latency between the beginning of the disturbance and the change in cortical cell firing was of the order of 30 ms and the direction of the effect in cells which normally fired before a flexion or an extension movement suggested to these authors that the cortical effect had a role in load compensation. It was indicated that the discharge of some flexion-related cortical cells was enhanced by limb displacements which tended to stretch flexor muscles. But not all the neurones studied behaved uniformly.

It remains to be demonstrated that the increased cell firing about 30 ms after the introduction of a disturbance during movement is causally related to the muscular reactions to this disturbance. It has been pointed out already that precise relationships between PTN discharge and muscle contraction have been difficult to define. For a very small proportion of cells it may be possible to deduce that increased discharge would inevitably be associated with increased contraction in some muscle with the motoneurones of which the cortical cell made specific and powerful connexion. But for most cortical neurones this relationship between cellular activity and muscle action required to move a load or overcome a resistance is not so clear cut. Hence it is not possible to deduce that a particular change in PTN discharge would lead to a particular muscular response.

The early responses of cortical neurones to a sudden disturbance of movement in the experiments of Conrad *et al.* were not affected by cooling of the dentate nucleus, but later responses, associated with oscillations in the movement following the disturbance, were greatly attenuated. Moreover, the oscillations in position of the limb were reduced in frequency following dentate cooling.

Even the influence of an abrupt disturbance of position on PTN may be capable of being modified depending on the instruction for response given to a monkey. Evarts and Tanji (1974) have trained a monkey to make one of two responses (to push or to pull a handle) according to a coloured light signal that indicated the direction of the movement to be made. The animal was taught to make the response immediately after a sudden

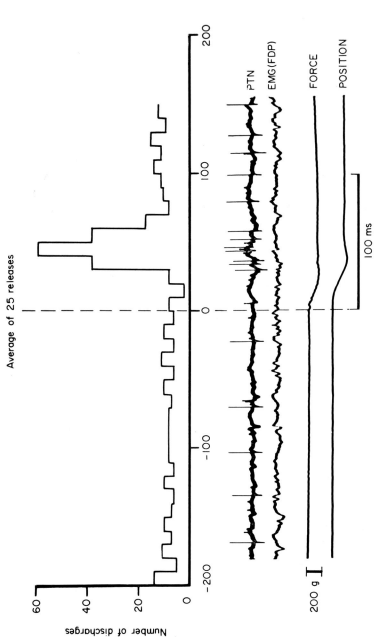

FIG. 7.16. The response of a cortical neurone to sudden finger flexion. While the monkey pulled with the tips of the fingers and generated force by almost isometric contraction of the long finger flexors, the lever was suddenly released to allow the fingers to flex. Time measurements relate to the release. The position record gives only an approximate indication of the time-course of the movement. Activity is recorded from a neurone (PTN) which could be stimulated antidromically from pyramidal electrodes (conduction velocity 56 ms⁻¹). EMG activity is recorded from within a part of *flexor digitorum profundus*. Above, and on the same time scale, is a histogram to show the total number of action potentials recorded in each 10 ms period before and after 25 consecutive releases of the lever. (Porter and Rack, 1976.)

disturbance of position of the handle was imposed either in the 'push' or the 'pull' direction. The short-latency responses of PTN to this sudden disturbance depended not only on the direction of the disturbance but also on the instruction about the movement to be made. Hence a neurone could be shown to produce a burst of impulses 20 to 40 ms after the hand was displaced in the push direction provided that the instruction had been for the animal to pull when the signal arrived. With the alternative instruction to push, the same disturbance failed to produce the burst of impulses or resulted in a smaller response. So the afferent limb of the 'cortical loop' could be made operative (closed) or inoperative (open) depending on other influences conveying aspects of an instruction for movement to the PTN.

The nature of the receptors responsible for the early response of PTN is not at present clear. As described in Chapter 6, muscle spindle afferents and joint afferents have been implicated in the production of excitation of PTN in monkeys (Albe-Fessard and Liebeskind, 1966; Fetz and Baker, 1971; Rosén and Asanuma, 1972; Lemon and Porter, 1976). Since muscle spindle afferents, shown to be conducting impulses during isometric contractions of hand muscles in man (Vallbo, 1970) would be influenced by the manipulations used by Evarts (1973), Wiesendanger (1973) and by Porter and Rack (1976) in their experiments, it is possible that muscle spindle afferents with access to PTN concerned in the innervation of alpha and fusimotor neurones for their muscle may provide a means of compensating for disturbances in load during movement performance (Phillips, 1969; Wiesendanger, 1973). It is possible that complex inter-actions between muscle spindle afferents and others (from joints and skin) occur to determine whether or not the output of PTN in response to a peripheral disturbance becomes effective in activating muscles (see Marsden et al., 1972).

Changes in muscle spindle discharge have been shown to occur during isometric contraction of finger muscles in man (Fig. 8.12, p. 352: Vallbo, 1970) and during contraction of intercostal muscles of the cat during breathing (von Euler, 1966). During locomotion, hindlimb muscle spindles in the cat have been shown to change their firing with the step cycle (Severin et al., 1967) and during chewing, muscle spindle afferents from the cat's jaw muscles demonstrate changes in activity (Taylor and Davey, 1968; Taylor and Cody, 1974). Changes of firing of muscle spindle afferents from jaw-closing muscles of the monkey have been demonstrated during mastication (Goodwin and Luschei, 1975). But, at least in the last case, the muscle spindle afferent discharge was greatest when the motoneurones of the muscle were inactive and the muscle was being stretched.

In a number of these examples, muscle spindle afferents were active during active movement when muscles were shortening (suggesting fusimotor drive) and also during passive lengthening of the muscle as the converse movement was produced by contraction of antagonists. For some muscle spindle afferents, at least, fusimotor bias during active movement was insufficient to overcome the unloading effect of rapid shortening of the muscle. What use the central nervous system makes of this afferent input is still an open question. But the input from spindles could be one source of projections to PTN.

7.7 Discharges of corticobulbar neurones associated with movements of cranial musculature

Because of the complexity of most arm movements which inevitably involve postural changes and muscular contraction in many parts of the body in addition to the moving limb, the observed relationships between neuronal discharge and the execution of a movement task are difficult to evaluate. Some self-initiated movements are mechanically much simpler and involve contractions of fewer muscles, whose activities can be described completely and quantitatively. The discharges of cortical neurones have been sampled during such movements (e.g. of the eyes and of the jaw) and some of the cortical units so studied have been shown to send their axons into the corticobulbar tracts.

Bizzi (1968) examined the behaviour of neurones in the cortex of the frontal eye fields from which conjugate movements of the eyes have been elicited by electrical stimulation. One group of cells (his type II), which all showed antidromic responses to stimulation of the cerebral peduncle, were found to produce a steady discharge when the eyes were directed to a particular position in visual space. The steady discharge stopped during saccades but the cells continued firing during slow pursuit movements of the eyes and during the slow phase of nystagmus provided these movements carried the eyes through the position at which discharge during fixation occurred. The range of eye position over which steady discharge was seen was of the order of 30° and, within this range, increasing degrees of deviation of the eyes were associated with increasing steady discharge. In all cases, the discharge tended to occur *after* the appropriate position had been reached rather than before the movement to this position. But the discharge was seen even in complete darkness: so it did not depend upon visual feedback. No discharge with the slow phase of nystagmus occurred if the rate of nystagmus was high. Bizzi therefore suggested that the response was probably not due to proprioceptive feedback from the eye muscles. But, in these chronic monkey preparations, the exclusion of eye muscle proprioceptors as the initiators of the discharge was not possible.

A second group of neurones in the frontal eye fields (type I of Bizzi's classification) most of which could not be shown to send their axons into the cerebral peduncle, discharged each time a saccade in a particular direction occurred. These cells showed no discharge when the eyes were still, irrespective of eye position. Like the neurones previously mentioned, these cells also fired *after* the saccadic movement and they could be seen to fire after the fast phase of nystagmus providing this occurred in the direction for the saccade to which the cells responded. Smooth pursuit movements in the same direction, however, were not accompanied by discharge of the type I units. These relationships between discharge and the kinetic phase of fast eye movements were also preserved in complete darkness.

In all the above experiments, the animals were able to move their eyes but the head was fixed. Bizzi and Schiller (1970) therefore re-examined the behaviour of frontal eye field neurones in relation to eye position when the head was free to be moved also—a more natural circumstance in which movements of the head and eyes were coordinated for direction of the gaze. Under these conditions, an object in the visual field first caused a fast saccadic movement of the eyes. Then a slower movement of the head in the same direction occurred while the eyes slowly moved in the head in the reverse direction, maintaining fixation of the gaze on the object. The characteristic firing patterns of the two groups of frontal eye field neurones (type I and type II) were maintained under these conditions. Type I neurones showed bursts of activity only during saccades in their preferred direction and type II cells discharged steadily in relation to characteristic positions of the eyes in the head.

The functions of cells in the frontal eye fields could not be deduced from these experiments. One group had discharges associated with the position of the eyes and the sustained contractions of the muscles producing this position. They recorded the direction of vision in slow pursuit movements while the other group was associated with the direction of saccadic movements. No neurones responded early enough to cause the movements and Bizzi suggested that they might be cells involved in corollary discharge recording the commanded movements of the eyes and the position specified.

In addition to the 'eye movement' neurones, a separate group of cells was identified whose discharges were associated with head turning. Most of these cells could be activated antidromically from the cerebral peduncle and they discharged before and during particular movements of the head. Some discharged before movements of the head to the right, others before movements to the left and some discharged irrespective of direction of movement. These cells were not affected by eye movements and they could have been related to the contractions of neck muscles in a manner analogous to the PT discharges with arm muscle contractions already described (Bizzi and Schiller, 1970).

Luschei *et al.* (1971) recorded from neurones in the 'face area' of the precentral gyrus of monkeys which had been trained to carry out a bite on a lever which allowed characteristics of the contractions of jaw muscles to be measured. Some units (37 of 61, none of which were identified according to the course of their axons) were found which discharged a burst of impulses about 50 ms before the development of force in the jaw-closing muscles but were not consistently related to the amount of force generated or its rate of change, or to the displacement achieved. During the development of maintained force they usually became silent. A further 17 of the 61 units decreased their firing rates or stopped firing prior to movement. All of the units with responses before the movement showed no detectable discharge to sensory stimulation of the mouth, tongue or face and showed no changes in discharge with movements of the tongue or face. The only consistent relationship found was between the time of change in discharge of some of the cells and the time of initiation of the jaw movement.

7.8   Discharges in other regions of the brain associated with movements of the limb

A comparison may be made between the discharge characteristics of PTN and those of cells in other regions of the central nervous system which could influence or be influenced by the motor cortex during movement performance. Reference has already been made to the fact that cells in the primary receiving cortex of the postcentral gyrus of the monkey tend to discharge after the completion of a learned movement response, although they are affected by sudden perturbations imposed on the learned movement before PTN in neighbouring regions of precentral cortex (Evarts, 1972a, b, 1973). Cells in other regions of the cerebral cortex may also show discharges related to the performance of movement tasks. Kubota and Niki (1971) examined the behaviour of neurones in prefrontal cortex during the performance of a delayed alternation task involving the use of each hand to press spatially separated levers alternately. Two groups of units were identified. The first group, comprising two-thirds of the sample of 49 responsive units, became active about 200 ms before the performance of the delayed movement response and this activity was associated regularly with the movement response itself. The second group of neurones discharged during the delay period between the signal and the movement response. Discharge was maintained for the duration of the delay and was then reduced when the animal pressed the lever. Both groups of unit activity were recorded whether the response was made with the ipsilateral or the contralateral hand. Interpretation of the meaning of these results will depend on further elucidation of the particular associaions of discharges of histologically identified neurones whose connexions can be defined with some particular aspects of this complicated behaviour.

A study of the activities of neurones in area 3a during voluntary movements was conducted by Yumiya et al. (1974). The cells studied were situated deep in the central sulcus and could be discharged at short latency (4 to 7 ms) after weak shocks were delivered to the median nerve at the wrist. Although 55 units were isolated, the responses of only 13 which could be influenced by displacements of the hand are discussed. These 13 responded to 'passive extension of the wrist and tapping in the flexor muscle' in addition to the stimulation of the median nerve. Six of these 13 neurones discharged impulses during extension of the wrist whether the monkey made these movements actively or the experimenter extended the wrist passively. It was considered that an input from muscle spindles, caused by stretch of the flexor muscle in both the active and the passive conditions, must be responsible for this discharge. Five other neurones discharged when the animal made flexion movements actively, even though passive extension of the wrist caused them to respond. These five neurones were considered to receive inputs caused by fusimotor drive to flexor muscle spindles during active contraction as well as from passive stretch of these same spindles. The remaining two units showed 'mixed behaviour'. The effect of requiring the animal to carry out the movement against increasing loads was tested for 7 neurones. All units discharged more in relation to active movements against an added load.

Mountcastle *et al.* (1975) examined the discharges of a large number of neurones in the posterior parietal association cortex (areas 5 and 7) of monkeys trained to produce movement responses to a series of sensory cues. The receptive fields and discharge characteristics of these cells were examined. About two-thirds of the neurones in area 5 were activated by passive rotation of joints, but a large proportion was more strongly influenced when the same joint rotated during active movement of the animal. In area 7, these investigators located a number of cells which appeared to discharge in relation to visual fixation or which were active during arm projection or hand manipulation. The patterns of discharge of these cells varied little with large modifications of direction or speed of movement. Hence they could not have been specifying detailed aspects of movement performance. Moreover, the discharges of cells in both areas 5 and 7 tended to follow movement performance rather than precede it.

Brinkman and Porter (1976) examined the discharges of a large number of neurones in the supplementary motor area on the medial surface of the monkey's cerebral hemisphere. The majority of these cells showed modulation of their activity during particular movements of the ipsilateral and the contralateral limbs. These particular movements with which discharge was associated were often symmetrical, e.g. wrist flexion on either side. Activity could be associated with spontaneous, self-initiated movements of either proximal or of distal joints of these limbs. Although most neurones discharged in relation to movement of both limbs, a few were found to be active only during contralateral or only during ipsilateral movements. Only a small proportion (5 per cent) of neurones in the supplementary motor area whose activity changed with voluntary movement could be demonstrated to send their axons into the pyramidal tract, and only a small proportion (15 per cent) was found to receive afferent inputs from peripheral receptors in the limbs.

The significance of recordings from cortical regions before and during movement can only be assessed when the connectivity between the neurones and the motor cortex or other neural systems concerned in movement or its related 'sensations' is known. Even in those circumstances where the regional connexions have been described, the precise topographical arrangements of these connexions and the delicate modifications of excitatory and inhibitory effects produced by them have not been evaluated in detail. It will be these specific influences which determine the significance of particular cellular activity in one region for the responses of receiving cells in another region.

Cells in parts of the cerebellum have been studied to assess the changes in their discharges during movement (Thach, 1970a, b). Monkeys were trained to hold a lever against a stop with the wrist in a flexed position until they were given a signal to move. The monkeys were then rewarded for executing a sudden movement to an alternative stop and holding the wrist in an extended position. Each of the positions of the wrist was held until the signal to move was presented and the animal could be made to produce alternating abrupt flexion and extension movements with repeated presentations of the signal. Recordings were made of the discharge of cells in the *nucleus dentatus* and *interpositus* and of Purkinje cells in folia of the anterior lobe of the cerebellum. Most of the cells in the dentate nucleus showed changes in discharge which preceded the execution of the fast movements by 50 to 100 ms, but over half of the cells in the interpositus nucleus changed their firing after the performance of the brisk movements. For many neurones, the discharges accompanying the dynamic phase of movements in one direction differed from those accompanying movement in the reverse direction, but most often the discharge during maintained flexion did not differ from that during the maintained extensor posture. The simple spikes of Purkinje cells in the intermediate zone of the anterior lobe of the cerebellum were related to movement in a manner exactly like that of the interpositus neurones to which this part of the cerebellum has been shown to project (Thach, 1970a, b).

Grimm and Rushmer (1974) studied the discharges of 350 neurones whose depth and position in the cerebellum would have placed them in the dentate nucleus. The activities of these cells were correlated with only brief parts of a complex motor task involving the sequential touching of three horizontally arranged touch-buttons. For example, some cells discharged during movement of the ipsilateral hand to one button, but not during quite similar movements to the other two.

Harvey *et al.* (1976) examined the discharges of Purkinje cells in a restricted region of the intermediate zone of the cerebellum just rostral to the fissura prima. Large responses were evoked in this limited region by electrical stimulation of forelimb nerves. The majority of Purkinje cells showed a marked modulation of their simple-spike activity in relation to movement performance with the ipsilateral forelimb. Although some of these Purkinje cells were demonstrated to have receptive fields on the skin of the moving limb, movement of joints did not affect the firing of the cells and disturbances of movement performance did not influence the Purkinje cell discharge.

Thach (1975) attempted to discover whether or not the discharges in the dentate nucleus (in relation to a brisk movement) preceded the discharges of neurones in the cerebral motor cortex in relation to the same movement. The timing of discharges of the two populations of neurones overlapped, and the experiment did not allow a clear definition of the temporal order of activity in these two regions.

De Long (1971) recorded from cells in the lateral portion of the external and internal segments of the globus pallidus which showed phasic discharges with the performance of movements using the contralateral arm. In a later, brief report (De Long and Evarts, 1971) it was stated that pallidal neurones changed their discharge prior to the beginning of movement and in this behaviour were similar to the units in *nucleus ventralis lateralis* (VL) of the thalamus to which some, at least, of the pallidal neurones project. But the possibility of projection of the sampled cells to this site was not tested. Evarts (1970) found that increases or decreases in activity of VL neurones preceded movement by as much as 100 ms. He and his colleagues have interpreted these findings in a number of central nervous structures as evidence for the involvement of the cerebellum and the globus pallidus, both acting through neurones in the ventrolateral nucleus of the thalamus, in the regulation and modification of PT activity during movement. But it will require very accurate measurements of the timing of the discharges of connected neurones during the performance of motor tasks to evaluate this concept adequately. The evidence available at present could not distinguish effects of the motor cortex on the thalamus (or the basal ganglia or cerebellum) from influences of those structures on the cerebral cortex with which reciprocal connexions exist. More recent experiments by De Long and Strick (1974) implicate neurones of the striatum in ramp movements rather than in ballistic movements (see Kornhuber, 1971).

That the dentate nuclear cells, at least, may be involved in the relationship between PT discharge and movement performance has been suggested by Brooks *et al.* (1972) who cooled the dentate nucleus during movement performance in a monkey from whose precentral cortex recordings of neuronal discharge were being made. The cooling of the dentate nucleus increased the velocity at which conditioned movements were performed. But, for a given movement against a set load at a particular velocity, less neuronal discharge was recorded in sample precentral neurones after dentate cooling. The meaning of this effect cannot be evaluated without more evidence about the nature and detailed connexions of the cells from which recordings have been made.

7.9   Recordings made during voluntary movements in man

It has not been possible to sample the activities of identified PT neurones in man and to record their discharges during voluntary movement. But some recordings of electrical activity of the cerebral cortex during movement performance have been made. Jasper and Penfield (1949) recorded the potential changes occurring over the exposed precentral gyrus and failed to find any clear characteristic variation in the potentials which preceded movements. The rhythmic waves of potential change which were seen in precentral regions (beta waves) were suppressed during voluntary hand movement. This suppression occurred only upon the initiation and termination of a movement and the beta waves returned during the maintenance of a continued posture (e.g. clenching the fist). On some occasions blocking of the rhythmic waves of potential was also seen with preparation for movement and before it was actually begun.

Dawson (1947) used the technique of summing many events, first by superimposition of photographic records and later by means of a specially constructed storage device utilizing capacitors (an early averaging computer), to improve the detection of small signals occurring within the on-going EEG activity of human subjects. He was able to show that, in a subject with myoclonic epilepsy, a large cerebral electrical response could be detected over the scalp after a tap on a tendon or after electrical stimulation of a peripheral nerve. This potential response was maximal over the contralateral precentral gyrus. Similar potential changes in this situation occurred about 15 to 40 ms before the onset of sudden, involuntary jerk-like contractions of skeletal muscle in this myoclonic patient. Much smaller changes in potential (like the evoked potentials recorded from the exposed cortex of lightly anaesthetized animals) could be revealed by using averaging methods and following electrical stimulation of peripheral nerves in normal subjects (Dawson, 1950).

Bates (1951) used superimposition of EEG recordings obtained from the scalp of subjects instructed to make a succession of abrupt grips of the hand on a 4 cm diameter cardboard cylinder at a rate of about 10 a minute.

The EEG recordings accompanying the repeated voluntary hand movements were superimposed with the instant of increased muscle action of
the grip lined up for each record. In some subjects, the instant of motor
performance tended to be related to a particular phase of the EEG alpha
rhythm. But more consistently, a small potential change in the region of the
contralateral central sulcus appeared 20 to 40 ms after the onset of movement. The timing of this potential change and that occurring when the
same muscles were made to contract by an appropriate electric shock were
very similar and it was suggested that the regular potential change accompanying movement was caused by afferent impulses arriving from the
periphery. No clear potential changes were detected in the scalp recordings
preceding the beginning of movement.

The availability of electronic averaging computers enabled Gilden *et al.*
(1966) to examine in more detail scalp EEG records obtained during repetitive movement performance. Voluntary contractions (making a fist) were
performed with the left or right hand and voluntary self-paced abrupt
dorsiflexions of the foot were also studied. These authors identified a
characteristic response ('motor potential') in all their 11 subjects. A slow
negative shift of the baseline began approximately one second before the
onset of EMG activity in the muscles being used. Then, 50 to 105 ms
prior to the onset of contraction, this negative shift was terminated by a
small positive deflection followed by a larger negative wave which increased
during the development of the EMG response. Fifty ms or so after the
onset of contraction another positive wave (possibly similar to that recorded
by Bates) was seen. The motor potential accompanying movements of the
foot was maximal near the vertex. With movements of the hand, although
the potentials were still large at the vertex, they could be recorded more
laterally and were especially prominent over the contralateral hemisphere.
It was considered that the sudden change in potential 50 to 150 ms before
the onset of movement might reflect activation of corticospinal pathways
associated with the initiation of movement.

Deecke *et al.* (1969) averaged the EEG records accompanying repeated
quick voluntary palmar flexions of the right index finger and small quick
abductions of the right arm. Potential changes preceding movement were
found in all the sixteen subjects studied, but the authors considered that the
term 'motor potential' should be applied to that part only of the total
response which was closely related in its spatial distribution to the zone
over the region of motor cortex which was active in a specific movement.
Accordingly, they divided the potential changes into three phases. A slowly
increasing negative 'readiness potential' began about 850 ms before the
onset of the mechanical displacement ('contingent negative variation' of
Grey Walter). It was followed by a rapidly increasing additional negativity
(the true 'motor potential') which began with a mean latency of 87 ms

before the mechanical response (and 56 ms before the beginning of EMG activity). A sudden positive deflection ('pre-motion positivity') began with a mean latency of 117 ms before the mechanical response (86 ms before the EMG). These individual components were differently distributed over the scalp. While both the readiness potential and the pre-motion positivity were recorded bilaterally and over wide regions of the scalp, the motor potential was restricted in its maximum amplitude to the zone over the contralateral precentral representation of the moving limb.

Kato and Tanji (1972) examined the relationship between averaged potentials recorded from the scalp and the discharge of individual motor units in *abductor pollicis brevis* or *opponens pollicis* muscles during voluntary contractions performed by human subjects. It was clear that systematic potential deflections were evident in association with the individual spikes of a motor unit's discharge and that these potential changes were not produced by visual or auditory feedback related to the muscle contraction. The records showed a triphasic (or biphasic) wave of potential. When the first negative wave occurred, it began about 500 ms before the first EMG spike from the motor unit. The spike then occurred at the bottom of this negative potential or immediately afterwards on the upstroke of the positive wave. By far the most prominent response was the second negative wave which followed well after the discharge of the motor unit. If these responses are to be equated with those of Deecke *et al.* the first negative wave must have contained the motor potential.

It has been suggested (Gerbrandt *et al.*, 1973) that these cortical potentials preceding movement are never sufficiently well localized to be used as an indication of specific cortical activity associated with the movement performance. While all the waves they recorded were similar to those reported by Gilden *et al.* and by Deecke *et al.* and while they were all larger over the contralateral than the ipsilateral hemisphere, they were not restricted to the scalp overlying the motor strip. Moreover, the second negative wave or motor potential most commonly occurred *after* the beginning of EMG activity in the movement performance. The usefulness of these averaged potentials in the analysis of the neural correlates of movement performance remains to be further evaluated.

Potentials evoked by peripheral stimuli have been demonstrated in the exposed human precentral gyrus (Goldring *et al.*, 1970) and these responses were most pronounced when afferent fibres from the limb represented in that part of the precentral gyrus were activated. In man, stimuli applied to other afferent systems were much less effective in producing precentral evoked responses. It is, therefore, of some interest that the prominent component of some of the potentials recorded from the human scalp during movement performance was the large deflection after the beginning of movement. It could be a response to activation by the movement of receptors in the moving limb.

Li and Tew (1964) recorded the discharges of individual neurones in the precentral gyrus of conscious human subjects undergoing surgery for epilepsy or Parkinson's disease. They reported that the discharge frequency of such precentral units was often altered by voluntary contraction and relaxation of the contralateral fingers. Moreover, in a single electrode penetration of the cortex, discharges of a number of cells could sometimes be sampled simultaneously. In such cases, reciprocal discharges of these cells with contraction or relaxation of the fingers were often seen. Goldring and Ratcheson (1972) extended these observations. They recorded from 30 cells in the hand motor area of five subjects undergoing craniotomy for treatment of epilepsy, but the focal epileptic region did not include the area studied with microelectrodes. Only sixteen of the thirty cells were responsive to the tests applied (passive flexion and extension of the wrists and of the digits, tactile stimulation of the skin with a cotton wisp, active movements of the hand on command); the others were not influenced. No sensations were produced by the presence of the electrodes in the motor cortex.

Although the number of observations is limited, it is important to examine the results obtained in conscious human subjects carefully. Although most of the cells responded only to contralateral stimuli, four of the 16 cells responded to physiological stimuli applied to either hand. (The local evoked potentials in this region were produced only by contra-lateral median nerve stimulation.) Two of these cells which were activated by passive flexion of the fingers also discharged during active closure of the hand to make a fist (finger flexion) and the increased firing continued while the active flexion was maintained. The opposite movement, of opening the hand, suppressed the discharge of these units. The discharge increased *before* the onset of electromyographic evidence of active movement and, in the example cited, where the cell had a receptive field for joint movement in each hand, the discharge also occurred with active movement of either hand.

Only active or passive movements of the hand influenced the sixteen responsive cells; they did not discharge in response to light tactile stimula-tion of the skin or to clicks. Some cells discharged during sustained closure of the contralateral hand and some were silenced by this active movement; and all the cells associated with hand movements had local receptive fields in the contralateral hand alone or in both hands. Cells situated so close to one another that their activity was sampled simul-taneously with a single position of the recording electrode could either behave in a reciprocal or in a similar manner during alternating opening and closing of the hand. Goldring and Ratcheson considered that their observations indicated a kinaesthetic (movement-sensing) input to cells in motor cortex, with some cells receiving this input from both pisilateral and contralateral limbs and sending an output to the motor systems of both.

Similarities between the findings in these neurones and those in identified PTN in monkeys are obvious. Although it has not been possible to identify the cells in the human precentral gyrus with respect to the destination of their axons, it is clear that some cells from which recordings have been made behave very much like identified PTN in monkeys. It is still necessary to seek evidence to implicate either muscle or joint receptors in the responses of these cells to passive movement, and it is conceivable that both may be involved. The collection of even a limited number of observations in man could be of the greatest importance in understanding the relationship of the function of cells in the precentral gyrus to voluntary movement performance. It would be of great interest, for example, to study the behaviour of precentral neurones in man in relation to a task such as that used by Marsden *et al.* (1972) in studying the servo-control of movement. A tracking task involving the generation of a ramp of force or position could be perturbed suddenly during its performance and the relationship of cortical cellular discharges to the task and to the disturbance could be examined. Such a study might make it clear whether or not a cortical loop is involved in the focusing of central nervous output on to appropriate alpha and fusimotor neurones during automatic load-compensating adjustments.

7.10 Motor potentials during natural movement performance in monkeys

Vaughan *et al.* (1970) recorded motor potentials from epidural or transcortical electrodes over the precentral gyrus of monkeys trained to close a switch at regular intervals by carrying out sudden wrist extension movements. These potentials had the form of a surface-negative wave before muscle contraction and a later positive wave. The timing of the negative wave varied from trial to trial but typically preceded the onset of movement by about 100 ms. A positive deflection sometimes preceded this negative wave and a more variable slow negative shift, beginning as much as two seconds before the movement was also seen sometimes—but, like the similar potentials in man, these were inconstant. The movement-related negative wave was more prominent over the contralateral precentral gyrus, but ipsilateral responses could be detected.

It is of considerable interest that monkeys with a forelimb which had been completely deafferented by dorsal root section could be retrained to carry out movements with this deafferented limb (Chapter 8). The EMG records accompanying the movements were modified—for example, the build-up of electrical activity and of force in a wrist extension task occurred more slowly than preoperatively. The shape of the motor potential in the precentral gyrus was said not to alter after deafferentation but a quantitative assessment was apparently not made. All the components were present and they appeared of similar size to the preoperative recordings. But the negative wave of the motor potential, which was most constant in the contralateral precentral gyrus and which normally preceded EMG activity by 80 to 250 ms was now found to begin 200 to 500 ms before the onset of the EMG response and contraction. The positive component also tended to occur earlier and was less constantly associated with the end of movement performance.

It was suggested by Vaughan *et al.* that the protracted development of EMG activity and the increased delay between the beginning of the motor potential and the onset of EMG activity in the monkey reflected the withdrawal of tonic excitatory effects normally converging on spinal motor centres from limb afferents. More temporal summation of corticospinal and other descending influences would now be required to produce a motor output. The lack of influence of deafferentation on the later components of the monkey's motor potential was put forward as evidence for a lack of influence of kinaesthetic feedback on motor cortex activity during movement performance. The positive component of the motor potential near or after the end of movement performance was conceived as an influence of feedback through central re-entrant circuits in the brain (Chapter 4) rather than from peripheral receptors. It was suggested that the influences of peripheral receptors, which may be demonstrated clearly with passive movements in the normal animal, may be blocked during active movements. As yet there are inadequate tests of these suggestions using recordings from central nervous system units. Moreover there are likely to be important alterations in neural function during the fairly prolonged retraining periods (about three months) necessary to restore movement performance after deafferentation. The findings of Evarts (1973) and Porter and Rack (1976) would surely appear to reveal the operation of a competent feedback from the peripheral receptors to PTN operating during the execution of a movement at least in relation to postural tasks.

Brindley and Craggs (1972) recorded signals from over the precentral cortex of baboons. The potential difference between electrodes 2 mm apart was passed through a filter which selected frequencies from 80 to 250 Hz. These filtered signals were amplified and when they were monitored on a loudspeaker, 'the rushing sounds in the loud speaker would come and go like the sea over a shingle beach' when the contralateral limbs were moved and then rested. Moreover, the signals reliably appeared in the arm or leg area of the cortex in association with movements of the appropriate contralateral limb. If the animals were restricted in the movements they could perform and if the characteristics of the filters were sharpened, when the animal moved it was possible to detect a signal envelope from the filtered recordings ('processed mapped voluntary movement signal') which, even in single trials, was a reliable event associated with muscle activity. By selecting an appropriate threshold for this voluntary movement signal, a prediction accuracy for the occurrence of movement of better than 90 per cent was obtained; in the other 10 per cent of cases, the cortical signal occurred but no movement was observed.

The most reproducible part of the signal envelope was the rising phase. This rising phase of the processed signal always occurred before movement, leading movements by a period of the order of 100 ms or so. The processed signal also survived spinal transection and, although the shape of the signal changed over a period of about one month following spinal transection, the rising phase remained unaltered. This led Craggs (1975) to suggest that such processed signals could perhaps be used to control movements in paraplegic patients. It also indicated the independence from peripheral feedback of the activity in the motor cortex which underlies the processed signal recorded in this way. Obviously, this transformation which does not require averaging over large numbers of trials, offers advantages over conventional EEG recording techniques in the search for neurological correlates of movement performance. Its timing in relation to movement suggests that it may indicate the changes in activity of populations of cortical neurones associated with movement performance.

Tanji and Evarts (1976) reported that the discharges of PTNs could increase well in advance of the performance of a movement if the animal was given 'instruction' about the direction (push or pull) of a future movement but required to wait upon a later signal (a perturbation of the lever itself) before executing the movement. More PTNs (75 per cent of 122) showed this change in firing in 'preparation' for future movement than did non-PTNs (65 per cent of 137) in the motor cortex or post-central neurones (23 per cent of 186) and the magnitude of the effect was greatest in PTNs. The PTNs began to change their discharge 200 to 500 ms after the instruction was provided, but this change in firing was not accompanied by any change in EMG activity. It was only after the perturbation signal was given, indicating that the time for carrying out the movement had arrived, that the appropriate muscles for the push or pull movement were called into contraction. The effects of the prior instruction about the direction of movement were differential, i.e. a neurone whose firing rate increased during the period ahead of a pull movement would show decreased firing after an instruction to prepare for a push movement.

This activity which Tanji and Evarts associated with an 'intention' to move, was found to be in parallel with changes in the dynamic stretch reflex tested by sudden perturbations of the lever to pull on muscles. An instruction for the animal to prepare to pull, only after a perturbation which stretched the biceps muscle was applied, led to an increase in the size of the short latency (24 ms) reflex caused by this sudden stretch. An instruction for the animal to prepare to push caused a reduction in the size of this particular stretch reflex. The activity of PTNs caused by the instruction could be having the effect of setting the subcortical and spinal centres in preparation for the trigger to move and the influences on the stretch reflex were taken to indicate a focusing of fusimotor drive to appropriate muscles by the PT activity. It has already been pointed out in section 7.6 that the input to PTNs from peripheral receptors is also capable of being modified ('gated') by prior instruction about a response to be made.

Although the monkeys in Tanji and Evarts' experiments were over-trained, and made few errors, it was of great interest to note that when the wrong movement did occur in response to the trigger signal for movement, this wrong movement was invariably associated with an 'incorrect' preparatory response of the unit. If the usual response of a PTN was to increase its firing after the instruction to pull, a pull movement occurred when the perturbation signal was given, even on those rare occasions when the animal made an error and the instruction preceding the increased discharge was to push.

The other finding of great interest was that, if the instruction and the perturbation followed one another with a very brief interval, the effect of the instruction had not been developed in the motor cortex before the arrival of the perturbation signal. Under these conditions the presentation of the signal to move 'was usually associated with a grossly impaired motor response'. Although this result is not discussed in detail, a function for the motor cortex activity following the instruction is implied: to prepare the motor centres in the brain and spinal cord for *appropriate* future action when the trigger signal is presented.

7.11 Summary

Pyramidal tract neurones and other cells situated in the motor cortex change their activity in relation both to conditioned movements and to voluntary movements of the contralateral musculature. The discharges of these cells precede the occurrence of specific movements about particular contralateral joints. Although a few neurones have been shown to code, by the amount of their discharge, the amount of force required to produce the movement, the majority of PT neurones are not so clearly associated with any one aspect of movement performance. It has been suggested that force of voluntary action may be graded by recruiting appropriate numbers of PTNs and it has been the clear observation of all workers that PT discharge is clearly associated with the timing of muscle contractions in voluntary movement, an important component of skill and precision. But the beginning of the discharge of individual PTNs precedes the beginning of movement by a period of the order of 100 ms.

Neurones in a variety of other cortical regions have also been shown to change their activity in relation to movement performance. Moreover, discharges in the cerebellar cortex, the deep cerebellar nuclei, the thalamus and basal ganglia may all precede movement. The relationships of these discharges to the organization of movement, to its initiation or to its control and coordination have not been discovered by the tests that have been performed so far. The structures in which discharges preceding movement have been registered are connected in a reciprocal manner with the motor cortex by synaptic linkages of various lengths. None of the observations allows a distinction to be drawn between influences of the motor cortex on these structures or its converse. So it is not possible to evaluate the concept of programming of movement in basal ganglia and cerebellum for subsequent instruction of the motor cortex by way of the ventral thalamus. This concept could not, however, provide the whole explanation of programming of the motor cortex because lesions of the ventral thalamus do not deny primates the ability to execute programmed movements.

The relationship between PTN and muscle contraction or movement performance is capable of modification in a variety of circumstances, both those which influence re-entrant circuits in the CNS, for example by cooling of the dentate nucleus, and those which modify the peripheral feedback from receptors in the moving limb. Moreover the general circumstances which surround the movement performance, the instructions about it and the rewards which will result from its accomplishment can all influence the PTN activity associated with the movement.

The potentials which can be recorded over the motor cortex in man also have a component which precedes the beginning of a brisk movement by a time of the order of 100 ms. These potentials could represent the recruitment to action of PTN and other neurones which precedes initiation of the movement. But, even these activities of the 'middle level' cells, most closely connected by direct synapses with the motoneurones of the final common path at the 'lowest level', discharge well before the onset of movement. This makes it unlikely that they would be providing the immediate signal to move unless the special properties of these synapses confer a priming function on the early impulses in their bursts and allow some later part of the discharge pattern (perhaps that part with the highest instantaneous frequencies of response) to initiate motoneuronal discharge.

8
The role of corticospinal neurones in 'least automatic' movement

8.1   Introduction

We return in our final chapter to the problem areas which we outlined in our first. We must now try to bring together the separate streams of research which we have been following in the intervening chapters. Two of the streams, those of microanatomy (Chapter 4) and electroanatomy (Chapters 2, 4 and 5) have contributed a wealth of structural data, which have led to speculations about function. Thus, in the cat, the synaptic endings of the PT are in the dorsal and intermediate regions of the grey matter, near to the incoming sensory inputs and the interneurones of spinal reflex arcs. There are also many synapses in the dorsal column nuclei, as in all mammals. In the primate series, an increasing proportion of the tract ends in the ventral horn, particularly in relation to the moto-neurones of distal musculature. These facts have suggested that it has three kinds of functions: (1) controlling the afferent input to the spinal cord, fore-brain and cerebellum; (2) controlling motor output, selecting parts of the segmental motor patterns in appropriate combinations and, in primates, by-passing these and engaging the motoneurones directly; and (3) interacting with ascending systems at sites at which motor 'commands' and the tactile and kinaesthetic inputs which result from movements can be compared, especially, perhaps, in the process of tactile and stereognostic exploration.

The contemplation of microanatomical structure has always been a major source of ideas about function. The great classical neuroanatomists, for example Ramón y Cajal (1909, 1911) and C. J. Herrick (1948), always sought to interpret the facts of clinical neurology and of human and animal behaviour in the light of their microscopical studies. It seems worthwhile to stress that the logical status of electroanatomical data does not differ from that of microscopical data. Because the techniques of electrical

stimulation and recording have won so much understanding of the functions of nerve and synapse, it seems sometimes to be supposed that they are
also capable of 'explaining' the 'higher' functions of the brain. It is true
that electrophysiological *methods* have gone beyond the mere supplementing
of microanatomical methods in the unravelling of connexions: they can
measure the relative quantities of excitation and inhibition (Chapter 4)
and can provide quantitative data about optimal impulse frequencies
(Chapter 3). But these are all aspects of anatomical connectivity. If we
share Polanyi's view (1968) that living systems are organized in hierarchical levels, and that each level imposes 'boundary conditions' on the
operations of the level below it, we should not expect to be able to deduce
the facts of motor performance from the structure and properties of
neuronal networks, any more than we should expect to be able to deduce
the properties of neurones from the principles of action at the molecular
level. Thus, accounts of performance that are based on electroanatomical
experiments, for example, Eccles' account (1967) of the operations of the
cerebellum and motor cortex in the 'dynamic loop' control of movement,
may be properly regarded as essays in imaginative inference in the tradition
of Cajal and Herrick.

From the behavioural side, attempts have been made to interpret
behaviour in terms of hypothetical assemblies of neurones (Hebb, 1949),
though the extent to which such hypothetical assemblies differ from black
boxes might well be argued. Only recently has it become possible to
relate the activities of neurones to specific performances in studies in which
both aspects can be observed simultaneously (Chapter 7). This approach
is already giving insights into the operation of the sub-routines of movement, and into the timing of the commands issued by their high-level
programmes (Chapter 7).

'At higher levels it has been possible to infer function only from the
negative effects of brain lesions.' (Denny-Brown, 1966.) We have deliberately deferred to this last chapter our considerations of this final
stream of research: the effects of destruction of the PT and of the motor
cortex, both in frustrating the exteriorization of the high-level programmes
of behaviour and in disorganizing the sub-routines of movement.

8.2 The hierarchical organization of 'sensorimotor processes representing movements'

8.2.1 HUGHLINGS JACKSON'S IDEAS ON THE CONTROL OF MOVEMENTS BY THE BRAIN

In Chapter 2 we tried to disentangle Hughlings Jackson's discoveries about
the localization of the projections that are available for selection by intracerebral 'processes representing movements' from his ideas and discoveries

about the physiology of movements. We were concerned at that stage only with his work on 'convulsions beginning unilaterally', due to 'discharging lesions', and not with his complementary work on the paralysis of different categories of movement by 'destroying lesions' of the brain.

From these complementary studies of the effects of 'discharging' and 'destroying' lesions, Jackson concluded that cerebral function is organized in hierarchical levels, and that every part of the brain 'represents' impressions and movements, linked in 'sensorimotor processes' (Phillips, 1973). 'I carry the doctrine of sensorimotor constitution of the nervous system further than anyone else, so far as I know, since I urge that the highest cerebral centres (the "organ of mind" or anatomical substrata of consciousness) represent parts of the body as certainly as that of the lumbar enlargement does', he wrote in 1889 (1932, p. 399). By 'sensorimotor processes' he implied the idea, which he had taken from Laycock, that the brain is subject to the laws of reflex action (1874; 1931, p. 167). In 1869 he had defined 'the unit of constitution of the nervous system' as including 'the skin impression, the sensory nerve, the centre, the motor nerve, the sensory nerves from the moving muscles, and from tracts of the skin stretched or relaxed by the movement' (1932, p. 235). 'The term "impression" includes all cases where a peripheral effect . . . disturbs a nervous centre, and the term "movement" is used in an unusually extended sense, to cover not only effects produced by nerve centres on muscles (including arterial coats, muscular fibres of intestine etc.) but on glands and effects by inhibitory nerves.' (1876; 1931, p. 136.)

The idea that 'sensorimotor processes' are organized in hierarchical levels, and undergo 'dissolution' from above downwards (the reversal of evolution) in disease, he credited to Herbert Spencer, to whom 'I should make more detailed acknowledgements were it not for the fear that I might be attributing crudities of my own to this distinguished man.' (1887; 1932, p. 92.) 'In the lower centres there is a direct adjustment of few and simple movements to few and simple peripheral impressions. In the very highest centres also there is a similar adjustment, but then it is of exceedingly special movements (representing movements of the whole organism) to the most special impressions from the environment. . . . In the lower reflex action some particular movement is fatally necessary and occurs rapidly after some particular impression. But in the highest centres it may be that there is not this absolute connexion . . . the sensory and motor elements which enter into the physical side of what is, psychologically speaking, our perception of the statical and dynamical qualities of objects, can be, so to speak, transposed, can enter into new combinations.' (1872; 1931, pp. 60–61.) The higher the level, the less directly are the 'sensorimotor processes' coupled via lower levels, to their appropriate peripheries; the looser also are their mutual interconnexions.

His studies of hemiplegia, and of the temporary and reversible paralysis (Todd's paralysis) which sometimes follows a focal epileptic fit, and which he supposed to be due to the temporary exhaustion of the cells which had been discharging paroxysmally, convinced Jackson that it is not muscles that are paralysed but rather movements that are lost. Not only can such muscles take part in some movements but not in others; they can also be involved in convulsions. 'To speak of a part as being both paralysed and also as being movable by the patient, is not even unusual in ordinary clinical language. . . . We should not speak of paralysis of *muscles* from central lesions. Nervous centres do not represent muscles, but, or except as, movements. Hemiplegia appears as loss of power in certain muscles, but really is a loss of a number of movements of the parts paralysed. . . . From a small destructive lesion of a centre a few movements of muscles may be lost, and many other movements of the same muscles be retained; the hemiplegic man, who cannot easily button his waistcoat, and yet can lift a chair, has only lost some power in the muscles of the arm, in the sense that he has lost some of the most special or "delicate" movements of this limb. Similarly there may be loss of some of the most special or "delicate" movements all over the body, with retention of very many more general or "coarser" movements all over the body.' (1880; 1931, p. 323.) 'The nervous centres represent movements, not muscles; chords, not notes. This is evident from the effects of destroying lesions of the corpus striatum.' (*sic :* see Chapter 2.) 'From a *small lesion* of this body there does not result paralysis of a *small part* of the arm, nor of any such group of muscles as flexors, or extensors; there results *partial paralysis of the whole arm*, the most special parts of it suffering most. There is a loss of a certain number of movements of the limb.' (1873; 1931, p. 113.) 'Movements of a single muscle, except perhaps in the face, are, as Duchenne insists, only producible artificially—that is, by galvanism.' (1873; 1931, p. 67.)

Recalling Jackson's 'unusually extended sense' of the term 'movement', we are not surprised to find him including inhibition in his account. 'Taking only the case of rigidity in perfect hemiplegia for illustration and limiting illustration to the hand, we see that there is loss of some movements of muscles of the hand and over-development of other movements of those muscles; there is, or is in effect, loss of all the complex cerebral movements of it and over-development of all the simple spinal (lowest level) movements of it (possibly the cerebellum is also concerned in this over-development).' The 'over-development' is due to release from inhibition. 'When we speak of representation of movements we tacitly take into account motor elements of centres empowering inhibitory nerves; they effect what may be called negative movements. . . . So, then, centres represent positive and negative movements, and positive and negative impressions; this qualification is always to be understood when the expressions "loss of movements" and "loss of impressions" are used.' (1888; 1931, p. 373.)

The most severe loss is of what Jackson at first called 'most voluntary', in contrast with 'most automatic' movements. (In later years, remembering that he was a dualist, he always used 'least automatic' instead of 'most voluntary'.) 'It is not to be implied that there are abrupt demarcations betwixt the two classes of movements; on the contrary, there are gradations from the most voluntary to the most automatic.' (1873; 1931, p. 63.) 'That parts suffer more as they serve in voluntary, and less as they serve in automatic operations, is, I believe, the law of destroying lesions of the cerebral nervous centres. . . . It must be added, that degrees of hemiplegia are not simple degrees; that is to say, they are not either degrees of more or less loss of power only, nor degrees of more or less range, only but of both. They are Compound Degrees. For example, if there be paralysis not only of the *most* voluntary parts of the body—face, tongue, arm and leg—but also of those next most voluntary, *viz.* loss of certain movements of the eyes and head and side of the chest, we find that the most voluntary parts (face, arm, leg) *are very much paralyzed.* In other words, the graver the lesion not only the more are the most voluntary parts paralyzed, but the further spread to automatic parts is the paralysis.' (1873; 1931, pp. 63–64.)

Jackson regarded the 'compound order' of spread of convulsion in cases of 'discharging lesion', and the 'compound order' of loss of movements in cases of 'destroying lesion', as being related to the normal functional associations between 'less automatic' and 'more automatic' movements, the former being expressed, especially though not exclusively, through the distal parts and the latter through the proximal parts of the body. Their differential engagement in health he illustrated by a description of lifting weights. 'Ignoring for convenience the possibility that any effort in lifting even a small weight requires a new equilibration of all the muscles of the body, we shall note only the striking sequences of movement in lifting weights made gradually heavier. The words of our description will imply that there are distinct intervals in the movements as they spread, really they glide into one another as the weight becomes heavier. If we lift a slight weight with the right hand we use only the muscles of the hand and forearm; if it be made gradually heavier, we bring into play those of the shoulder, next those of the right side of the spine, leg, then of the jaws and chest.' On the opposite side of the body, 'What must happen first is stiffening of the muscles of the left side of the spine, next stiffening of the upper part of the left leg, next that limb is lifted off the ground in extension and away from the body, and a little in advance of it. Then the arm is raised, the forearm being in extension; the hand is extended, the fingers being straightened out. . . . This spreading shows well the compound sequence. The heavier the weight, not only the more the arm is used, but the further does movement spread to automatic parts.' (1876; 1931, pp. 271–272.)

It is now difficult to accept Jackson's interpretations of convulsions due to 'discharging lesions' as 'the strong development of many movements at once, or rather, as a contention of many movements' (1882; 1932, p. 29); or a '"clotted mass" of innumerable movements.' (1875; 1931, p. 39.) In Chapter 2 we have cited evidence which supports a different interpretation: that 'sensorimotor processes representing movements' would be disrupted by 'an excessive, sudden and abrupt cerebral discharge' which would, however, fire the projection pathways and so convulse the periphery. Faradic stimulation of the human motor cortex always paralyzes voluntary movement, whether or not it also activates the periphery (Penfield, 1958). As Walshe (1953) observed: 'This abnormal mode of activating the cortex has given a glimpse of a *structural* pattern related to the projection pathways efferent from the cortex, but not any glimpse of the *functional* patterns of pure cortical activity. Structural patterns are fixed, but functional patterns are not, and the two must not be confused.' We have seen (Chapter 2) that the parts which are preferentially involved in focal convulsions are the same parts which are preferentially accessible to cortical stimulations. They are the parts whose motoneurones receive the densest projections from the cortex; the parts which are especially employed in 'least automatic' movements, that is, in the movements which suffer most severely in cases of 'destroying lesions' of the cortex and of its projection pathways.

'Destroying lesions' of the cortex need not deprive their victims of all 'sensorimotor processes representing movements', and we need not assume that these 'processes' would normally have been confined within the area of cortex that has been destroyed. Some of the 'processes' which might be localized in other cortical areas or in cerebellum, basal ganglia and thalamus, might merely be deprived of their channels of expression by a destroying lesion of the motor cortex which disconnected them from the 'lowest level'. Jackson's striking phrase 'Convulsion beginning Unilaterally, the Mobile Counterpart of Hemiplegia' (1873; 1931, p. 67) is therefore ambiguous about mechanism, admirably though it sums up the results of his brilliant clinical investigations.

His ideas were founded on intensive and detailed study of his patients' disabilities; couched as they were in esoteric and often obscure terminology, they remained, perhaps, imperfectly understood by his contemporaries and have been largely ignored by his successors; but they are by no means without value today. To make the point we have only to substitute, for 'sensorimotor processes representing movements' at 'higher' and 'lower' levels, terms such as 'programmes', 'sub-routines', 'closed loop operation' which are now in common use. We distinguished 'highest', 'middle' and 'lowest' levels in Chapter 1, Fig. 1.4 (p. 18), and have presented our whole survey of corticospinal projections in terms of connexions between 'middle' and 'lowest' levels. 'So far as I know, no one agrees with me in dividing the brain proper into middle and highest centres.' (We have already noted Ferrier's disagreement with the notion of a spatially separated 'highest level' in Chapter 1.) 'But I take it for granted that at least two levels of the central nervous system will be admitted by all.' (1889; 1931, pp. 373–374.)

It is remarkable that Jackson appreciated the importance of the cerebellum in relation to the 'middle level' (Fig. 1.2, p. 8). He had adopted Gowers' hypothesis that 'the cerebellum exerts a restraining influence on motor centres of the cortex cerebri' (cf. Chapter 6) 'and that the cerebellum coordinates movements by intermediation of these centres'. But he also cited Lowenthal and Horsley who had discovered that cerebellar stimulation causes contraction of biceps and relaxation of triceps in the decerebrate dog, and imagined that 'the cerebellum in coordinating movements acts in two ways on the cord, directly and round by the cortex cerebri' (1897; 1932, p. 425).

On the details of the coordination of movements he could make little headway without graphical recording and analysis, and had to confine himself to generalities. 'Harmony of movements is space coordination— the coordination of simultaneous movements; melody of movements is time coordination—the coordination of movements in succession.' (1876; 1931, p. 272.) 'It is, I think, of great importance to distinguish the two kinds of coordination. It will not, at all events, suffice to speak of "co-ordination" as a separate "faculty". Co-ordination is the function of the whole and of every part of the nervous system. And although each part co-ordinates different impressions in different time-relations, no doubt the process in every part is fundamentally the same—in breathing, walking and thinking. We are, I think, studying co-ordination in its simplest aspects when we work at regional palsy and sequence of spasm.' (1870; 1931, p. 36.)

8.2.2 ANALYSIS OF MOVEMENTS AND OF THEIR CONTROL

Graphical recording of human movements was begun by Muybridge, Marey and Braune and Fischer at the end of the last century, first by cinematography, later by chronophotography. Chronophotography was improved, made three-dimensional, and combined with measurements of the masses and centres of gravity of the limbs and of the body as a whole, by N. A. Bernstein of Moscow. The combination of measurement of the range and velocity of movement (cyclograms, Fig. 8.1) with calculation of mechanical forces made it possible to describe the work done by the muscles and to draw conclusions about the motor output of the CNS

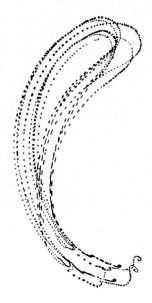

FIG 8.1. Superimposed cyclograms of a succession of finger-pointing movements, showing the different trajectory and velocity of each. The spacing of the dots indicates velocity. (Bernstein, 1967.)

(in so far as this is directly measurable in the work of the muscles and is not complicated by their variable mechanical properties: cf. Nichols and Houk, 1973). Bernstein's own selection of his papers, which began to appear in the 1920s, has only recently been made available in English ('The Co-ordination and Regulation of Movements', 1967). He was evidently a laboratory genius as well as a sagacious mathematical inter-preter of his measurements and a fertile source of stimulating ideas. He appreciated what his predecessors had been trying to do. 'As often happens during periods of scientific quarrying, glimpses of the new ideas and general forecasts may now be noted in the work of the older classical physiologists (Bell, Sechenov, Jackson).' It requires an effort to remember that the second chapter, 'The problem of the interrelation of co-ordination and localization', with its modern neuropsychological and neurophysiological insights, was first published as long ago as 1935. In a short survey it is not possible to do justice to this fascinating and readable book. Beginning with studies of the centre of gravity of the whole body in walking and running in order to help in the design of foot bridges, Bernstein became interested in the structure of the movements of locomotion and of some 'less auto-matic' movements, and in the formulation of general principles of the control of movement by the central nervous system. Prominent among these is the conception of hierarchical levels of control: first, the overriding engram, 'motor problem', 'motor image' or 'programme of a movement' (Bewegungsformel, Bewegungsgestalt), which is organized in advance, and which is *simultaneously* present *in toto* in the CNS; and the subordinate engrams of the 'operational stages' which intervene, in their correct *sequence*, in the 'ecphoration' of the movements. He writes of the integrity and structural completenesss of a movement, 'which makes it impossible to treat it as an arbitrary collection of successive reflex elements'; of its specific four-dimensional 'morphology', and of its 'structural physiology'; and notes that the neuropsychology of movement has lagged behind that of perception, with the neurophysiology of movement in third place. In the skilled use of a hammer, his experiments showed that 'the direction of the trajectory of the elbow (forwards or to the side) gives a close correlation with such phenomena apparently far removed from the elbow as the relationship of the maximal velocities of the head of the hammer in the movements of raising and striking, the angle of inclination of the hammer to the horizontal in raising, the relationship between the length of the trajectories of the hammer and of the wrist, and so on. It seems to me that the effects of changes in tempo on the whole construction of a movement are relevant here, as I have discussed in other studies on striking piano keys and on locomotion. A movement never responds to detailed changes by a change in its detail; it responds as a whole to changes in each small part. . . .' The 'motor image' is of the 'motor field' or 'motor space', not of muscles and joints. 'The hypothesis that there exist in the higher levels of the CNS projections of space, and not projections of joints and muscles, seems to me at present (1935) more probable than any other.' 'The fact that the habit of movement is not engraphed in those centres in which the muscles are localizationally represented is at once demonstrated by the fact that an acquired habit may exist while incorporating very different muscles in various combinations.' We recall that in the early 1920s Lashley (1950) had excised the 'motor' areas from monkeys and found that they had retained their previously learned ability to open problem boxes despite the clumsiness of their movements. In their projection into the 'motor field', the localizational pattern in the higher centres of the brain 'is none other than some form of projection of external space'. It 'must be congruent with external space, but only topologically and in no sense metrically'. (The term 'topological' is not here used in its strict mathematical sense.) The detail of a movement need not be repeated exactly. 'It is quite sufficient to be acquainted with cyclogrametric records of the movements of pointing with a finger at an object, carried out with optimal skill and accuracy, to become convinced that N successive gestures by the same subject are made through N non-coincident trajectories which only gather, as at a focus, in the vicinity of the same required point which is being indicated' (Fig. 8.1). Paillard (1960) has noted that no two repetitions of a movement are electromyographically identical. In writing on a horizontal paper or on a vertical blackboard, with different limbs or with his mouth, an individual's handwriting remains recognizably his own.

The successive 'ecphoration' of the 'elementary engrams' as the movement evolves is brought about, Bernstein believed, partly by the programme
and partly by triggering by feedback from the parts of the movement set
going by the elements nearer the beginning of the chain. Since the records
and calculations show that the movements start from different initial
postures and take place in different and unpredictable fields of external
forces, the 'motor impulse' for a stereotyped movement cannot itself be
stereotyped. These factors must be allowed for in ballistic movements,
for example, throwing a dart or jumping a ditch; or in moving to intercept a moving target at a predicted point and instant. In movements in
which correction is possible during their course, feedback plays an essential role. The required excitation E of a muscle must be a function of time,
position and velocity:

$$\frac{I \mathrm{d}^2 a}{\mathrm{d}t^2} = F\left[E\left(t, a, \frac{\mathrm{d}a}{\mathrm{d}t}\right), a, \frac{\mathrm{d}a}{\mathrm{d}t}\right] + G(a), \qquad \text{(Bernstein's equation 3c)}$$

where I = moment of inertia of the limb, a = angle of articulation,
t = time, F = momentum of muscle with respect to joint, G = gravity.
   'In this way we have stated in the basic equations of movement a super-
position of two cyclical connexions of different orders and related to
different topics. The first cyclical connexion is the mutual interaction of
the position a and the momentum F, and exists purely mechanically. . . .
The second connexion, constructed on the first one, is a similar interaction
between the position a (and also of the velocity) and the degree of excitation
E; this connexion is effected by means of reflexes and is related to the
activity of the central nervous system.' During its course, the movement
may encounter irregular and unpredictable forces which require 'adaptive
restructuring' of the programme by information from the receptors.
   Bernstein's minimal requirements for the black boxes of a 'closed
circle' control system are shown in Fig. 8.2. He treats the process of
coordination of a movement in terms of 'micro-intervals of its track and
time'; the command Sw ('Sollwert') represents the 'continuous planned
path or process of movement', its factual course being represented by Iw
('Istwert'). The threshold values of deviations 'which are more or less
accurately corrected during the course of the movement' are represented
Δw. This is a *tracking system*, in which Δw does not steadily diminish, as
in a *stabilizing system* (e.g. for mean arterial pressure), but oscillates. The
comparator (Fig. 8.2, 4; cf. Oscarsson, 1971; Chapter 4) would have its own
specific thresholds, one for its responses to deviations from the prescribed
course, and another for its responses to deviations from the prescribed
velocity. The existence of the velocity-sensitive primary endings of the
muscle spindles was not known to Bernstein; he thought there were no

velocity sensors in the body, and he was therefore obliged to assume that velocity was measured by comparison of the momentary position of a moving part with a 'fresh trace' of its momentary position at a preceding interval of time Δt. This led him to think that correction would be discontinuous, and to wonder about the relation of the threshold value of Δt to Reaction Time.

Of the interaction, at the periphery, between the central nervous output E, the changing mechanical situation, and the resultant afferent input, Bernstein wrote in 1940: 'This functional area deserves a metaphorical description as a peripheral synapse . . . the co-ordinational reflex is not an arc *but a closed circle with functional synapses at both ends of the arcs.*' The conception of peripheral closure of the ring has been strengthened by the subsequent discovery of the centrifugal control of the muscle spindles by fusimotor neurones (the 'gamma loop') (Chapter 4), and of the coactivation of fusimotor and α motoneurones in human voluntary movement (see overleaf).

Foerster's map of the human cortex was already available in 1935, and Bernstein was well aware of the multiplicity of corticocerebellar and

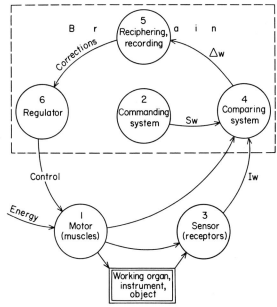

FIG. 8.2. Bernstein's 'simplest possible block diagram of an apparatus for the control of movements' (1957).

1, Motor output; 2, command system or control element specifying required value Sw (Sollwert) for time-course of 1; 3, receptors which detect *factual* time-course Iw (Istwert) of 1; 4, comparator which measures magnitude and sign of mismatch (Δw = Iw−Sw) between 2 and 3 (cf. Oscarsson, 1971: Chapter 4); 5, coding of correction signals for transmission to 6, controller of 1.

cerebrospinal connexions, all of which ultimately converged on the same system of muscles and joints. 'The pallidum is concerned with the same musculature as the brain cortex; it is not the objective but the manner of excitation which is specific.' He recognized also the multiplicity of projections to the CNS from the periphery. Bernstein's equation (above) 'is quite different from our usual, qualitatively simple models of the interaction between the centre and the periphery; when, however, we are obliged to confront their complex interaction as a result of the mutual activity of entire systems of organs which, anatomically and clinically, display varying degrees of independence, then the resulting great structural complexity becomes more obvious still'.

In 1935 it would have been generally believed that the same central output a always produced movement A, and b always produced B, 'from which it is easy to proceed to a representation of the motor area of the cortex as a distribution panel with push-buttons'. But what if (because of the changing situation at the periphery) the outputs which generate movement A are never identical. Bernstein's statement of the dilemma is worth quoting in full:

Let us suppose that the cells of the gyrus centralis are in reality the effector centre for the muscles. Let us further suppose that the activity of these cells must be (as is inevitable with the given hypothesis) sharply different from instant to instant on the multiple repetition of a given movement, in relation to changes in the external force field and to proprioceptive signals. If we suppose for clarity that we may represent each excited effector cell in the cortex as lighting up like an electric bulb at the moment when its impulse is transmitted to the periphery, then under such an arrangement the effecting of every movement will be visible to us on the surface of the cortex as a zig-zag discharge. The absence of one-to-one correspondence and all the considerations which have been described above as consequences of equation (3c) will be obvious in this case because on every repetition of a given movement the zig-zag discharge will be visibly different. Now suppose that this repetitive movement is an automatized act, the realization of a habit of movement, in other words, a conditioned motor reflex. From the discussion above it follows as an inescapable deduction that the conditioned reflex of movement operates each time through a new zig-zag—through new cells; in other words, we arrive at the conclusion that the hypothesis of cellular localization of muscles necessarily leads to a denial of cellular localization of conditioned reflexes. One of the two chess pieces must here be taken, and it is here a very pertinent question which of the two the old-fashioned localizationist would rather sacrifice. (1935.)

Forty years on, the reality seems less stark than the inescapable sacrifice of the knight or the bishop. The gyrus centralis is not made up of isolated push-buttons which operate isolated pools of motoneurones, but of overlapping areas which project to subcortical and spinal interneurones as well as to motoneurones (Chapters 2 and 5). Thus there could be some variability of the 'zig-zagging' even for outputs to similar groupings of motoneurones. We still have to admit our continuing ignorance of the locations and structure of even the simplest motor programmes, whether in the neuropil of the motor cortex itself or in that of other cortical areas, or in the basal ganglia, neocerebellum and thalamus, and of the 'zig-zagging' process by which these programmes select the appropriate groupings of muscles and suppress the activity of 'unwanted' muscles. But we can claim to be investigating directly the actual variability of response of PTN in stereotyped conditioned movements (Chapter 7) and also their responses to inputs from the periphery (Chapter 6).

Bernstein's definition of 'co-ordination of a movement' is 'the process of mastering redundant degrees of freedom of the moving organ, in other words its conversion to a controllable system'. Granit (1973) has also remarked on the embarrassing wealth of degrees of freedom and on the need for 'teleological constraints in order to narrow down the number of possibilities in a sensible manner'. For Bernstein, 'automatization' involved transfer of corrections to lower levels of control, with disappearance from the field of consciousness. 'In higher organisms (and in man in particular) there exists a rich and multisided sensorily equipped hierarchical system of co-ordinational levels involved in circular control. . . . This is clearly a consequence of the enormous number of degrees of freedom of the motor apparatus . . . (which can only be controlled by a system as complex as we find here). This is also the underlying biological mechanism which permitted organisms having such a powerful central apparatus for motor control to develop their organs of movement during phylogenesis without being limited by the number of kinematic and dynamic degrees of freedom involved.'

If we have reviewed Bernstein's contribution at some length it is because we are aware of it only from this book; we have not seen it cited or discussed in Western literature. Our hope is that others will be encouraged to read it, and we imagine that specialists will find valuable material in the original monographs and papers (mostly in Russian) on which it is based. Bernstein's comments are always penetrating: for example, that in cybernetics the time may have come to look for *differences* rather than only for similarities between living organisms and artefacts, and that, in modelling, authors tend to 'project their models on their material', so that it is not surprising that they are 'invariably satisfied with the accuracy of their analogies'.

8.2.3 NEUROPSYCHOLOGICAL STUDIES OF MOVEMENT

The programmes of elaborate sequences of movement, built up by learning over the course of many years, are not yet on the agenda of practical neurophysiology. Experimental psychology has been much concerned with relatively simple movements, such as keyboard tasks and tracking tasks, and Welford (1974) has suggested that the simplest of these may now be ripe for collaborative study by both disciplines, even though they comprise 'larger functional units than those normal in physiological studies'.

In movements which are directed to the tracking of a moving visual target, the minimum 'functional unit' or programme whose properties can be investigated is limited in its time-span by the visual reaction-time (about 300 ms). Pre-programming is therefore necessary, based on prediction of the position of the target at the time the movement should reach it: if the target suddenly deviates to either side of the predicted course, the pre-programmed movement cannot be modified in less than one visual reaction-time; it is therefore ballistic (Welford, 1974). The spatial extent of the minimal functional unit is determined by the minimum field of musculature that is needed to operate the manipulandum. It is a 'timed and phased sequence of muscular contractions and relaxations' which is initiated as a whole. The results of many experiments have been generalized in the concept of 'single channel operation', in which three separate serial processes can be distinguished. The first is the analysis and short-term storage of the visual input, the second is the selection of the appropriate response, and the third is its execution. Process I is supposed to be the setting-up of a 'unified instantaneous pattern'; Process II, the issue of 'an instantaneous set of orders for a programme of action', which Process III then transforms into a 'temporal sequence of detailed, spatial actions', that is, into a 'differentiated pattern of activity in the motor areas such that some muscles are activated and others are not'.

If a second deviation of the visual target occurs during the reaction-time to the previous deviation, the reaction-time of the second response is prolonged. This is interpreted as due to the interposition of a 'gate' between Processes I and II. The gate is supposed to remain shut until the single channel is once more disengaged, that is, until 'feedback signifies that the responding action has begun'. Hence the need for short-term storage in Process I. Direct access of a visual error signal to Processes II and III does not seem to occur to a significant degree; but the results of preliminary experiments with mechanical and electromyographic recording of the motor response (mainly at the shoulder) to a second visual input are complex, and much more work will be needed to discover the extent to which such access is possible, and to measure the shortest latency of the effects. When a stationary visual target jumps abruptly to one side and then, 50 to 100 ms later, makes a second jump in the same or in the opposite direction, the initial effect, in either case, is a speeding-up of the movement in progress, even when this is in the direction opposite to the required response (Megaw, 1974).

Neurophysiological interest has for some years been settling on Process III. Leksell's discovery of the centrifugal control of the muscle spindles (1945) led to Merton's fertile hypothesis (1951) of the initiation of some movements by fusimotor activation, operating the segmental stretch-reflexes as a follow-up length servomechanism. This was followed by Granit's hypothesis of coactivation of skeletomotor and fusimotor neurones ('αγ linkage', 1955) and by Matthews' hypothesis of the servo-assistance of movement (1964, 1972). The electroanatomical discoveries that signals from the muscle-spindles are transmitted to the cerebellum (Oscarsson, 1965; Jansen and Rudjord, 1965) and to the cerebral cortex (Chapter 6) have raised the possibility that the output from the fore-brain, as well as that from the spinal motoneurones, may also be subject to servocontrol and to monitoring by feedback from the moving muscles. The cerebral and segmental loop-times are about 50 ms and 25 ms respectively in the case of human hand-movements (see section 8.3.6). Both are short enough to operate repeatedly during a single visual reaction-time. They are also shorter than a single kinaesthetic reaction-time (about 150 to 200 ms; Welford, 1974). Both may be important in sustaining the 'timed and phased sequences of muscular contractions and relaxations which are initiated as wholes' by the successive visual stimuli in the course of a tracking task, keeping the movements on their visually programmed course in the face of changes in the peripheral force-field which would tend to make them deviate from it. We do not know whether this type of correction, of which neuropsychology has, as yet, taken relatively little note, operates continuously, or whether it operates intermittently as is evidently the case in the visual correction of tracking errors. In the most rapid movements, for example those of the fingers of a concert pianist at about ten per second (Ching and Hartridge, 1935) there would hardly be time for it to operate: these are ballistic movements *par excellence* (see below).

8.2.4 COMBINATIONS OF MUSCLES IN MOVEMENTS

Most movements are brought about by the actions of several muscles, but we know little about the way in which these combinations are selected by the central nervous system. Several relatively stereotyped patterns have been familiar to clinical neurologists since their first description by Duchenne (1867) and Beevor (1904). Duchenne (1867) may have been the first and Bernstein (1967) only the latest, to point out that a simple antagonistic relationship can only occur between muscles which operate a single hinge joint. In the case of muscles acting across more than one joint, or at joints with more than one degree of mobility, the relationships become more complex, and must shift, perhaps from reciprocal inhibition to coactivation, during the 'melody' of a complex movement. Beevor gave classical descriptions of such patterns as the fixating action of the dorsi-flexors of the wrist during flexion of the fingers. Every clinician is familiar with this stereotyped pattern, which survives in patients with cortical or capsular lesions who cannot make the wrist extensors contract when they wish to dorsiflex their wrists. During a strong grasp, triceps also contracts as a fixator, although its voluntary use as an extensor of the elbow is impossible. Some movements are antagonized by gravity. Others are not, and in one of these, voluntary flexion of the fingers, Duchenne's hypothesis that the actions of the prime movers ('associations musculaires impulsives') are moderated by co-contraction of the antagonists ('associations muscul-aires modératrices') has been upheld by simultaneous electromyography of the finger flexors and extensors (Long and Brown, 1964).

Beevor also described such varying combinations as those of interossei, lumbricales, flexor sublimis and flexor profundus digitorum and extensor digitorum communis in the separate movements of individual phalanges; and of biceps and triceps in different movements of the elbow and shoulder. Thus, in the movement of supination of the forearm, in which biceps is a prime mover, elbow flexion is prevented by co-contraction of triceps. In the movement of adduction at the shoulder, in which the long head of triceps is a prime mover, extension of elbow is prevented by co-contraction of biceps. Only in flexion and extension of the elbow are the actions of biceps and triceps reciprocally related: the pronators must then oppose the supinator action of biceps. Reviewing the clinical and experimental evidence that was then available, which included much of Sherrington's (Chapter 2), Beevor (1904) concluded that the neural arrangements for such relatively stereotyped combinations of muscles were laid down in the spinal cord, and extended along more than one segment. Later came the theory of Leyton and Sherrington (1917) of the breaking-up by the cortex of 'compounds already constructed by lower centres' and of the possibility of 'varied compounding' of the differentiated 'local items of movement' that could be elicited by liminal faradic stimulation (Chapter 2). We still do not know whether the selective 'compounding' of cortical outputs is a property of the neuropil of the motor cortex, or of thalamocortical connexions, or of both. It is tempting to suspect the presence of 'command neurones', analogous to those which have been found in invertebrates (Kennedy, in Evarts et al., 1971), which would link up the outputs to specific groups of muscles in stereotyped patterns, but there has so far been no evidence of them in mammalian brains.

8.3 Engagement of the segmental motor apparatus in man: its possible control by corticospinal projections

8.3.1 METHODS OF INVESTIGATION

In Chapter 7 we describe experiments on conditioned movements in sub-human primates. We must now look at the results of some experiments on the simplest voluntary movements in man, for example the sudden movement of a pointer from one target to another, or the steady pursuit of a slowly moving target. Neurophysiological study of the segmental response to commands emanating from man's brain is necessarily limited to measuring the resulting changes in reflex excitability of populations of α motoneurones, as in the H reflex; to electromyographic recording of the discharges of populations of motoneurones with gross electrodes applied to the skin overlying a muscle; and to recording the discharges of a few or of single motor units with fine electrodes buried in the substance of a muscle. The responses of single afferent axons from the muscle spindles can also be recorded by thrusting fine tungsten electrodes into the peripheral nerves (Hagbarth and Vallbo, 1969). The movement itself can be recorded at the same time by a potentiometer whose spindle registers the angular displacement and velocity of a single joint acting in one plane. Alternatively one can record the force developed in isometric contraction. Investigation is usually limited to a pair of muscles which function as agonist and antagonist in the particular movement, and which are samples of the possibly large assemblage of muscles which take part in the movement. One can then try to interpret the findings in terms of the segmental components on which corticospinal axons are known to project: skeletomotor (α) and fusimotor (γ) neurones, Ia-inhibitory interneurones, etc. (see Chapter 4). The shorter the reaction-time (RT) of the response to the moving stimulus, and the briefer its duration, the greater the likelihood that it is mediated by corticospinal rather than by the less direct cortico-rubro-spinal, cortico-tectospinal and cortico-reticulo-spinal pathways. About this there can be no certainty. Significant advances will depend on the results of work which is only now beginning to gather pace, in which normal patterns of response will be compared with the abnormal patterns that will be found in patients with specific lesions of the brain and spinal cord, whose size and location will eventually be definable at autopsy.

8.3.2 PRIORITY OF INHIBITION

Such experiments have discovered that the earliest cerebrospinal action is inhibitory. Hufschmidt and Hufschmidt (1954) set human subjects the task of extending the elbow as soon as possible after they felt a tactile sensation evoked by a weak shock to the median nerve in front of the elbow. While awaiting the stimulus they kept the biceps tonically contracted. The EMG of biceps was usually silenced about 50 ms before the onset of activity in triceps. The shortest RT for the action on biceps was 40 ms. Accepting Dawson's measurement of 18 ms for the transmission time from nerve to cortex and estimating 12 ms for efferent transmission from cortex to muscle, the Hufschmidts were left with a minimum of 10 ms for the central inhibitory process. Hallett *et al.* (1975a) set subjects a pursuit task which required flexion of the elbow in a horizontal plane (eliminating gravity) on a surface lubricated with talcum powder. The average RT from the sudden jump of the visual target to the onset of the EMG biceps was 200 ms. When flexion was aided by a load, the initial angle of 90 % at elbow had to be maintained by tonic contraction of triceps. When the target jumped and the subject responded, the silencing of EMG activity in triceps preceded the onset of activity in biceps by 0 to 50 ms (Fig. 8. 3A). A similar relationship between inhibition of antagonist and excitation of agonist has been observed in rapid voluntary extension of the thumb (Fig. 8, 3B: Marsden *et al.*, 1977).

The prior inhibition of the antagonist is evidently determined by a central programme. Experiments on subhuman primates will be needed

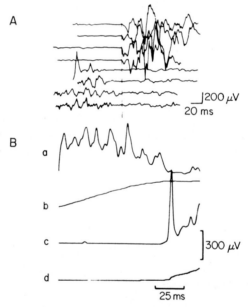

FIG. 8.3. A. Inhibition of tonic triceps activity before a fast elbow flexion. This is a composite of four individual records from one subject. The first line is a tracing of the biceps activity and the fifth line is a tracing of the triceps activity of the same trial. Lines 2 and 6, 3 and 7 and 4 and 8 are related similarly. The tracings are arranged so that the vertical line denotes the onset of biceps EMG recorded with surface electrodes. (Hallett *et al.* 1975a.)

B. Antagonist inhibition prior to a ballistic movement in man. The subject flexed the top joint of the thumb against a resistance (0.16 Nm). On a signal he extended the thumb as quickly as possible. The EMG records (taken with fine electrodes inserted into the muscles), are: a, rectified EMG; b, rectified and integrated EMG from flexor pollicis longus; c, rectified EMG; d, rectified and integrated EMG from extensor pollicis longus. The average of 16 trials is shown.

Note that ongoing EMG activity in flexor pollicis longus begins to silence about 25 ms prior to the burst in extensor pollicis longus. (Marsden *et al.*, 1977.)

to discover whether the effect is due to active inhibition of PTN which had been driving the antagonist, or to the mere abrupt withdrawal of excitation from them. The result, in either case, would be withdrawal of excitation from the antagonist's motoneurone pool. Alternatively or additionally, the effect might be due to excitation, by the programme, of PTN which actively excite spinal interneurones which then inhibit the motoneurones. Here we recall the firing of PTN 50 to 100 ms in advance of movement (Chapter 7). If this proves to be the explanation it will be necessary to find out if the spinal inhibitory interneurones are the Ia-inhibitory inter-neurones which are monosynaptically excited by CST axons (Jankowska and Tanaka, 1974), and which apparently remain 'switched off' in man unless their excitability is increased by voluntary motor activity (Tanaka, 1972: see Chapter 4).

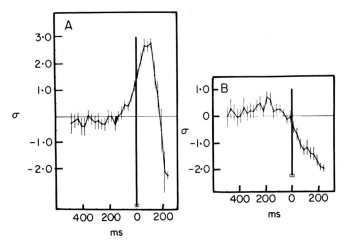

Fig. 8.4. A. Subjects of this experiment were instructed to plantarflex the ankle as soon as possible after hearing a click. The earliest EMG response in every trial has been lined up at zero time on the abscissae, so that all events are referred to this time. The ordinates measure the amplitude of the H reflex of soleus, one of the agonist muscles, tested at different times before and after the onset of the EMG in response to the click, and expressed as multiples of the control amplitude (zero of ordinates). Each point on the curve is averaged from eight subjects and the vertical bars give the limits of confidence of the means ($p = 0.05$). Up to 0.5 s before the earliest EMG response there is possibly a slight *reduction* in the excitability of the soleus motoneurones; the *increase* in their excitability begins more than 100 ms before the onset of the response to the click. Although the instruction called for as brief and as rapid a movement as possible, the increase in excitability of the motoneurones was not sudden, but progressive over at least 100 ms.
    B. Subjects of this experiment were instructed to dorsiflex the ankle as soon as possible after the click. The triceps surae muscle, whose H reflex amplitudes are plotted in the graph (same conventions as in A; averaged responses of 8 subjects), was therefore one of the antagonists to the demanded movement. Note that the changes of excitability of triceps surae motoneurones are the reciprocal of those which were measured when that muscle was a prime mover in the movement of plantar flexion.
    (Coquery and Coulmance, 1971.)

Another method of detecting prior inhibition is by measuring changes in the excitability of the H reflex. Since this reflex can most easily be elicited in the calf muscles, there is a temptation to narrow the scope of experiment to voluntary movement at the ankle. From 0.5 to 0.1 s before the onset of a sudden voluntary plantar-flexion of the foot, the amplitude of the H reflex of soleus is slightly depressed, but during the final 0.1 s its amplitude increases (Fig. 8. 4A: Coquery and Coulmance, 1971). Voluntary dorsiflexion causes reciprocal changes in the reflex excitability of soleus motoneurones (Fig. 8. 4B). It is not clear whether these changes in excitability of the motoneurone pools of the agonist and antagonistic muscles are specific or whether they are merely part of a more widespread preparatory response. Thus, when the subject suddenly closes his *fist*, the *soleus* motoneurone pool shows an increase in reflex excitability which begins 50 to 100 ms before the EMG of the finger flexors (Coquery and Coulmance, 1971).

8.3.3 BALLISTIC MOVEMENTS

When the elbow is flexed rapidly in pursuit of the sudden jump of a visual target, the initial inhibition of the antagonist triceps is followed by a rapid excitatory alternation between biceps and triceps (sometimes called 'bang-bang') which was discovered by Wachholder and Altenburger half a century ago. This is not modifiable by external events and is evidently ballistic and pre-programmed (Hallett *et al.*, 1975a). The diagram of Fig. 8.5 shows the first burst of activity in biceps which begins about 130

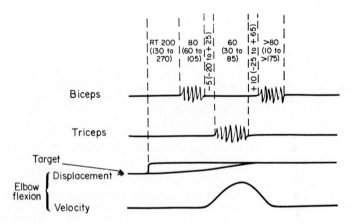

FIG. 8.5. Diagram showing sequence of electromyographic and mechanical responses when the elbow is suddenly flexed to bring a pointer as rapidly as possible on to a target which has suddenly jumped. Figures give averaged values from 18 normal subjects (ms). Figures in brackets give the largest and smallest averages from the individual subjects. (Modified from Hallett *et al.*, 1975a.)

to 270 ms after the movement of the target. A silent period in the EMG of biceps is accompanied by a burst of activity in triceps. The silent period is followed by a second period of activity in biceps: this is the earliest part of the response which is sensitive to external perturbations, or to 'the subject's appraisal of whether he is over- or under-shooting the mark'. Figure 8.5 gives an indication of the variability of timing of this minimal programme from one subject to another; the measurements are also 'moderately variable from trial to trial for a single subject', though no measure of this variability is given for the 18 normal subjects. The variability may make it difficult to prove whether Welford's Process III is, or is not, accessible to feedback, either from the muscles and joints of the moving limb or from a second jump of the visual target during the RT of the first (cf. Megaw, 1974).

Hallett et al. (1975a) have proved that the burst of discharge into triceps is part of the centrally programmed response and is not due to a stretch reflex evoked by the contraction of biceps. Figure 8.6A shows records of the type illustrated in the diagram of Fig. 8.5 but with balanced weights opposing both flexion and extension. In Fig. 8.6B the weight which had been opposing extension was detached electromagnetically during the RT. The other weight then forcibly extended the elbow and *shortened* triceps, but this did not prevent the burst of discharge into triceps. When the subject was holding the pointer to a stationary target,

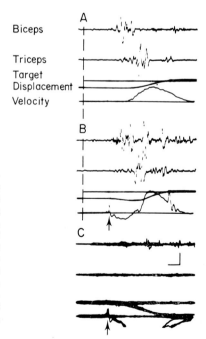

FIG. 8.6. The effect of passive elbow extension on the fast flexion pattern. The tracings in each part of the Figure are similar to Fig. 8.5. A illustrates the EMG pattern with a 2 kg weight on each side of the arm. In B, the weight pulling in the direction of elbow flexion is dropped at the time noted by the arrow. In C, no voluntary movement is requested: the subject merely matches the baseline and the weight is dropped as in B. The record shows three superimposed trials. A small stretch reflex is seen in biceps, but triceps is quiet. Calibration: 50 ms, 500 μV. (Hallett et al., 1975.)

sudden forcible extension of the elbow had no excitatory effect on triceps
(Fig. 8.6C). Another piece of evidence that the triceps burst was centrally
programmed and was not due to a stretch reflex was furnished by the
occurrence of the normal B-T-B sequence in a patient with severe pan-
sensory familial neuropathy whose arm was effectively deafferented.

A similar sequence of agonist–antagonist activity has been recorded by
Marsden *et al.* (1977) in ballistic flexion of the thumb (Fig. 8.7). They gave
their subjects the task of rapid flexion through different angles and againts
different loads imposed by a printed motor attached to the lever they had
to move. The range of durations of the bursts of activity in the agonist
(flexor pollicis longus) and antagonist (extensor pollicis longus), and the
duration of the associated silent period of the agonist, were unaltered by the
different angles and loads; only the amplitudes of the bursts were altered.

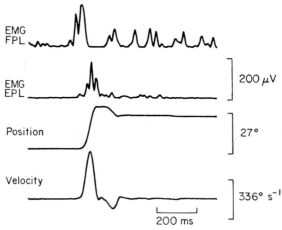

FIG. 8.7. Fast ballistic movements of the thumb in man. The subject flexed the interphalangeal joint of the thumb through 20°. The records, from above down, are: EMG,
FPL, rectified EMG activity in the agonist, flexor pollicis longus; EMG, EPL, rectified
EMG activity in the antagonist, extensor pollicis longus; position; and velocity. (Marsden
et al., 1977.)

The distance moved depends mainly on the amplitude of the pre-programmed agonist burst and on the opposing mechanical constraints: the
amplitude of this burst is linearly related to the required accelerative force
(Fig. 8.8). Though the pre-programmed burst in the antagonist would
have a braking effect, its amplitude is not systematically related to decelerative force (Fig. 8.8). The second agonist burst is variable in duration
as well as in amplitude, and Marsden *et al.* agree with Hallett *et al.* that
this is the earliest part of the performance whose *duration* is susceptible to
modification: by feedback, or by knowledge of results, or both? Marsden
et al., however, find that stretch of the agonist, appropriately timed to

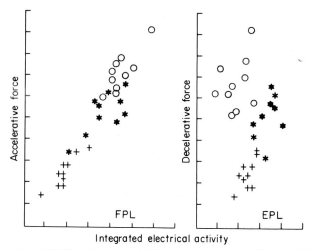

FIG. 8.8. Relation of EMG activity in initial burst in the agonist (flexor pollicis longus—FPL) and antagonist (extensor pollicis longus—EPL) in ballistic thumb flexion movements to the accelerative and decelerative forces generated.

Data for one subject are shown. A series of fast thumb flexions (as shown in Fig. 8.7) were made through 5° (+), 10° (*) or 20° (o). The forces produced were calculated from records of acceleration and are shown in arbitrary units. The integrated EMG activity from the two muscles was measured directly and is also shown in the same arbitrary units. (Marsden et al., 1977.)

precede the ballistic flexion, can increase the amplitude of the initial burst, and that a similarly timed unloading of the agonist can reduce it. The antagonist burst responds similarly to stretch or release of the antagonist. Thus the response of the spinal motoneurones to a pre-programmed cerebrospinal discharge is modified by input from the muscles. Is this effect exerted on PTN, or at the spinal level, or at both? It is interesting that in the baboon those motoneurones of distal muscles which receive the largest quantities of monosynaptic excitation from the CST receive also the largest quantities of monosynaptic excitation from the muscle spindles (Clough et al., 1968); if a similar arrangement obtains in man, such motoneurones would be focal points in the interaction between the stereotyped programme and the loading or unloading of the muscle. The accurate measuring-out of a ballistic movement, that is, the pre-programmed generation of the force that will be necessary to cover the required distance at the required speed, must be determined, in large part, by prediction (Bernstein's 'motor image' or 'motor problem'). Marsden et al. draw attention to the surprise that is felt when one jerks an unexpectedly empty suitcase with a force that would be appropriate to lift it if it were full. But Marsden et al. find that the simplest ballistic movements cannot be executed accurately by patients with lesions of the dorsal columns. As well as the central programme, inputs from the periphery are therefore necessary. Information of the initial angles of joints, initial lengths of muscles, and actively maintained static forces prior to the onset of movement, would be available in signals entering by the dorsal roots; their central actions could be enhanced or diminished by the activity of collaterals of CST axons in 'relay' nuclei (Chapter 4). The motor output responsible for maintaining the pre-existing posture in the face of the prevailing external forces could also be monitored internally.

Evarts and Granit (1976) have shown that people can pre-programme themselves to produce a sudden movement in response to a mechanical stimulus to a hand with a RT of less than 100 ms. In their experiments the subject's elbow was kept at 90°, and the hand gripped a handle which could be jerked by a torque motor in the direction of pronation or supination of the forearm. In this posture, biceps is stretched when the forearm is passively pronated, and unloaded when it is passively supinated. In some trials the subject was given the prior instruction to pronate, and in others to supinate his forearm as soon as he felt the jerk.

When the signal was a jerk which stretched biceps, and the subject had pre-programmed to supinate, the earliest EMG response of biceps was that due to the segmental myotatic reflex. The second EMG response would have been due in part, and might have been due entirely, to a 'trancortical reflex' response to muscle stretch (see section 8.3.6 below). That the response was not entirely due to muscle stretch was proved by trials in which the stimulus-jerk was in the direction which unloaded the muscle-spindles of biceps. The initial, segmental EMG response was now absent, but the intended voluntary contraction was still present, with $RT < 100$ ms. Whether the stimulus was from skin, or from joints or deep receptors other than muscle receptors, is not yet known. Inhibition of a prevailing isometric voluntary contraction of biceps could be evoked with a similarly short RT, regardless of whether the muscle was stretched or unloaded by the signal.

8.3.4 'RAMP' MOVEMENTS

In those experiments of Hallett *et al.* (1975a) in which the subjects were tracking a slowly moving target (in what is often called a 'ramp' in contrast to a 'ballistic' type of movement: Kornhuber, 1971), the alternating biceps–triceps–biceps activity was not seen. Since the flexion of the elbow was in a horizontal plane and on a slippery surface, the effect of gravity was eliminated, and biceps usually responded alone. Sometimes, however, there was coactivation of triceps, recalling Duchenne's 'associations musculaires modératrices'. In ramp movements of the thumb, Marsden *et al.* (1977) found that the initial ballistic sequence was present at first, the second agonist burst being prolonged into a smooth output; after some practice, the initial ballistic hump could be smoothed down so that the movement appeared as of ramp type from the beginning (Fig. 8.9). It is probable that a ballistic element is present at the outset of every 'ramp' movement. Ramp movements are highly responsive to servocontrol by feedback from the moving parts (see below). They include all movements other than throwing, jumping, striking the keys of instruments, etc.

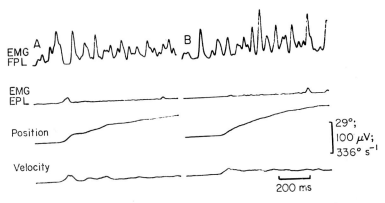

FIG. 8.9. Attempts to generate slow ramp movements of thumb flexion for comparison with the fast ballistic movement in the same subject shown in Fig. 8.7. As shown in A, such movements may begin with initial ballistic bursts in the agonist (FPL) and antagonist (EPL) but with practice it was possible to obtain a relatively smooth onset of contraction with asynchronous activity in the agonist (FPL) and little activity in the antagonist (EPL). The calibration is 200 ms and 100 μv, 29° or 336°s⁻¹. (Marsden *et al.*, 1977.)

8.3.5   RECRUITMENT OF α MOTONEURONES IN VOLUNTARY MOVEMENT

The manner of engagement of α motoneurones by central programmes can be readily investigated by electromyography of single motor units. In their engagement in reflexes, much importance has come to be attached to what is known as the 'size principle' (Henneman *et al.*, 1965; Kernell 1966a), which states that the 'small', 'slow' or 'tonic' motoneurones in a pool (those with the slowest axonal conduction velocity, the highest membrane-resistance and the largest EPSPs) are the first to be recruited in a gradually increasing response; and that the 'large', 'fast' or 'phasic' motoneurones (Granit, 1970) are the last to be recruited, though these latter may fire one or two impulses at the sudden onset of a reflex. Such an orderly sequence of recruitment has also been reported in voluntary contractions in man, in experiments in which the subjects have been asked simply to increase their output of force, for example in isometric contraction of the first dorsal interosseus muscle (Milner-Brown *et al.*, 1973; Freund *et al.*, 1975) or extensor indicis (Freund *et al.*, 1975). The last-named authors found that in contractions which were increasing linearly at a rate of 50 g s^{-1}, orderly recruitment was the rule, with different units coming into action at their own 'tonic thresholds'. In stepwise increments of tension many units fired phasically during the rise of the step, but only those whose tonic threshold-tension was reached by the step continued to fire during the plateau. No units behaved exclusively as tonic or phasic units.

Grimby and Hannerz (1968), who worked on the ankle dorsiflexor, tibialis anterior, concluded that the order of recruitment of motor units in voluntary contraction was not determined by an invariant, stereotyped mechanism, but could be modified by changing afferent input. Thus, in a sudden voluntary contraction, the units sampled at a single position of the needle electrode may include a phasic unit (A) which gives an initial discharge, single or double, and a tonic unit (B) which continues to fire as long as the contraction is sustained. If the sustained contraction is increased a second tonic unit (C) joins in, but if the contraction is then weakened, B may drop out and C may continue. If the contraction is begun just after stretching the muscle, C may fire first, but if the muscle is unloaded during the contraction C may drop out and B may take over. When voluntary contraction was begun during unloading, B fired at a high frequency but C was not recruited. These sequences could not be influenced by voluntary effort. Again, if vibration (which selectively excites the primary endings of the muscle spindles) was applied for 15 s before the start of voluntary contraction, this began with C instead of B. During co-contraction of other muscles of the same leg, C fired first. Injection of 1 per cent lidocaine into the region of the motor nerve, which did not block the skeletomotor axons but would have blocked the fusimotor axons, made B dominant as before. Grimby and Hannerz (1968) commented: 'As a matter of fact the concept of a hierarchy of motor units entirely dependent on the size of the cells and thus competely stereotyped has not been borne out by the results obtained in most human experiments.'

It is readily imaginable that under a general barrage of excitation, whether of reflex or of cerebral origin, the order of recruitment of motoneurones in a pool would be determined by relative densities of synaptic connexion and by the sizes and membrane properties of the cells, and would be relatively if not completely stereotyped. The question next arises, are the cerebrospinal projections capable of addressing the individual α motoneurones more selectively than this? The upper limit of such capability would presumably be conferred by the monosynaptic corticomotoneuronal projection (Chapters 4 and 5).

Basmajian (1963) and Basmajian et al. (1965), who cited earlier experiments by Harrison and Mortensen, reported that if people were presented with auditory or visual feedback of the discharges of single motor units in their muscles, they could train themselves to discharge selected units at will. Most experiments were done on *m. abductor pollicis brevis*. Some subjects having once characterized the unitary potentials by their sounds in the loudspeaker or by their shapes on the screen of the oscilloscope, could even learn to discharge a single motor unit without the aid of the auditory or visual feedback. They found it hard to explain how they did this without any help other than the experimenter's assurance, after the event, that their effort had been successful: they 'thought about' a motor unit as they had seen and heard it previously (Basmajian, personal communication to Phillips 1966). At first sight, these results appear to be in conflict with the size principle, and at a symposium on the control of movement and posture, Henneman stated that he and his colleagues had been unable, in human subjects, to vary the order of recruitment of voluntarily activated motor units, and in particular, 'to cause an easily recruited unit to cease firing while maintaining discharge in a unit recruited later than the first' (Granit and Burke, 1973). Kato and Tanji (1972) found that large units (those with large extracellularly recorded action potentials, which discharged only during strong contractions) could not be singled out by voluntary effort. But they also found that the units that were recruited in gentle voluntary contractions could be selected with a high degree of accuracy by subjects provided with visual and auditory feedback. Their intramuscular electrodes could sometimes record from 10 units at a single locus. They said to their subjects 'Now I will ask you to discharge only this tall unit', or 'Now stop the activity of all motor units except this one'. Any unit which the subject could not learn to control in a period of 30 minutes they classified as uncontrollable. They collected 286 units from 14 subjects from the following muscles (Table 8.1).

TABLE 8.1

Muscle	Number of units	Controllable	Uncontrollable
Opponens pollicis	143	104	39
Abductor poll. brev.	80	59	21
Extensor digitorum comm.	49	34	15
Extensor carpi. radialis	10	9	1
Extensor pollicus brev.	3	2	1
Abductor poll. brev.	1	1	0

Basmajian (1963) had also reported that some subjects, when provided with auditory feedback, could regularly reproduce particular rhythms of discharge in a unit they had selected. Kato and Tanji (1972) found that subjects could reproduce some given frequencies better than they could reproduce others. Each of the frequencies to be reproduced was presented for 10 s on both loudspeaker and cathode-ray screen. The subject was then

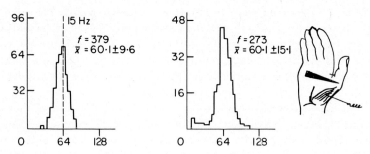

FIG. 8.10. Comparison of discharge frequencies of volitionally isolated motor unit during conscious effort (left histogram) and during reflex discharge (right histogram). The motor unit was picked up from *M.abd.poll.brev.*; direction and place of pressure stimulation are shown in the diagram on the right. *Ordinates*: frequency of occurrence. *Abscissae*: interspike intervals (ms). f = total frequency of occurrence. $\bar{x}$ = mean $\pm$S.D. (Kato and Tanji, 1972.)

asked to sustain that frequency for 30 s. After 3 to 5 repetitions the next frequency was presented, and so on. Forty-three volitionally isolated motor units were able to sustain discharges at 8, 10, 11 and 15 Hz, but were less successful with 2, 3, 4, 5 and 25 Hz. There was a strong tendency to discharge at 15 Hz, in reflex as well as in voluntary contractions (Fig. 8.10). In experiments on the tonic stretch reflex there was some interesting evidence of interaction between the driving from the periphery and from the brain (cf. the interaction between CM and Ia inputs to motoneurones: Clough *et al.*, 1968). There was no response to any unit to peripheral stimulation unless the muscle was sustaining a gentle voluntary contraction, and no response to cutaneous or painful stimulation. The adequate stimulus was pressure on the tendon. The subjects were asked to arrest the firing of a volitionally isolated unit but not to relax. They then closed their eyes and the loudspeaker was switched off. In 28/30 experiments the unit was restarted by pressure at the appropriate location and direction (Fig. 8.10) without the subject knowing that it was firing. The frequency could be varied by adjusting the stimulus, but not below 5 Hz or above 30 Hz. This experiment could be continued for up to 10 min after the subject had been asked to arrest the unit but not to relax the muscle.

Somjen (1972) commented as follows on these results in relation to the size principle:

The relationship we have found is that, in the overwhelming number of cases, motoneurones with axons of smaller calibre fired before larger ones, no matter what kind of synaptic drive excited the motor nucleus . . .

Neither these findings nor their interpretation preclude exceptions to the general rule. Very powerful inputs channelled to a large neurone may well excite a cell so singled out in preference to other, innately more excitable, smaller cells. Equally possibly, inhibitory synapses could suppress highly excitable small neurones under circumstances in which the larger cells in a nucleus remained excited . . . It is also conceivable that deliberate, voluntary effort on the part of an experimental subject can so concentrate the flow of excitatory input, or demarcate it by surrounding inhibition, as to activate one large cell out of a motor pool selected at will.

Such special arrangements serve to emphasize the more general case in which input to a pool of neurones is distributed at random and, other things being equal, the smaller members of the population are regularly called into action before the larger ones.

Kato and Tanji had also recorded motor cortical potentials in 12 subjects from the scalp approximately overlying the finger area (cf. Deecke *et al.*, 1969). The subjects were asked to discharge up to 50 impulses at self-paced intervals of about 5 to 10 s. The scalp records were subsequently lined up on the first action potential of the unit, and averaged. For 21 motor units of opponens pollicis, the amplitude of the cortical motor potential was compared with the motor potential associated with pressing a key by a movement of opposition of the thumb. The potentials were similar in size in the two cases. The discharge of an equally large population of cortical neurones in the case in which only a single spinal motoneurone was to be discharged is interesting in the light of Somjen's suggestions of a focusing of excitation on a target motoneurone and of a projection of inhibition to other motoneurones: such selection might well require a considerable corticofugal discharge. The monosynaptic CM projection, which is most powerful to the finger muscles, and the disynaptic corticospinal inhibitory projection (Chapter 4), come naturally to mind. Such selective addressing of the spinal motoneurones would be expected to differ from the less direct corticospinal excitation of spinal reflex arcs (Chapters 2 and 4) in which the input to the motoneurones might be distributed at random, so that their recruitment order would be determined by the size principle.

8.3.6 $\alpha\gamma$ COACTIVATION AND THE SERVO-ASSISTANCE OF RAMP MOVEMENTS

In Chapter 4 we have given evidence that the CST can excite and inhibit the fusimotor neurones as well as the α motoneurones. We now come to evidence that both types of neurones are coactivated in voluntary movement.

Merton's (1953) original hypothesis of the initiation of movement by servo-action has been an extremely powerful stimulus to thinking and experimentation in the physiology of motor control. He proposed that posture can be changed, and movements initiated and carried out, by cerebral commands directed solely to the fusimotor neurones, which would operate the length-measuring muscle spindles and α motoneurones (Fig. 4. 14, p. 130) as a follow-up length-servo (Hammond *et al.*, 1956). At any preset equilibrium position, the segmental 'stretch reflex' network, which was outlined in Fig. 4.14, would operate to maintain the existing posture. Any displacement by external forces would stretch some muscles, whose α motoneurones would be excited by the increased input from their spindles. In order to move to a new position, the brain would excite the fusimotor neurones which innervate the spindles of the required prime movers. The resulting increase in the firing of the length-measuring receptors would excite the α motoneurones of the prime movers and shorten these muscles to the new, 'demanded' length, that is, to the precise length at which the barrage of impulses from the receptors would be brought back to the initial level. The hypothesis was supported by a reinterpretation of the well-known 'silent period' in the electromyogram of a steadily contracting human muscle which follows an interjected twitch, which momentarily unloads the spindles and suspends the reflex drive (Merton, 1953); and on experiments on postural mechanisms of the cat's hindlimb (Eldred et al., 1953). At that time it was believed that the monosynaptic excitatory feedback from the spindles of any muscle was directed only to the α motoneurones of the same muscle and to those of its closest synergists. J. C. Eccles et al. (1957) then discovered, in the cat, that the feedback was not thus narrowly focused, but reached, in some cases, the motoneurones of muscles operating across different joints. In discussing this unexpected result Lundberg (1959) concluded that precisely circumscribed movements could hardly be initiated by the fusimotor route. Clough et al. (1968) found a similar situation in some muscles of the baboon's hand.

In his original statement, Merton (1953) considered the probability that urgent movements would be initiated by directly addressing the α motoneurones, which would save about 50 ms in moving the human hand. The resulting contraction would shorten the spindles and cut off the feedback. Matthews (1964) proposed that voluntary movement could be initiated by the α route without losing the advantages of servocontrol, if 'employed in conjunction with sufficient fusimotor activity to prevent any decrease in spindle discharge occurring during the contraction; this would be achieved if the relative amounts of α and γ activity were adjusted to be appropriate for the velocity of shortening "expected" . . . then if shortening proceeded faster than "intended" by the higher centres it would be slowed by servo-action, and if shortening were hindered by some unexpected load it would be speeded up by servo-action'. This conception, which Matthews (1972) has called 'servo-assistance of movement', is illustrated in Fig. 8.11. His monograph in the present series, and also the review by Stein (1974), should be consulted for a more detailed and rigorous treatment of the servo-loop and of its gain.

Granit (1955, 1968) introduced the concept of '$\alpha\gamma$ linkage' to encourage investigation of the coordinated distribution of suprasegmental motor

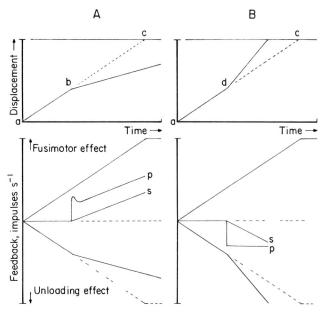

FIG 8.11. $\alpha\gamma$ coactivation in a ramp movement. Explanation in text. (Phillips, 1969.)

output between the α and γ routes, and to describe their coactivation in reflexes. In the special case of the respiratory movements, Corda *et al.* (1965) showed that the α and γ motoneurones of the intercostal muscles are indeed coactivated, and that obstruction of the airway causes increased feedback from the spindles which evokes a compensatory increase in α discharge. And in experiments on voluntary isometric contraction of flexors of the human forefinger, Vallbo (1970, 1971, 1973) found that single spindle afferents, recorded from the median nerve by the method of Hagbarth and Vallbo (1969), were silent when the finger was at rest, but began to discharge at about the same time as the muscle began to contract (Fig. 8.12A). This is evidence for $\alpha\gamma$ coactivation in this willed movement, and against the original follow-up length servo hypothesis in this specific case. In spite of the difficulty of maintaining contact with a single axon when movement is allowed, Vallbo (1973) has also been able to show that the spindle discharge can be sustained when the muscle is allowed to shorten freely in a ramp movement (Fig. 8.12B). If the isotonic shortening is rapid enough (as it would be in a ballistic movement) Vallbo finds that the rapid unloading of the spindle does reduce their discharge (Fig. 8.12D).

In the slow isotonic ramp movement of Fig. 8.12B, it is remarkable that the spindle frequency rises abruptly to about 25 Hz and then oscillates around the same value throughout the movement. Vallbo (1973) comments on the absence of 'a systematic change which was closely related to the muscle length. Thus it seems that the sense organ was relatively insensitive to the muscle length. An alternative interpretation is that there was a continuous increase in the fusimotor outflow which compensated for the muscle shortening.' Such a 'continuous increase' was suggested in the diagram of Fig. 8.11, to which Vallbo's beautiful result now gives encouraging support. In Fig. 8.12C, the lower record is derived from part of a ramp record like that of Fig. 8.12B. It shows the velocity of the

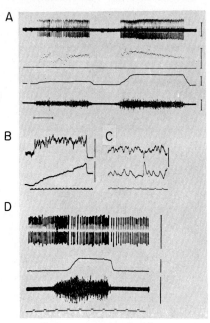

FIG. 8.12. A. Afferent unitary discharge associated with two successive voluntary contractions, without external shortening, of the flexor muscles acting on the index. From above are shown the unitary nerve impulses, the instantaneous impulse frequency, the torque due to the muscle contractions, and the EMG activity recorded with surface electrodes over the flexor muscles 10 cm distally to the medial epicondyle of the humerus. Straight line indicates zero impulse frequency. *Vertical calibrations* (from above down): 60 μV; 30 impulses per second; 0.2 Nm; 0.2 mV. *Horizontal calibration:* 2 s. (Vallbo, 1970.)

B, C. Response of a spindle primary ending during an isotonic contraction. B. Relation to joint angle. The top trace represents the impulse frequency of the single unit and the lower trace the angle at the metacarpo-phalangeal joint when the subject slowly flexed his ring finger. The events associated with the second half of this contraction are also illustrated in C. Calibrations: 0 and 25 impulses per second, 155° (bottom) and 145° (top). Time signal: 1 s. (Vallbo, 1973.) C. Relation to speed of joint movement. The upper trace shows the single unit impulse frequency and the lower trace the time derivative of the joint angle signal, i.e. it represents the speed of the joint movement. Calibrations: 0 and 25 impulses per second. Time signal: 1 s. (Vallbo, 1973.)

D. Response of a spindle primary ending to an isotonic contraction. From above downwards, the single unit impulses, the angle at the metacarpo-phalangeal joint and the EMG activity when the subject flexed his ring finger. The flexion was opposed by a load corresponding to a torque of 0.1 N m at the metacarpo-phalangeal joint. Calibrations: 100 μV, 150° (bottom) and 140° (top), 0.2 mV. Time signal: 1 s. (Vallbo, 1973.)

irregularities of the ramp record. The upper record is of the frequency of discharge of the spindle afferent. As Vallbo comments: 'The two signals go in opposite directions in most instances, implying that the faster the muscle was shortening, the lower was the discharge rate and *vice versa* . . . this finding indicates that the excitatory drive on to the skeletomotor neurones decreases immediately when the movement progresses faster and increases when the movement progresses slower. In this way any variations in the speed of movement—which could be due to a variation of the load, a variation in the frictional resistance or an irregular skeletomotor output— would be reduced in amplitude and the result would be a smoother movement.'

Thus, if a ramp movement, commanded by $\alpha\gamma$ coactivation, were slowed by unexpected resistance, as in Fig. 8.11, there would be an error signal in the form of increased activity from the primary and secondary endings of the muscle spindles. This should operate to provide servo-assistance at the segmental level (Granit, 1975). It is true that the input from the primary endings is not focused exclusively on the motoneurones of their own muscles, and, in the case of the baboon's hand, that its mono-synaptic excitatory power is not as great as that exerted by the spindles of triceps surae on triceps surae motoneurones in the cat (Clough *et al.*, 1968). But Clough *et al.* measured the largest quantities of monosynaptic action in those α motoneurones which also received the largest monosynaptic actions from the CST. This property would improve the selectivity of cortical control by $\alpha\gamma$ coactivation: any spindle feedback directed to motoneurones other than those selected by the CM projection could well remain subthreshold, and need not blur the precision of the movements. The output of the motoneurones thus selected could be servo-assisted by marginal changes in a cortically sustained spindle feedback, reinforcing or withdrawing support from the CM input in response to changes in peripheral load. Nothing is yet known of the central effect of the secondary endings of the muscle spindles at the segmental level in man and other primates. Evidence that they, too, may contribute to tonic stretch reflexes in the cat (Matthews, 1969, 1970) has been challenged (Grillner, 1970), but there is evidence that they can monosynaptically excite α motoneurones of intercostal muscles and of triceps surae (Kirkwood and Sears, 1975).

The existence of the powerful CM projection in primates, coupled with Evarts' (1967) demonstration that the discharge of movement-related PTNs was increased when the movement was resisted by an added load (Chapter 7), led to the suggestion that servo-assistance might operate at the cortical as well as at the spinal level (Koeze *et al.*, 1968; Phillips, 1969). Possible routes by which the spindle input could be brought to bear on the PTN have been discussed in Chapter 6. The exact timing of the effects of sudden perturbations on movements in monkeys has been described in

Chapter 7: the timing of the first and second EMG responses was appropriate for transmission across a segmental and a transcortical loop respectively. The timing of the responses of postcentral and precentral neurones was appropriate for transcortical transmission of the second EMG response.

In human experiments, whose importance was not widely appreciated at the time, Hammond (1956, 1960) required his subjects to maintain a steady isometric contraction of the elbow. They were instructed either to 'resist' or 'let go' when the elbow was suddenly and forcibly extended, several seconds after the instruction was given. In either case, the EMG of biceps showed a burst of discharge which began about 18 ms after the sudden pull (Fig. 8.13A, B). This response, on which Hammond did not comment, occurred at a latency appropriate for transmission across the monosynaptic stretch-reflex loop. When the prior instruction was 'resist', a second burst appeared in the EMG, about 50 ms after the start of the pull (Fig. 8.13A). The prior instruction 'let go' often abolished the second burst and the associated contraction of biceps (Fig. 8.13B). We know now that the latency of 50 ms is appropriate for a transcerebral (possibly a transcortical) 'stretch reflex'. It is shorter than the RT to a tap on the wrist (Fig. 8.13C), so the subjects could not possibly have taken any decision during the interval between the pull and the response. This long (possibly transcortical) loop must therefore have been 'closed' by the subjects when they received the prior instruction 'resist', and 'opened', more or less successfully (Fig. 8.13B), when they received the prior instruction 'let go', several seconds before the pulls. Hammond assumed, reasonably enough in 1956, that the response was a spinal reflex whose mechanism could 'be preset by nervous activity from the brain'. Marsden *et al.* (1972), however,

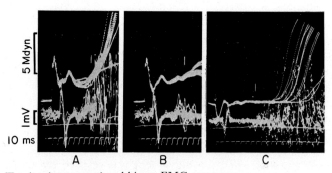

Fig. 8.13. Tension (uppermost) and biceps EMG responses.

A. Sudden extension of forearm, 40 cm s^{-1} at wrist. Ten superimposed records. Subject instructed to resist impending pull.

B. As in A, but subject instructed to let go when pulled.

C. RT to taps at wrist. Subject instructed to pull hard as soon as he feels the tap. (Electrode connections reversed compared with A.)

(Experiments of Hammond, 1956; reproduced from Hammond *et al.*, 1956.)

have pointed out that the loop time of 50 ms is in good agreement with the latency of the myoclonic jerks which can be evoked by peripheral stimulation in rare cases of myoclonic epilepsy, in which the precentral cortical mediation of the jerks is well established. In one such case, investigated by Carmichael (1947) and Dawson (1947), the adequate stimulus for the jerks was stretch of muscle. The main lesions were found postmortem in the cerebellum (unpublished report by the late J. G. Greenfield cited by Marsden et al., 1972). It is tempting to speculate that an intact cerebellum allows the normal subject to open the transcortical loop when he is asked to prepare to 'let go'.

In Hammond's experiments the subjects were trying to maintain a steady isometric force; their responses to perturbation gave valuable measurements of loop times. We come now to the experiments of Marsden et al. (1972) on the servo-assistance of linear ramp movements performed by the flexor of the distal phalanx of the thumb. The manipulandum incorporated a printed motor which opposed the movement with an initially constant force. In the control trials this force was constant throughout the movement, and the records of angular displacement of the distal phalanx, and of the integrated EMG of the flexor muscle, showed constant slopes (Fig. 8.14, records C in A, B, C, D). In the other trials the movement was disturbed, 50 ms after its onset, in one of three ways: 1, by sudden forcible extension of the thumb (records S); 2, by suddenly halting the movement (records H); or 3, by suddenly reducing the background force, so that the movement accelerated (records R), as in Fig. 8.11B. The latency from the moment of disturbance to the change in the integrated EMG was the same for all three types of disturbance: it was about 60 ms in one subject and about 50 ms in the other (whose arm is shorter). These times are consistent with a transcortical pathway: notice that the records show no earlier response that would be consistent with the monosynaptic spinal pathway (as in Hammond's isometric experiments). Marsden et al. regard the response to forcible extension of the thumb (record S) as a stretch reflex, possibly mediated transcortically. They consider that 'the response to halting (records H) is, in effect, a stretch reflex without muscle stretch. It is the best piece of evidence we have for the original servo theory because, from the animal evidence, it is difficult to see how it could arise except by contraction of the spindles stretching the sense endings on them . . . it can be calculated that the misalignment signal calling for more contraction must have left the muscle when its degree of shortening was only some 50 μm less than it would have been if the muscle had gone on shortening unimpeded.' Finally, the response to unloading the movement (records R) 'is the negative of the stretch reflex and it demonstrates that the muscle must have been receiving excitation *via* the stretch reflex arc at the moment of release. (This argument is essentially the same as the original argument from the silent period which led to the servo theory: Merton 1953.)' 'The misalignments which turn the muscle completely off must be of the same order of magnitude' as those involved in the responses to halting (records H). 'The detection, within milliseconds, of these minute misalignments in an actively shortening muscle many centimetres long represents a considerable feat of sensory discrimination and we begin to see why muscles require the profuse and elaborate sensory apparatus they have long been known to possess and which has always hitherto been something of a mystery.'

The gain of the servomechanism is measured by the muscle power turned on by a given misalignment; it turns out to be proportional to the force that must be exerted to sustain the movement. In Fig. 8.14B the initial resistance is ten times greater than in Fig. 8.14A. Such an increase of gain with load is not a property of engineers' servomechanisms. In the CNS it presumably involves recruitment of more α motoneurones in proportion to the initial resistance. In addition to automatic compensation for load, there is also automatic compensation for the effects of fatigue (Fig. 8.14C, D). In these first experiments, the functioning of the servomechanism was depressed by local anaesthesia of the thumb, which would not have affected the belly of the long flexor in the forearm which contains the spindles. The tentative explanation of this result was that the input from the skin and joints (which converges on PTN: Chapter 6) serves two functions: first, to adjust the gain of the loop; second, to focus the input from the spindles on to the α motoneurones that are needed for the movement. The matter has become more complicated now that the two principal subjects, after six years' experimenting on their thumbs, are finding that local anaesthesia 'no longer strikingly depresses such servo responses, but if the subject is now rendered ataxic with alcohol, anaesthesia does abolish them' (Marsden *et al.*, 1977). They consider the possibility that they have been learning to focus cerebral control on their thumbs in the absence of sensation, and that this learning can be temporarily abrogated by alcoholic disruption of cerebellar and cerebral function.

The extent to which the CST is involved in any or all of the foregoing experiments remains, strictly speaking, unknown. We have already suggested that if the latency of any response is short enough, its mediation can be ascribed with greater confidence to the CST. This brings us to the need for ablation experiments. Further investigation requires that we compare the performances of patients and animals with anatomically verified lesions of the CST with the performances of normals. The simpler the performances the better, so that their altered timing, velocity and displacement can be more accurately specified and compared. We shall see that rigorous quantitative work of this fundamental kind has scarcely begun.

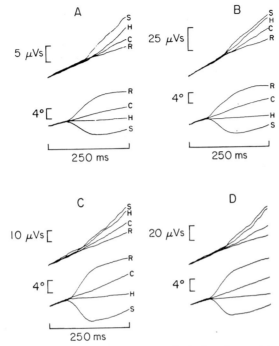

FIG. 8.14. A. Servo-type responses from the muscle flexing the top joint of the thumb. During the course of a tracking movement against an initially constant resistance, the movement may either be reversed (S) eliciting a stretch reflex, or halted (H), or allowed to accelerate by a reduction of the opposing resistance (R). In the control trials (C) none of these things happen. The initial resistance was a torque of 150 g cm (about 2 per cent of the maximum torque that the subject could exert). The top records are the integrated electromyogram of the flexor muscle, the slope of the trace giving the degree of activation of the muscle. The bottom records give the angular position of the terminal phalanx of the thumb. Each trace is the average of sixteen trials, formed in a Biomac averaging computer.

B. As in A but with the movements against a ten times greater initial resistance.

C, D. Gain compensation during fatigue. The initial force in this experiment was low, the same as for A. C. Fresh muscle. The muscle was then fatigued by applying maximal shocks to the median nerve at the elbow at 50 Hz for 60 s. Recovery was prevented by a blood pressure cuff on the upper arm, arresting the circulation. D. Muscle fatigued. The electrical responses are of the same form as before fatigue, but scaled up by a factor of roughly 2, as shown by the calibrations. Force records (not illustrated) showed that the forces developed in the half and in the other responses were the same as before fatigue. In these experiments each trace is the average of eight trials. The period of circulatory arrest was too short to cause ischaemic nerve block.

(Marsden *et al.*, 1972.)

8.4   Effects of disconnexion of CST outputs on performance

8.4.1   SCOPE AND LIMITATIONS OF ABLATION EXPERIMENTS

Many people will find it surprising that we have chosen to devote a small part only of our book to the subject of ablation experiments, and to defer that part to a mere subsection of our final chapter. The traditional textbook approach has always treated ablation as the complement of stimulation, and has devoted roughly equal attention to both. In Chapter 1 we noted the remarkable asymmetry between the dramatic results of cortical stimulation and the relatively insignificant results of section of the PT in the dog. The reasons for this asymmetry are not far to seek. The superficial resemblance of the cross-section of the medullary pyramid to a peripheral nerve was misleading; our awareness of the complexity of its morphology and distribution is relatively recent (Chapter 4). Cutting it is not like cutting a peripheral nerve which permanently paralyses specific muscles, those that would have contracted if the nerve had been stimulated. The function of the nerve is obvious; it can be defined equally by either method, and confirmed by dissection of the dead body. But the function or functions that are mediated by the PT cannot be thus simply subtracted from an animal's total behaviour, and read off as performances of which it has been rendered permanently incapable. The loss includes inhibition as well as excitation. As the animal recovers from the operation we are brought up against the marvellous adaptive power of the surviving parts of the brain, which evidently enable the animal to learn to produce appropriate behaviour when deprived of the PT outflow. The deficits seen in the acute stages may be compensated more or less completely. Such compensation is found to be most complete in young animals, for example, in infant monkeys deprived of precentral cortex (Kennard, 1938), whose brains are still actively building up internal models or schemes of their bodies and of the environment and enlarging their repertory of 'least automatic' movements. The higher the mammal, the more the brain is concerned with learned performances, and the larger the repertory it can build up during its lifetime. The possibility of compensation seems less surprising to the neurophysiologist of today, who knows better than his predecessors that the PT is not the only outflow from the motor cortex, and that this is not the only cortical or subcortical area that is concerned in movement. Even if the 'compensated' performance is relatively rich, we have no right to assume that the PT, if it had remained intact, would not have been mediating much or all of it.

The acute effects of ablation are therefore important, but they are unfortunately complicated by a temporary enlargement of the lesion, beyond its intended and final dimensions, by local oedema and locally spreading spasm of blood vessels; an unknown part of the process of compensation is thus due to shrinkage of the lesion to its eventual, histologically verifiable location and size. For many kinds of experiments the ideal lesion would be acute, temporary and reversible. The value of focal cooling for this purpose was pointed out by Trendelenburg in 1910 (Brooks, 1975). Modern cryoprobe technique has only recently begun to be exploited for such work, by Brooks and his colleagues in the cerebellar nuclei (references in Brooks, 1975) and in the parietal cortex of monkeys (Stein, 1976). It will be important to implant cooling discs in contact with the ventral aspect of the uninjured medullary pyramids, where cortico-spinal transmission can be interrupted with minimal disturbance of other structures, and to record the reversible effect of temporary interruptions on the execution of simple learned performances and on the elemental patterning of ballistic and ramp movements. To the extent that progress can be made in these directions, the asymmetry between the amount of 'positive' and 'negative' information that can be obtained from ablation experiments and from other modes of experiment will be reduced.

In developing classical chronic ablation experiments, the practical problem is to invent specific tests which are sufficiently refined to reveal subtle degrees of disability. Such tasks must be based on detailed knowledge of the normal abilities of the species in question. Adequate motivation by reward is essential. Everything that can be learned from casual observation of the spontaneous behaviour of cats and monkeys with lesions was learned long ago. It is essential to establish which abilities, if any, are permanently lost. In principle, parts of the body that remained capable of *movement* might be rendered incapable of executing, or of re-learning, specific *performances*.

8.4.2   SECTION OF THE PT AND LESION OF THE MOTOR CORTEX IN ANIMALS

The effects of pyramidotomy differ in severity in the few mammals which have been subjected to it, and are roughly related to the state of develop-ment of the corticospinal component (Chapter 1) and to the degree of elaboration of the cortical motor map (Chapter 2).

Bilateral pyramidotomy in the marsupial phalanger or brushtail possum, *Trichosurus vulpecula* caused relatively minor disability, even in the acute stages (Hore *et al.*, 1973). In this animal the corticospinal tract ends in the cervical region (Chapter 2). The possum is a nocturnal arboreal animal, with well-differentiated digits which can grip alternatively with soft pads or with hard, sharp claws. Whenever possible it reaches for food with its mouth, but it will grab at a distant morsel with one or both forelimbs, opening and closing all the digits together. On a tree which we erected in the laboratory our normal possums climbed and moved gracefully collect-ing and eating the morsels of food that were hung from the branches, sometimes clamping the pelvis with hindlimbs and prehensile tail while moving the head and forelimbs freely in space. After bilateral pyramidotomy there was no abnormality in posture or gait as the animal stood or scam-pered along the floor. In the tree, the normally graceful and flowing move-ments were impaired by a difficulty in placing the limbs accurately on the branches. A pendant limb would grope several times for a hold, and might even take hold of another limb. When holding a food morsel in its cage, the digits of the forelimbs sometimes got intertwined and then seemed difficult to disengage. There was little improvement in 80 days. We could not make observations in darkness and do not know if the disability would then have been more severe.

In the rat, unilateral pyramidotomy caused transient paresis lasting up to 20 days, worst in the contralateral forelimb and worst in the digits (Barron, 1934).

The cat seems, at first sight, remarkably little affected by cutting one PT. Posture and locomotion appear normal after the first few days, though attentive observation reveals slight circumduction of the contralateral hindlimb, with occasional dragging of the foot. Severe weakness and clumsiness of the limbs opposite to an acute unilateral lesion last for a few hours at most. For a few days, weakness of flexion of the fore-claws is evident in grasping a ball of paper in play, and in climbing a wire mesh. On a slippery floor the affected limbs may slide passibly into, and remain for some moments in, abnormal attitudes. Considerable disability is obvious only in locomotion along a horizontal ladder, but this improves over a period of months. This disability is more severe if both pyramids have been cut. Tactile placing, the normal ability of a blindfolded cat, suspended in air, to place a paw promptly on the surface of a table on being brought into contact with its edge, is lost permanently (Liddell and Phillips, 1944). This is probably the functional consequence of the intimate and localized relation between cutaneous input and motor output in the motor cortex (Chapter 6). All observers agree that flexion reflexes are deficient (recalling the effect of the PT on reflex arcs, Chapter 4); but Marshall (1934) and Liddell and Phillips (1944) found a positive exaggeration of extension reflexes whereas Tower (1935) and Laursen and Wiesendanger (1966) did not.

A more refined test, and one which revealed an important new aspect of disability, was devised by Laursen and Wiesendanger (1967). They found that cats with incomplete PT section, and after complete recovery of walking, jumping and climbing, were still able to press a lever (to obtain fish) as rapidly (no change in simple RT) and as frequently as before operation. One cat still always used the same paw for pressing the lever in spite of a contralateral PT lesion. But if cats had to discriminate correctly between two lights in order to be rewarded for pressing the lever, their choice RT was lengthend from 0.1 to 0.8 s as compared with their preoperative averages: the larger the lesion, the slower the response. This might mean that the cerebral organization involved in the learning normally has a more direct access to the PT than to other output pathways; alternatively, or additionally, that the available alternative routes of transmission from brain to spinal motoneurones are slower. Laursen and Wiesendanger suggest that the speed conferred by the PT would be important for the survival of the cat as a predator of fast-moving prey.

In monkeys, the disability resulting from unilateral section of the PT is far milder than that of spastic hemiplegia due to capsular lesions in man. The effects on posture and locomotion are minimal (Denny-Brown, 1966), but prehension of objects by the contralateral hand, as distinct from its prehensile use in locomotion, is impaired, and its normal reactions to contact are lost. Tower's (1940) pioneer description has never been bettered. The monkeys prefer the unaffected arm for grooming and feeding, and will not use the disabled arm for these purposes unless the normal arm is restrained. 'Instead of the normal movement which culminates in the opposition of thumb and index to pick up small objects', there is 'a highly stereotyped reaching-grasping act involving the entire body-half, similar to the reaching-grasping act of the newborn monkey . . . the hand is brought down on the object in half-pronation and scoops it into the ulnar side of the hand . . . the transfer to the mouth is effected by bringing the mouth to the hand where the lips then remove the food between the fingers which themselves do not open. The act is quite incapable of modification so as to take food from between the observer's fingers, or from any except an unobstructed surface. It is unsuccessful with small objects such as kernels of grain. Aim is achieved by orientating the entire body.' Even after three years, all discrete usage of the digits is utterly and permanently eliminated. Use of the affected hand in running and climbing is indistinguishable from normal from an early stage of recovery from the operation.

Bilateral PT section is more instructive than unilateral, first, because it completely denudes each side of the cord of pyramidal synapses; secondly, because the animals cannot rely on a normal hand and are more strongly motivated to overcome their disability. Maximum compensation is important if one is seeking to identify some performance of which the animal remains permanently incapable, and for which, therefore, the PT is uniquely necessary. Lawrence and Kuypers (1968) tested the hands by offering food morsels in different sized holes drilled in a board. A normal monkey winkles out the morsels from the smallest holes with index finger alone, which it extends independently of the other fingers which remain semiflexed. This performance was impossible after bilateral PT section unless some PT axons had been spared. For the first 4 to 6 weeks 'reaching for food consisted of a circumduction of the arm at the shoulder with the elbow slightly flexed and the fingers loosely extended and abducted. At this stage closure of the hand tended to be part of a total movement of the arm' (cf. the 'whole arm control' of Prosimians, Chapter 1). The ability to open and close the hands without movement at proximal joints returned later. The pronated hand could now be placed quickly and accurately over a food morsel, without circumduction at shoulder or orientation of the body as a whole: it could be steered to its target through a transparent tunnel. But food could be taken only from the largest holes in the board—'the fingers closed together to pick up the food and take it to the mouth'. There, the difficulty in voluntarily relaxing the grasp, first noted by Tower (1940), remained severe for the whole follow-up period of 5 months, although there was 'no difficulty in releasing the grip when climbing or clinging'. From the earliest days the monkeys had been able to run and climb rapidly and without obvious abnormality. It seems, there-fore, that the independent activity of index finger, the use of the precision grip of thumb and index, and the ready letting-go of small objects from the grasp, are performances for which the PT is essential. Infant monkeys subjected to bilateral pyramidotomy within 4 weeks of birth never learned these abilities, although a control infant companion was performing them normally by the age of one year (Lawrence and Hopkins, 1976).

Some conflict of evidence still awaits resolution. Bucy *et al.* (1966) cut the PT bilaterally in monkeys at the level of the cerebral peduncles, but not always completely. Although they state generally that 'the fully recovered animal, in addition to his ability to walk, climb and jump well, was able to use the thumb and index finger alone to pick up small seeds', some in-dividuals showed 'nil' recovery of the hand to pick up food (after 6–20 months); some 'used hand as a unit'; others 'used thumb and fingers slowly'. Tower (1940) and Lawrence and Kuypers (1968) were sure that there was no recovery of independent use of the digits; the latter authors were able to correlate such recovery with sparing of some PT axons by the lesion.

Hepp-Reymond and Wiesendanger (1972) and Hepp-Reymond *et al.* (1974) re-trained monkeys to squeeze a transducer between thumb and index after unilateral or bilateral pyramidotomy. The experiments showed that after recovery from the initial paralysis (2 to 4 weeks), and under strong motivation, monkeys can re-learn to produce an isometric 'precision grip' (Napier, 1956, 1960); but their ability to learn to produce independent movements of thumb and index in other situations was not assessed.

In the one monkey with bilateral (but sub-total) PT lesions, the reward was given only when a pressure of 50 g was attained as rapidly as possible after the presentation of the signal light (Hepp-Reymond *et al.*, 1974). The animal was unable to squeeze the transducer until four weeks after the operation. Reaction times were measured to the onset of EMG and to the instant of attaining 50 g. Pre- and postoperative values for the right hand are given in Table 8.2. It can be seen that RT $_{50g\ pressure}$ never re-gained its preoperative level. RT $_{flexor\ EMG}$ recovered, but the difference between the two RT, which measures the slowed development of force, remained elevated; the two abnormal measurements 'could therefore represent irreversible deficits due to pyramidotomy'.

TABLE 8.2

	Mean RT $_{\text{flexor EMG}}$ (ms)	Mean RT $_{\text{50g pressure}}$ (ms)
Preoperative	161$\pm$38	249$\pm$36
Postoperative		
2–3 months	227$\pm$112	395$\pm$122
5–6 months	178$\pm$41	305$\pm$48
10 months	153$\pm$32	294$\pm$33

This lengthening of simple reaction-time in the precision-grip experiment stands in contrast to the results obtained by Laursen (1970), who found in monkeys, as Laursen and Wiesendanger (1967) had found in cats, that simple RT is unaffected but choice RT is lengthened. In Laursen's experiments the monkeys responded with movements of the whole arm. The lengthening of simple RT in the thumb-index experiment may be the specific consequence of sub-total or total deprivation of these 'distal' motoneurones of their corticomotoneuronal synapses.

Denny-Brown's (1966) studies have emphasized the loss of reactions to contact with the hand. The loss of tactile placing had already been described by Tower (1940). Visual placing recovers, with surviving but impaired ability for prehension under visual guidance. There is loss of the 'instinctive grasp reaction', a complex, automatic response to contact over an area extending to the dorsal and lateral aspects of hand and wrist which, by well-adjusted movements of extension, flexion, pronation etc., serves to bring the object into contact with the palm, when the fingers will close upon it in a 'grasp reflex'. The instinctive grasp reaction is lost but the grasp reflex is exaggerated by PT section. This reflex depends on skin contact as well as on stretch of the finger flexors, which, like the muscles acting at the wrist and elbow, are mildly spastic, with increased tendon jerks. This slight spasticity is not to be compared with the severe dystonia resulting from exaggerated labyrinthine and body-contact reflexes: the PT is not much involved in restraining these. But postural support is an essential foundation for the spatially oriented and delicate behaviour of the hands, and Denny-Brown and Evans (Denny-Brown, 1966) found evidence, from electrical stimulation, that it can be mobilized bilaterally by spread of activity forward from area 4 to activate 'extrapyramidal' cortex. Denny-Brown (1966) sums up by saying that the PT is concerned 'with those spatial adjustments that accurately adapt the movement to the spatial attributes of the stimulus. Thus grasping is adapted to the shape of the thing to be grasped, whether a particle of food, a pin, or a surface.' Prior opening of the hand is essential in the formation of the appropriate pre-hensiveness patterns, and for this, the preferential corticomotoneuronal accessibility of the finger extensors is presumably important (Phillips, 1971).

Since the PT is not the sole projection from pre- and postcentral gyri, it is not surprising that their destruction in monkeys causes more severe disability than does section of the PT: 'a severe and permanent defect in all delicate spatial adjustments of movements of the hand, and to a lesser extent of the foot and mouth. The small eversions, abductions, rotations that enable precise palpation and exploration or withdrawal, depend on the integrity of pre- and postcentral gyrus. The defect is exaggerated by blindfolding, when palpating exploration is deprived of visual guidance.' (Denny-Brown, 1966.)

The full extent of the disabled monkey's dependence on vision is revealed by its behaviour when blindfolded. It sits immobile, with flexed limbs; it makes no response to light touches on its hands, and makes no attempt to remove its blindfold (Denny-Brown, personal communication).

Figure 2.5 (p. 33) shows the area from which Leyton and Sherrington (1917) evoked primary movements of a chimpanzee's elbow, wrist, fingers, index and thumb. The terminal degeneration of PT axons resulting from ablation of this area was described in Chapter 4. Within hours of the operation the animal which was feeding and active, seemed surprised by the disability of its contralateral arm. The shoulder was slightly weak, the elbow more so. There was wrist drop. The fingers could be moved a little, the thumb and index hardly at all. It could not grasp the vertical bars of the cage. Next day it was not attempting to use its hand—'seems to have learnt its disability in regard to that hand, and to do without it'. A month later, the shoulder and elbow had recovered. The wrist was possibly drooping slightly. The three ulnar fingers were used well, but the index was not moved independently, and got on to the wrong side of the bar when grasping. The thumb, because of its relative shortness, had not been much used preoperatively (cf. Phillips, 1971). Five weeks after the first operation the lesion was re-excised, and the adjacent shoulder area was also excised (Fig. 2.5). The slight recrudescence of weakness of shoulder had recovered in a week. The condition of the hand was unaltered by the second ablation. From the day following it the animal was climbing, swinging, holding food as before.

That the precentral gyrus is not itself the repository, or is not the sole repository, of engrams of learned movements was shown by Lashley (1950). Monkeys were trained to open problem boxes containing food. When, after sufficient recovery from bilateral destruction of the motor areas the boxes were again presented, it was found that the monkeys had retained the learning and, in spite of their clumsiness, went correctly about the task of getting out the food.

8.4.3 LESIONS OF THE PT AND MOTOR CORTEX IN MAN

Pathological processes which are confined to the medullary pyramids are extremely rare. Brown and Fang (1961) reported the case of a chronic middle-aged man, psychotic and hypertensive, who suffered sudden onset of left hemiplegia, including the face, with paralysis of the right hypoglossal nerve. Twenty-four hours later, the left limbs were flaccid, the left arm 'more affected' than the leg (it was immobile); the left plantar response was extensor (the sign regarded since Babinski as pathognomonic of pyramidal disorder) and the right flexor. There was no sensory loss. Two weeks later the left facial weakness had recovered; the left abdominal and cremasteric reflexes were absent and so was the left ankle jerk. Eight months later he could walk with a limp; his left arm was 'weak . . . held in flexion'. There was therefore some spasticity. After 2 years the left limbs were slightly wasted, with 'hyperactive reflexes'; the left plantar response was still extensor. There was unfortunately no report on the function of his left hand at any stage. Five years from the onset he died suddenly. There was a cyst in the right pyramid at the pontomedullary junction which also involved the hypoglossal nerve, with a loss of pyramidal axons and myelin sheaths caudal to the lesion. Some large cells survived in the precentral gyrus; the number of cells in laminae III and V seemed depleted, but no counts were made. There was an old small cyst in the head of the left caudate nucleus. Meyer and Herndon (1962) reported a case of tetraplegia of sudden onset in a middle-aged man, without sensory loss. Vision and eye movements were normal, he could clench his jaw, but there was weakness of pharyngeal and tongue muscles. He needed tracheostomy and, for a few days, assistance from a Drinker respirator. Eventually all tendon reflexes became hyperactive and both plantars extensor. He died after seven weeks without having recovered any voluntary movement of the limbs. Both pyramids were destroyed by a lesion which was joined by a narrow isthmus to another lesion in the dorsal paramedian pontomedullary reticular formation.

Neurosurgeons have sometimes divided the PT unilaterally at the level of the cerebral peduncle for the relief of the violent unilateral involuntary movements known as hemiballismus (Bucy, 1957). Since the indication for operation is a severe disorder of motor function, the situation is not comparable with experimental ablations carried out on normal animals. One such case, of a man aged 70, is of unique importance because the exact extent of the lesion was determined histologically (Bucy et al., 1964).

The severity of the hemiballismus made any preoperative assessment of the motor abilities of the left limbs impossible (the patient was right-handed). The immediate effect of operation was a flaccid left hemiplegia; the hemiballismus was cured permanently. After 24 hours the patient could move the left toes and could grasp with the left hand. From the third day, the left plantar reflex was extensor. On the 10th day the patient could stand alone and walk with assistance, and could lift the left arm above the head. 'Strength and range of voluntary movement returned more rapidly in the hand and fingers, and in the foot and toes, than at the more proximal joints . . . slightly more rapid in the lower than in the upper extremity'. There was no spasticity. By the 24th day he could get into and out of a chair without help. There was now slight spasticity of the left leg, and the tendon jerks were increased in arm and leg. On the 29th day he could walk unaided for a short distance, dragging the left foot. On the 32nd day, 'fairly good use of his left hand and upper extremity. He could execute fine movement of individual fingers fairly well. Voluntary movements of his left leg were quite good, and he could move his left foot and toes well.' The left tendon reflexes were 'moderately hyperactive' but 'resistance to passive manipulation was increased little if at all'. There was no sensory loss. There was moderate weakness of the left lower face. At 7 months it seemed that maximum recovery had been reached. There was no weakness of the face. The left handgrip was slightly weaker than the right. 'Fine, individual movements of the left fingers were only slightly less well executed than on the right side.' The left toes could not be moved 'quite as extensively as the right ones'. There was still no increase in resistance to passive manipulation of the left limbs, but the left tendon reflexes were 'a little more active'. The patient could hop well on either foot alone—a little better on the right than on the left. He died after $2\frac{1}{2}$ years from cardiac failure and malignant disease not involving the brain, which showed no abnormalities other than the surgical lesion and the degeneration resulting from it. DeMyer counted that 83 per cent of PT axons were lost from the sectioned PT. The uncrossed PT reached the mid-thoracic level, the crossed PT extended to the lowest level of the cord. It was estimated that at least 90 per cent of the largest PT ('Betz') cells were missing on the side of the lesion, presumably due to retrograde degeneration.

That any independent finger movement should have survived this lesion is remarkable enough. The survival of 17 per cent of PT axons (cf. Lawrence and Kuypers, 1968) may, however, have been important, as, also, the surviving uncrossed PT. Further, the mere ability to *move* the fingers may be functionally less informative than a catalogue of skilled movements that the subject could not perform, or learn to perform. In future cases, it would be valuable to make the fullest possible neurophysiological and neuropsychological studies of performance. It is already clear, however, as Bucy (1957) rightly insists, that patients after pedunculotomy are far less disabled than patients with haemorrhagic destruction of the internal capsule, and do not exhibit many of the signs designated 'pyramidal' in clinical neurology. The venerable Sign of Babinski, however, retains its significance as pathognomonic of injury to the PT in man.

For historical reasons, the observers of these rare cases were pre-occupied with the old problem of whether a lesion of the PT causes flaccidity or spasticity rather than with an exact specification of what movements are permanently lost or disordered, and of which performances, if any, can be re-learned and under what circumstances. Cases of focal lesion of the motor cortex and its underlying white matter are much more common, and have been collected for over a century by many acute clinicians beginning with Charcot and Hughlings Jackson (section 8.2). To the hazards of natural pathology must be added the small circum-scribed lesions resulting from penetration of the skulls of previously healthy people by small high-velocity missile fragments (Russell and Whitty, 1953). The general conclusions of such studies are embodied in every textbook of neurology (e.g. Walshe, 1973). What, therefore, it may be asked, remains to be added? The answer is threefold. First, there is much still to be learned from precise neuroanatomical study of cases with well-circumscribed lesions in which detailed clinical, neurophysiological and neuropsychological investigations were carried out during life, not only to specify the location of the lesion but also to trace, by modern techniques, the resulting anterograde and retrograde degeneration (Chapter 4). Since the human brain and cord are so large, such studies are bound to be extremely laborious. There is a further practical difficulty. The smaller the lesion, the longer the prospect of survival and the greater the likelihood that the patient will outlive the doctor. Special arrangements will therefore be necessary if this small but rich neuroanatomical harvest is ever to be reaped. This will apply with special force to the small focal lesions of World War II. Secondly, entirely new prospects have been opened up by the application to disordered movements of the analytical techniques and functional concepts which we have outlined in section 8.3; and substantial progress is to be expected in the next few years, compounded over a longer period if even a few well-investigated cases can be brought eventu-ally to proper neuroanatomical completion. Thirdly, introspective accounts of their own disabilities by neurologically trained observers have evidently much to contribute (Brodal, 1973) and should be a fertile source of sug-gestions for analytical experiment by the methods of section 8.3.1. These are people who are likely to have cultivated special manual skills, to cooperate in devising appropriate rehabilitation, and to be brave enough to wish to enrich science by analysing distressing symptoms which might otherwise represent an unmitigated personal loss. The whole field is one in which intensive work on small numbers of cases is likely to yield deeper insights than the collection of fragmentary data from larger numbers.

As an example of the possibilities of neurophysiological analysis of elemental movements in lesions of the sensorimotor cortex and underlying white matter we may cite the pioneering work of Adam et al. (1976), who investigated abnormalities in the servo-assistance of ramp movements. In the disabled hand, the responses of flexor pollicis longus to stretch, halt and release (section 8.3.6) were 'abolished or considerably attenuated'. In one case there was 'a small superficial tumour in the Rolandic fissure, and the responses largely recovered when this was excised'. After recovery of motor function was apparently complete there remained a mild degree of astereognosis and of inattention to bilateral simultaneous stimulation, although position sense and two-point discrimination had returned to normal, and the early part of the long-latency response to stretch remained 'relatively attenuated'. The evidence from these cases suggests that the early part of the long-latency servo-response is mediated by a trans-cortical loop, though it cannot distinguish between a loop in which the thalamus is directly linked to area 4 and one in which the thalamus is linked to area 3a with a transcortical linkage to area 4 (Chapter 6). The response is also diminished in cases of isolated lesion of a dorsal column (Marsden et al., 1973).

The effect of central lesions on the programming of elemental ballistic movements has so far been concerned with lesions of the cerebellum (Hallett et al., 1975b; Marsden et al., 1977) or with experimental alcoholic intoxication (Marsden et al., 1977) which since Flourens has been held to disrupt cerebellar function. The timing of the agonist-antagonist bursts is prolonged (section 8.3.3) and the servo-assistance of ramp movements is also impaired. 'Since many normal human limb movements comprise a mixture of a ballistic initiation and a ramp execution, these abnormalities must cause the cerebellar patient to start moving with the wrong muscles and be subsequently inaccurate in correcting for the initial errors.' (Marsden et al., 1977.) Presumably the disorder involves faulty programming of the motor cortex by the lateral cerebellum, and faulty control of transmission through the long cerebral servo-loops by networks of which the inter-mediate zone of the cerebellum forms part.

Quantitative analysis of graphic records of movements which are still relatively simple, though more complex than the elemental ballistic and ramp movements at a single joint, has, no doubt, much to offer, especially if combined with electromyography and especially in cases in which the cortical lesions and their corticocortical and corticosubcortical connexions will eventually be verified. The most brilliant graphical analyses so far have been those of movements disordered by pathological lesions and gunshot wounds of the cerebellum (Holmes, 1939). In these studies, which he began over half a century ago, Holmes measured the delay in the initiation and in the termination of movements, their slow and unsteady rise to maximum force, their diminished power, their erratic velocity, uneconomical trajectories and failure to arrive accurately at their goals. His use of stereophotography of a flashing light attached to a finger-tip (Fig. 8.15) makes an interesting comparison with Bernstein's records (Fig. 8.1) in which the light did not flash but was interrupted by a rotating shutter. Simple kymography of visual tracking movements in Parkinson's disease is now beginning to give valuable results (Cassel *et al.*, 1973; Flowers, 1976). Human patients can perform voluntary movements, whether healthy or disordered, without the need for the prolonged and laborious conditioning required by monkeys.

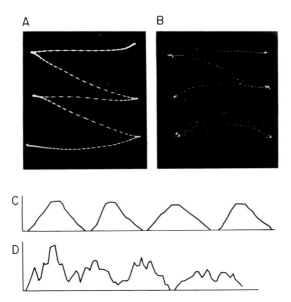

FIG. 8.15. A, B. Records obtained by photographing points of light attached to the tips of the forefingers as a patient with a lesion of the right side of the cerebellum attempted to move each finger slowly and accurately between series of luminous red points (not visible in the photographs) in a dark room. Each flash of light corresponds to 0.04 s. The range of each movement was about 75 cm. A is the record obtained from the left hand, B, that from the right. The irregularity in the rate and in the directions of movements of the affected hand, and the failure to arrest this finger accurately at the points, are well shown in B.

C, D. An analysis of four of the separate movements of each record in A and B, to show irregularity in the velocity of motion of the right hand (D). Horizontal distance between each dot corresponds to 0.04 s; the heights above the base lines represent the spaces between successive flashes of light and therefore the rate of movement at the corresponding points in space.

(Holmes, 1939.)

Jung and Dietz (1975) find that the RT to a click, measured to the earliest EMG response in a paretic contralateral limb, is lengthened by unilateral lesions of the motor cortex and internal capsule. If simultaneous bilateral response is required, the difference between the normal and paretic RT is much reduced. In explanation of this result the authors invoke the uncrossed CST.

Brodal's account of his own case (1973) shows the quality of the contribution to be expected when a patient with profound neurological insight analyses his own symptoms and observes and encourages his own progress to 'compensation' and recovery. A right-sided embolus from the carotid artery caused a left-sided hemiplegia with no somatosensory or visual-field impairment. Five days later there was some recovery of movement at shoulder, elbow, hip and knee, and of flexion of fingers and plantar-flexion of foot; extension of the fingers and thumb, and dorsi-flexion of the foot and toes, were still impossible. After two months he was buttoning his clothes and holding his fork at table, though slowly and clumsily, and tying his bow tie. In the earliest stages of recovery the nature of the muscular weakness was of special interest. 'Subjectively it was felt as if the muscle was unwilling to contract, and as if there was a resistance which could be overcome by very strong voluntary innervation. The greater the degree of paresis of such a muscle, the greater was the mental effort needed to make it contract and to oppose voluntarily even a very weak counter-force. On the other hand only a slight mental effort was needed to bring about a fairly good contraction of a muscle able to work with about half or a little less of its full force . . . . The expenditure of this mental energy is very exhausting, a fact of some importance in physio-therapeutic treatment.' Specially interesting also was the value of passive movements in rehabilitation. 'At the beginning it often happened that the patient, even with his strongest effort, was unable to make a voluntary movement of a particular joint . . . but when the proper movement had been made passively by the physiotherapist a couple of times, the patient was able to perform the movement, although with minimal force. Subjectively it was clearly felt as if the sensory information produced by the passive movement helped the patient to "direct" the "force of innervation" through the proper channels . . . it may well be that there are subtle neurophysiological mechanisms involved in this "facilitation" of movements. From introspection it appears, however, that the subjective information about the movement to be executed, its range and goal, is an essential factor. The phenomenon is probably parallel to the learning of all motor skills. Among an original multitude of more or less haphazard movements the correct ones are recognized as such by means of the sensory information they feed back to the central nervous system, and this information is later used in selecting the correct movements in the further training.' It seems that there is a sense in which it is fair to say that compensation is a re-learning of old performances with neural apparatus not previously used for those performances, and can be compared with attempts by an uninjured person to learn a difficult new skill in adult life.

The possibility that some degree of spasticity, presumably generated by fusimotor activity, is useful in ensuring an inflow of information from the muscle spindles to the brain is also important (cf. Chambers and Gilliatt, 1954). 'In the first weeks following the stroke, very little active movements of the fingers were possible. When the fingers had not been moved for some time, the patient, as is usual, had no feeling of his muscles in the hand and forearm and of the position of the finger-joints, but when making the first movements with the fingers, even very slowly, a feeling of resistance was obvious to him, giving the subjective impression of what could best be described as "stiffness". On repeating the movement this feeling increased as did the objectively-observed spasticity. This feeling, not being known to the patient before, was at first assumed to be derived from the joints or to be caused by slight oedema of the hand, and was not recognised as coming from the muscles. This became clear to the patient only later when he had some control of his finger movements. It should be noted that the joints were all freely movable, and the subjective feeling could be localized to particular muscles, for example particularly interossei.' The helpful effect of exciting the spindle primary endings by vibration (Hagbarth and Eklund, 1966) may be relevant here.

The distinction between the programme of a learned performance and its execution was striking in the early efforts, two months after the stroke, to resume the daily tying of a bow tie. Seven to ten attempts were necessary. 'The appropriate finger movements were difficult to perform with sufficient strength, speed and coordination, but it was quite obvious to the patient that the main reason for the failure was something else. . . . Subjectively the patient felt as if he had to stop because "his fingers did not know the next move". He had the same feeling as when one recites a poem or sings a song and gets lost. The only way is to start (again) from the beginning. It was felt as if the delay in the succession of movements (due to pareses and spasticity) interrupted a chain of more or less automatic movements. Consciously directing attention to the finger movements did not improve the performance; on the contrary it made it quite impossible.' The forty-year-old programme, perhaps, was intact, but, deprived of a sequence of feedbacks from successfully completed movements (in the manner envisaged by Bernstein (section 8.2)), following on one another within a critical period of time, somehow 'got lost' and failed to retain control of the performance.

Writing is a performance at an even higher level. The patient is right-handed, and was surprised to find in the acute stages that although there was no dysgraphia (and no dysphasia or dyslexia) his handwriting, with the normal right hand, was altered in the following ways: the lines uneven, oblique not horizontal, unequally spaced; the individual letters irregularly shaped, and less smooth; occasional dropping-out of a letter or unnecessary repetition of a letter; transposition of digits, e.g. 46 instead of 64. This raises the question of bilateral corticospinal control of the movements of the hand (in view of the absence of corticocallosal interconnexions of the cortical hand areas in monkeys: Jones and Powell, 1969) and of bilateral cerebrocerebellar representation of its higher functions. Brodal's (1973) review of the cerebrocerebellar interconnexions 'makes it clear that the common assumption of a cerebellar half controlling only the ipsilateral half of the body is an oversimplification', and that 'the right cerebral half acts not only on the left but also on the right cerebellar half through the pons and the inferior olive'. He reminds us that there are about 19 million corticopontine axons on each side in man.

Removal of parts of the motor cortex for the relief of focal epilepsy or of involuntary movements has often been practised, and is also a valuable source of observations, subject to the caveat that the brain was already abnormal before the operation: the effects of such excisions cannot strictly be compared with those of similar-sized lesions in previously healthy brains. Horsley (1909), however, was obviously correct when he concluded from his considerable experience of such cases that not all voluntary movements are 'alone generated by' the precentral cortex and its contained Betz cells. His patient Hn was a powerful young man who suffered from violent choreoathetosis confined to the left arm. Horsley mapped the right precentral arm area by faradic stimulation and then excised it all. The involuntary movements were completely cured. Powerful normal movements of the proximal parts of the arm were restored, but not those of the fingers. Horsley examined histologically the block of cortex he had removed and saw the Betz cells within it. Some of the parts which had responded to their stimulation had recovered the power of voluntary movement after their excision. Later evidence of bilateral cortico-reticulo-spinal projections to proximal muscle groups, which go far to explain this particular example of compensation, has been given in Chapter 4.

8.5 Effects of interference with inputs on performance and perception of movement

8.5.1 SECTION OF THE DORSAL ROOTS IN MONKEYS

Accurate movement requires feedback from the moving parts, continuously or intermittently checking the actual progress of a movement against the progress prescribed by the central nervous programme (Bernstein,

1967). The feedback is conveniently designated 'response feedback', to distinguish it from 'internal feedback' ('efference copy', 'corollary discharge', possibly mediated by collaterals of corticospinal axons (Chapter 4)) and from 'knowledge of results' (Evarts, in Evarts et al., 1971).

The relative importance of response feedback in movements of the monkey's arm has been assessed by cutting the dorsal roots. The experiment is subject to the general limitations of chronic ablation experiments in respect of compensation (section 8.4.1): brief, reversible deafferentations, which could be injected during elemental ballistic or ramp movements, whose execution could then be quantitatively compared in the normal and deafferented mode, would be invaluable. Again, section of the dorsal roots entails loss of input from skin and joints in addition to those from muscle spindles and tendon organs to which, in the present context, great interest is attached, and which it would be preferable to isolate if that were possible. Finally, the existence of unmyelinated axons in the *ventral* roots in man (Coggeshall et al., 1975), and the demonstration that some such axons are *afferent* in the cat (Clifton et al., 1976) is a complication, raised originally by Foerster in breach of the Bell–Magendie Law, which still obstinately refuses to go away.

Mott and Sherrington (1895) performed unilateral deafferentation of the cervical cord in monkeys. It caused virtual paralysis of the deafferented arm, although the responses to electrical stimulation of the cortex were unimpaired. Reviews of early literature by Nathan and Sears (1960) and Bossom (1974) have shown that there was uncertainty and disagreement about the range of movement that was possible. Sherrington (1931) later wrote of the 'striking contrast' between the monkey's use of its arm and its later responses to cortical stimulation: 'Willed movements are upset in the extreme. In the monkey the desensitized limb is practically useless, for prehension quite so. The animal soon treats it as useless and as an encumbrance worse than useless; it attacks it and would tear it away. . . . Wild incoordination under willed action; little or no abnormality under the action of the directly stimulated motor cortex.' It has since become clear that under chronic restraint of the normal arm, monkeys can *learn* to reach for food with the deafferented arm, but that the movements are abrupt in onset and exaggerated in range (Knapp et al., 1963).

On the second day after bilateral deafferentation of the arms, Denny-Brown's (1966) monkeys were able to move their arms in association with active, but not passive, movements of the neck; after three weeks, there was some recovery of visual placing reactions of the arms, and 'alternating progression movements appeared in the arms when the animal was running on the hind limbs'. This shows that the quadrupedal locomotor programme was reasserting its influence on the forelimbs. The animals could walk on all fours after three months. Monkeys bilaterally deafferented by Taub and Berman (1968) began to move their forelimbs after two weeks and their performance improved over a period of two to six months. They could walk and climb slowly, even when blindfolded.

The 'less-automatic' movements of reaching and prehension could eventually improve to the extent that some monkeys became able to pick up raisins with thumb and forefinger from a small hole in a board (Taub and Berman, 1968). At this point, it became clear that the process of re-learning to reach and grasp was favoured by a careful intradural division of the dorsal roots which spared the small blood vessels which run with them into the cord (Bossom, 1974), and thus avoided any local ischaemic damage to the spinal cord. The animals then 'attempted to use their arms to obtain grapes within hours after recovery from anaesthesia'. Bossom's observations on properly tamed monkeys show how heavily the movements of extension and grasping depend on visual control. 'The animal attends closely to his arm and spends much time observing attempts to move the arm. Moreover, we have not seen reaching movements soon after surgery unless the offered object and the hand were in simultaneous view.' Grasping is not possible at first: 'when the food is batted the animal pauses on it with open palm and must be helped to form a grasp. . . . The thumb is not seen to be used in the grasp and the fingers are opened, palm towards the mouth and the food either ingested, or, as occasionally happens, falls to the floor of the cage.' Bilaterally deafferented monkeys observed by Gilman et al. (1976) were sometimes successful in picking up food from a table-top after daily training for two weeks. 'After attempting to grasp the food, the animal often supinated its forearm and gazed at the supinated hand. If the hand was empty, the animal halted its beginning elbow flexion and started the task again.' The food though picked up in a 'clumsy shovel grasp' was usually held between thumb and forefinger. A single arm attempted the task; the opposite arm made mirror movements. The success rate at two weeks was 55 per cent and at five weeks 98 per cent. Gilman et al. (1976) plotted the trajectories and the dynamic characteristics of the movements from cine films, measured the lengths of the circuitous trajectories, and recorded their oscillations, multiple overshoots and the irregular, un-predictable combinations of low-speed and high-speed segments of the trajectories by which the monkeys moved their hands on to the target (Fig. 8.16); these contrasted with the relatively direct and undisrupted trajectories (not shown in the Figure) by which they brought the food to their mouths.

Bossom (1974) stresses that the movements remain permanently ataxic and dysmetric. 'This point has been lost in recent reports and requires reiteration. Although movement is not abolished and single components of a forelimb repertoire have been trained by various investigators, the elegance of normal movements is lost.'

Animal I CO Animal I DA 15 days Animal 3 DB 14 days Animal I DA 38 days DB 10 days

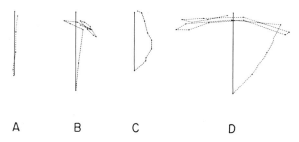

A   B   C   D

Fig. 8.16. Kinematic records of trajectory and velocity of movements made by monkeys reaching for food. The reaching movement was along a horizontal table-top and was filmed by a movie camera pointing vertically downwards. The location of the reaching hand was represented by the mid-point between the first and second metacarpo-phalangeal joints. Heavy dots mark positions of this point at intervals of approximately 63 ms. They are interconnected by dotted lines. The average distance of the food target was 15 cm; its direction was varied randomly between five positions. A. Normal monkey. B. 15 days after bilateral deafferentation (the relatively normal trajectory of the movement from target to mouth is not shown). C shows the different nature of the disorder of reaching produced by decerebellation, and D, the combined effect of deafferentation and decerebellation. (Gilman *et al.*, 1976.)

The cases of successful retraining in reaching and grasping have evidently depended on strong motivation, visual control of movements, and 'knowledge of results'. Crucial evidence that they have depended to any extent on internal feedback is still lacking, in spite of the wealth of anatomical structures (Chapter 4) that could provide for such feedback. Bossom (1974), however, cited unpublished experiments by Levine and Ommaya to the effect that deafferented monkeys could be trained to maintain a grasp of a demanded pressure in order to obtain a food reward. If this point is established it is very important, for it is most parsimoniously explained by internal feedback.

It is not clear whether it would be possible for a deafferented monkey to learn to move his hand on to a target at a standard distance and orientation from his body, and then to learn to repeat the performance after blindfolding. This would have to depend, it would seem, on memory of internal feedback, established during the visually guided training. Two alternative explanations would, however, need to be excluded: first, that the animals had learned to utilize some unidentified response feedback entering by unmyelinated axons in the ventral roots; second, as Bossom (1974) points out, that the movement might have become firmly linked with an associated movement of some normally innervated part of the body, which would generate a response feedback. 'Monkeys are quite capable of such subterfuges and suitable controls for them have not been incorporated into some of the behavioural tasks which have been used.'

A final source of error, that of regeneration of the sectioned dorsal roots, should always be excluded by postmortem examination including histology.

Dorsal rhizotomy cuts off all inputs from the forelimb indiscriminately, and it would obviously be desirable to be able to cut off, one at a time, the inputs from muscle, tendon, joints, skin, etc. Although, as is well known, different modalities of input travel in different spinal tracts on their way to the brain, it is, unfortunately, impossible to interrupt, selectively and completely, these different inputs from the forelimbs of monkeys by making lesions in the dorsal columns or in other ascending spinal tracts (Brown and Gordon, 1977).

8.5.2   VISUAL STEERING OF THE HAND AND FINGERS IN MONKEYS

Eye–hand coordination has played a central role in the evolution of primates Chapter 1), but details of the visuo-motor connexions are not yet fully worked out. Behavioural experiments, in which the cortical motor output to the hand is disconnected from its visual input, leave no doubt of their existence and importance.

Brinkman and Kuypers (1973) examined monkeys in which all the fore-brain commissures and the optic chiasma had been sectioned. They blindfolded one eye: suppose the right (Fig. 8.17). Then the only visual input was to the left hemisphere (and only from the right half of the field of vision). They then presented the monkey with a special recessed food-board on which the food was easily visible but difficult to palpate. The monkey could bring its left hand straight on to the food target. Its ability to do this is explained by the existence of bilateral cortico-reticulo-spinal

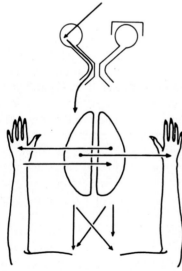

FIG. 8.17. A diagram to illustrate the experiments of Brinkman and Kuypers (1973) in which the forebrain commissures and the optic chiasma of monkeys were cut. When the right eye was temporarily blindfolded, the only visual input went to the left hemisphere. This controls the axial and proximal arm joints bilaterally, but the hand and fingers of the right forelimb only. The fingers of the left hand are 'blind'; tactile exploration by them depends on their somaesthetic input to the blind right hemisphere. Further details in text.

projections from the 'seeing' left hemisphere to the motoneurones which control the movements of the trunk and of the proximal joints of *both* arms (Chapter 4). If the right arm is free and the left is restrained, the right hand goes straight to the target and the thumb and index pick out the food. These digits are controlled by contralateral corticospinal and cortico-rubro-spinal projections from the 'seeing' left hemisphere (Chapter 4). If the right arm is restrained, the left arm (its proximal joints directed by the left hemisphere) goes straight to the food; but the left fingers, which are directed by the 'blind' right hemisphere, now explore dextrously over and around the food in a tactile search which may or may not happen to dislodge it from its recess in the board. The left arm, as it were, can 'see' but its fingers are 'blind'. If the right arm is set free its index and thumb pick out the food immediately.

Haaxma and Kuypers (1975) have taken the matter further. To test the visual steering of the movements of the fingers in a more refined way, they devised a different food target. The food was at its centre, flush with the surface of the board, and surrounded by radiating grooves wide enough to admit a monkey's finger. The cylindrical food pellet was partly encircled by a thin wall which separated it from all the grooves save one diametrically opposed pair; this pair, and the wall which partly enclosed the food, were brightly outlined in white, contrasting with the dark board. The white outline thus resembled a double keyhole, with the food in the hole. A finger placed in any groove outside the white outline could not pick out the food because it was protected by the thin wall. This whole target could be rotated to set the white outline at any desired orientation. A normal monkey's hand approaches this target with the plane of its thumb and index correctly orientated with respect to the white outline, whatever its orientation. Thumb and index thus enter the correct grooves without need for tactile guidance, and pick out the food.

In one series of monkeys, the left occipital lobe was excised and the two hemispheres were disconnected by section of midline commissures; in the other series, a deep parieto-occipital leucotomy disconnected the left visual from the left motor cortex, the two hemispheres being disconnected as well. Animals of either series could steer the right hand straight to the target, but could not orientate it correctly with respect to the white outline. The blind fingers (operated by the corticospinal projections from the injured left hemisphere) then embarked on a tactile exploration of the target (guided by inputs from the moving fingers) which often led the fingers into the wrong grooves but would eventually lead them into the correct grooves to loosen and dislodge the food. If the cylindrical food pellet projected above the plane of the board's surface it was immediately palpated and picked up at once. Elaborate control experiments showed that in hemispheres in which the visual and motor areas were disconnected, different orientations of the target could be discriminated perfectly. The loss of visual steering of the hand and fingers was therefore due to deprivation of the corticospinal projection of its visual input, and not to any damage to the geniculo-calcarine input to the visual cortex. The visuo-motor pathway reaches the precentral hand area indirectly, by way of the premotor and supplementary motor areas which distribute many fibres to the precentral gyrus (references in Haaxma and Kuypers, 1975).

In man, very small and accurate movements of the fingers are possible, guided by vision under the microscope. With a little practice, a person is able to position a slide accurately on the stage of a microscope using only his hand and visual control. A technician will soon find it possible to focus first on the centre of a single red blood cell viewed under high magnification, and then to move the slide so that the centre of focus is on the rim of that same erythrocyte. A delicate, controlled movement of only 3 or 4 μm has been executed with the musculature of the arms, hand and fingers. Accuracy requires external, visual feedback and the accomplishment of the precise movement performance is intimately linked with and dependent upon the sensory experience. We can also do fairly fine dissections under a dissecting microscope without recourse to a micromanipulator.

8.5.3 PERCEPTION OF EFFORT, MOVEMENT AND POSITION

People are perfectly aware of the positions of parts of their bodies in relation to one another and to the body as a whole, and of the movements they make; over monkeys they have the advantage that they can not only describe the positions and movements of a limb, but can also, and more conveniently for the investigator, imitate the postures and track the movements with the limb of the opposite side. Although their experience of passively imposed movements and postures is small in everyday life, healthy people, even when blindfolded, find no difficulty in describing them, or in imitating them by active movements of the opposite limbs, when asked to do so by a neurologist. It is well known that perception of passive movement is more delicate in the shoulder than in the fingers. We cannot go deeply into this important part of neuropsychology. These abilities depend on the building-up during infancy of an internal cerebral model of the body, the 'body image' or 'schema' (Head, 1920) to which current perceptions are referred. We must limit ourselves to the possible contribution of the CST to these abilities in the adult. We shall be concerned with the performances and perceptions of blindfolded people, and with abilities that must be most highly developed in people blind from birth.

Att he outset we can try to distinguish the perception of movement (kinaesthetic sense) by structures and processes that are common to active and passive movement from those that are specific to active movement. Common to both are the joints and the muscle receptors: of the latter, some will be stimulated by passive stretch, others unloaded by passive shortening. Active movements will be accompanied by fusimotor activation of the muscle spindles of the prime movers and by discharge of their Golgi tendon organs. In addition, there will be excitation and inhibition of the neurones of afferent relay nuclei within the central nervous system by corticonuclear axons and PT collaterals (Chapter 4).

We perceive position (postural sense) partly as a result of the memory of the movement that brought it about. Since we are never still for any length of time, but are constantly making small shifts of posture, it is difficult to be sure that awareness of position can be maintained solely by tonic inputs from slowly adapting peripheral receptors, for example, muscle spindles kept active by centrifugal fusimotor control. In finger flexor muscle spindles, resting discharge is insignificant (Vallbo, 1974). Clinical neurologists, in testing awareness of position, are accustomed to distract the patient's attention while they are 'passively' imposing a new posture on a limb, and not to ask him to imitate the posture until some time has elapsed; in cases of impaired position sense, an important 'behavioural' criterion is the patient's obvious surprise when he opens his eyes and sees his error (Holmes, 1946). In health, it is a fact that positions reached by active movement are more accurately perceived than those imposed on the subject by the examiner (Paillard and Brouchon, 1968). In hemiplegia, 'when the fingers had not been moved for some time, the patient, as is usual, had no feelings of his muscles in the hand and forearm and of the position of the finger joints' (Brodal, 1973).

Specific to active movement, and, it would seem, almost inevitably involving the CST, is something else which contributes to kinaesthesia, which has been variously described as 'sensation of innervation', 'sense of effort', 'corollary discharge' and 'internal feedback', and which probably includes separable elements. In his classic textbook, Gowers (1899) wrote: 'Our knowledge of active states of the muscle is due, at least in some measure, to the effects on consciousness of the activity of the nerve-structures causing the movement.' He offered three 'proofs' which we shall take up in what follows.

This 'knowledge' probably includes an element which is often called 'sense of effort'. This element may not be dominant in strong efforts in which consciousness may seem to be filled by unpleasant sensations arising from the pressures on and tensions within the trunk and limbs, but it is obvious to a hemiplegic who is striving by maximal 'force of innervation' to produce a flicker of movement (Brodal, 1973). Nothing is known of the origin of this sensation. It seems safe to assume that in hemiplegia, such awareness of 'force of innervation' is not aroused by the activity of PT collaterals, whose activity would be much reduced or abolished, but rather that it is associated with 'programming' processes upstream of the PTN. In normal subjects, however, there may well be an additional contribution from PT collaterals to the 'sense of effort' which has been invoked by McCloskey *et al.* (1974) as an important factor in the estimation of weights.

'Sense of effort' ought to be separated conceptually from 'perception of movement', for perception is accurate when 'effort' is minimal, as when the movement is unopposed by gravity or resistance and the muscles are not weakened by fatigue. Perception of movement might depend on 'internal feedback' (e.g. by PT collaterals) as well as on 'response feedback' from the moving parts (Evarts *et al.*, 1971). But we shall cite evidence that healthy subjects, temporarily deprived of inputs from the moving parts, but presumably still generating internal feedback, can make willed movements of whose occurrence they remain unaware. We do not know the extent, if any, to which subjects chronically deprived of response feedback by section or disease of primary afferent axons can learn to become aware of their active movements by internal feedback.

Internal feedback is sometimes used to include 'corollary discharge' ('efference copy'), and confusion is inevitable unless two distinct concepts are kept separate. Gowers' first 'proof' of the existence of an 'effect on consciousness of the activity of the nerve-structures causing the movement' was this: 'In palsy of an ocular muscle, objects seen are referred to the position (in relation to the body) that they would occupy if the movement corresponded to the innervation; it is the latter, i.e. the activity of the centre, to which the perception corresponds.' Thus, if the right external rectus muscle is paralysed, then when the patient strives to look to the right, objects in the field of vision appear to move to the right. If the retina had moved as willed, the visual world would have remained stationary (Helmholtz). In health, it is only passively imposed movements of the eyes that cause apparent movement of the visual field. Goodwin *et al.* (1972) have dispelled much confusion by distinguishing this process of compensation for the effects of displacement of a receptor surface, to which the concepts of corollary discharge and efference copy are strictly appropriate, from any process by which people perceive the occurrence of active movement by 'consciousness of the activity of nerve structures causing the movement': thus, in the case of movements of the eyes, the question in which we are interested, in terms of the present discussion, is whether internal feedback contributes to our knowledge of the range and direction of willed movement of our visual axes in the dark.

The perception of movement depends on inputs from joints, muscles, tendon organs and possibly skin folds. During active movement their first and second synaptic relays could be adjusted for optimum discrimination and sensitivity by centrifugal control within the CNS, presumably, in part at least, by the activity of PT axon collaterals (Chapter 4). At the periphery, the primary and secondary endings of the muscle spindles are under centrifugal control by the fusimotor neurones and these are excited and inhibited by the PT (Chapter 4). Their excitation during voluntary isometric movements and voluntary ramp movements of the fingers has been illustrated in Fig. 8.12. It is linked in time with the course of the movements. We now know that the inputs from the spindles, like those from the other receptors, reach the cortex (Chapter 6); those from the primary endings arouse sensations of movement (Goodwin et al., 1972). All inputs during willed movement, thus adjusted by the output, would presumably evoke sensory awareness which would be specific to active as distinct from passive movement. Such a concept of 'receptor sensitization' should perhaps be distinguished from the concept of efference copy, which may carry overtones of comparison of output with input, of cancellation of the effects of displacement of receptor surfaces, and of the detection of mismatch between demanded and actual performance (Bernstein's 'Sollwert' and 'Istwert').

These considerations have a bearing on another of Gowers' (1899) three 'proofs' of 'consciousness of the activity of nerve structures causing the movement': 'In some convulsions beginning locally, slight attacks may be attended with a feeling that the arm is raised above the head, or otherwise moved, when it is hanging by the side.' Though suggestive, such epileptic activation of an illusory perception of movement can be interpreted as a primary disturbance of a 'sensory' or 'memory' mechanism rather than as secondary to the sublimal activation of a motor output mechanism which is capable of generating internal feedback. We could not now accept it as proof that 'the central motor process is an important source of our knowledge'.

Having drawn his conclusion about the importance of the 'central motor process', Gowers (1889) went on: 'But to its effects must be added that of the impulses from the muscles. . . . Our knowledge of rest posture and passive movement must be derived from incoming impulses. These are not from the skin; the sense of posture may be lost when cutaneous sensibility is normal, and perfect when this is much impaired. . . . The chief source of these perceptions must therefore be the deeper afferent nerves, those of the muscles and joints, perhaps chiefly of the muscles.' The input from the joints would be common to active and passive movement of equal amplitude, direction and velocity, except in so far as the joint capsules might be subject to additional pressure and traction during the active movement, and their central relays subject to changing backgrounds of centrifugal inhibition and excitation. The muscle spindles, in passive movement, would signal length and velocity of passive lengthening. Their sensitivity would be subject to background levels of tonic fusimotor activity related to states of relative arousal of preparedness to move, as distinct from the phasic changes of fusimotor activity which occur in the prime movers during phasic movements (Granit, 1975).

Experimental and clinical observations which bear on these problems can be classified as follows: 1, effects on performance and perception of depriving subjects of inputs from the limbs; 2, illusions of movement created by vibrating the tendons of muscles, which selectively excites the primary endings of the muscle spindles; 3, absence of any illusion of movement when motor impulses are prevented from activating the muscles; and 4, observations bearing on the last of Gowers' (1899) three 'proofs': 'After amputation of a limb, a person who makes an effort to move the lost part seems to feel as if he did move it.'

8.5.3.1 *Effects of blocking inputs from limb*

Cutting the dorsal roots has often been practised for the relief of spasticity (Foerster, 1927), but the effects would have been complicated by the pre-existing neurological disorder. Foerster cut the roots from C_3 to D_3. Even in the acute stage, and without visual aid, these patients could voluntarily flex, extend, raise, lower and rotate their arms, and pronate, supinate, extend and flex their hands, but they often declared that they would be unable to perform these simple movements, and that they were unaware of the movements they had actually succeeded in making. Therefore any internal feedback was uninformative. The start of the movements was delayed, but they were prompter and more accurate if vision was allowed. Movements of the fingers were worst affected, whether or not under visual guidance. When the patient was asked to move an individual finger, the wrong fingers would respond, or if the correct finger were moved it would be accompanied by movements of other fingers or of the whole hand. With time and practice, there was an unspecified degree of improvement. We still do not know whether a patient with a chronically deafferented arm, who had taught himself to move his hand on to a target under visual guidance, would ever be able to reach it accurately when blindfolded; and whether the internal feedback which would be necessary to enable this performance would make him *conscious* of his visually programmed movement and would tell him when it had reached its goal.

Dorsal rhizotomy has the disadvantage that it cuts off all inputs indiscriminately. By injecting the base of a digit with local anaesthetic or by making the whole hand ischaemic by inflating a pressure-cuff round the wrist, the input from skin and joints can be cut off, leaving the extrinsic hand muscles unmolested in the forearm. In the former experiment, un-controllable seepage of the local anaesthetic may cause an unknown degree of blockage of input from the lumbricals and interossei of that digit: in the latter, the very considerable input from all the intrinsic hand muscles will be blocked. People differ in their ability to detect passive movement of a digit when the whole hand is anoxic and the extrinsic muscles are relaxed. Some fail to detect flexion and extension of 90° at the inter-phalangeal joint of the thumb (Merton, 1964; Goodwin et al., 1972) but others have no difficulty. Goodwin et al. found that all subjects could do so if their extrinsic muscles were under slight voluntary contraction, in which fusimotor coactivation would increase the input from the spindles; and Chambers and Gilliatt (1954) found in spastic patients that kinaesthesia was 'strikingly preserved' in the fingers of an anoxic hand. Goodwin et al. noted inability to detect lateral movements at the metacarpophalangeal joints, which do not stretch the extrinsic muscles and would normally be perceived by stretch of the interossei and of the joint capsules. The contribution from the joint receptors is dispensible, for passive flexion and extension of the metacarpophalangeal joints can still be perceived after these joints have been excised and replaced with flexible silicone-rubber implants (Cross and McCloskey, 1973). That there is indeed a contribution from receptors in the extrinsic hand muscles has been shown by Matthews and Simmonds (1974) in patients undergoing division of the carpal ligament under local anaesthesia. Single flexor tendons were pulled to and fro with fine forceps without moving the digits themselves. The subjects always felt a sensation of movement which they referred to the correct finger (or thumb).

With regard to the perception of active movements, Goodwin et al. found that these are not distinctly perceived, in the digits of an ischaemic hand, unless their amplitude is large enough. If this perception depended only on sense of effort or internal feedback then obstructing the movement without the subject's knowledge should result in the illusion that the movement had actually taken place. The subjects reported no such illusion. It may be concluded that the perception was due to the spindles of the extrinsic muscles, but without being able to assign responsibility to those of the prime movers or to those of the antagonists; and possibly also to the tendon organs of the prime movers which are exquisitely sensitive to active tension. Another experiment, in which the index finger of the left hand was anaesthetized by injection of lignocaine at its base, is illustrated in Fig. 8.18 (Goodwin et al., 1972). The blindfolded subject was asked to extend all the digits of the left hand, and then to imitate the resulting posture with the right hand. There was a striking failure to perceive that the proximal interphalangeal joint of the index had been successfully extended. The extrinsic muscle, extensor indicis, extends only the proximal phalanx; extension of the middle and distal phalanges requires the intrinsic interossei and lumbricals (Duchenne, 1867). The extent of diffusion of the local anaesthetic into the motor and sensory innervation of these muscles, and into the metacarpophalangeal joint, remains unknown. Certainly sense of effort or internal feedback was ineffective in informing the subject of his successful extension of both interphalangeal joints.

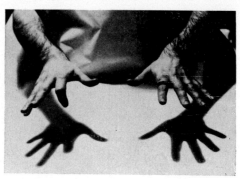

Perceived movement   Real movement
(normal finger)   (anaesthetized finger)

FIG. 8.18. The index finger of the left hand (marked with circle) had been ring-blocked by the injection of lignocaine at its base. The subject was asked suddenly to extend all the digits of the affected hand starting from a position of flexion, and then immediately afterwards to put the fingers of his other hand in the position into which he felt he had moved the affected hand. His position was then voluntarily 'frozen' and photographed. The insentient finger was felt to have failed to extend itself at all joints, though it actually succeeded in doing so. (Goodwin et al., 1972.)

In further experiments Goodwin et al. made the forearm ischaemic, as well as the hand, by a pressure-cuff above the elbow. The blindfolded subjects were asked to extend the index finger periodically and then to reproduce the movement with the index finger of the normal hand. Both movements were recorded (Fig. 8.19). As the time of complete paralysis approached, the subjects underestimated the extent of their movements, and finally made a few successful movements of which they were unaware. There was presumably a period of complete block of afferent axons from the spindles of the forearm muscles before the skeletomotor axons were finally blocked. A cuff was then applied at the wrist and the upper cuff was removed, so that the hand remained anoxic while the extrinsic muscles were allowed to recover. The movements of the index were partially restored, but their full amplitude was not perceived. Loss of input from intrinsic muscles and joints must have been at least partly responsible for this reduced perception; internal feedback and sense of effort created no illusion that the index had been fully extended, but a partial contribution to the reduced perception cannot be excluded.

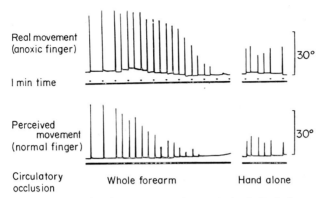

FIG. 8.19. Records demonstrating that on progressive paralysis of a limb the perception of movement may be more severely impaired than the actual ability to move. The top trace shows the movements at the metacarpo-phalangeal joint of the index finger of one hand at a time when the circulation to the arm was occluded; the interphalangeal joints were fixed in full extension by strapping. Periodically, the subject was asked to raise his finger to full extension and then to lower it again; in between the finger lay partly flexed under the action of gravity and a light spring. Immediately afterwards he was asked to make an equivalent movement with the index finger of his other hand, thus providing an objective measure of his perception of the extent of the movement which was being paralysed. In the first part of the record the circulation to the whole of the forearm and hand was occluded by a pressure cuff above the elbow. This eventually led to a complete paralysis of all the muscles involved, and to a complete loss of sensation. Even when he was paralysed the subject still continued to attempt the movement at half-minute intervals. In the second part of the record the pressure cuff had been shifted to the wrist so that the hand remained anaesthetized, but the muscles of the forearm had been able to recover. The upper cuff was inflated for 13 min before the beginning of the records shown. There was an interval of 14 min between the two sets of records. The recordings were made by connecting the fingers to freely moving potentiometers. The subject could not see either his hands or the recordings. (Goodwin *et al.*, 1972.)

8.5.3.2 *Illusions of movement resulting from vibration of tendons*

In the cat, longitudinal vibration of a tendon is a highly selective stimulus to the dynamically sensitive primary endings of the muscle spindles (Brown *et al.*, 1967). It is probable that transverse percutaneous vibration of intact tendons, the important method which Hagbarth and Lance and their colleagues (Hagbarth and Eklund, 1966; DeGail *et al.*, 1966) have introduced into clinical neurophysiology, acts similarly, and sends abnormally synchronized afferent volleys into the central nervous system from the muscle spindles, phase-locked to the sinusoidal vibrations. These volleys arouse illusions of movement. If the forearms are suspended in a horizontal plane so that gravity does not act on the elbow joint, vibration of the biceps tendon, whose frequency and amplitude are so adjusted as to cause no reflex contraction of biceps, arouses the illusion that the elbow is extending (as if the biceps were being lengthened). The direction of the illusory movement can be demonstrated by the blindfolded subject by tracking it with the opposite forearm which is similarly suspended (Goodwin *et al.*, 1972). The illusion is vivid, and 'could continue for a minute or more'; it is evidently a sensation which persists for too long to correspond to any possible real movement at the elbow at anything like the illusory velocity. This 'velocity' can be measured by requiring the blindfolded subject to duplicate it with a voluntary movement of the opposite arm (McCloskey, 1973).

If the vibration is adjusted so that it evokes a 'tonic vibration reflex' (Hagbarth and Eklund, 1966), we have a complex and intriguing situation which does not correspond to perception of either passive or active movement as we have so far considered them: namely, illusory perception of the course of an involuntary reflex movement and of the position to which it brings the limb. The systematic illusion is that the reflex has moved the joint through a smaller angle than it has done in reality: that the vibrated muscle is, at any instant, longer than it really is (Goodwin *et al.*, 1972). In Fig. 8.20, the tendon of the biceps of the relaxed right arm was vibrated, and the subject, who could not see his arms, was asked to track the reflex movement with his left arm. The recorded movements show that the tracking arm lagged behind the vibrated arm, showing that the rate and range of the reflex movement were being underestimated.

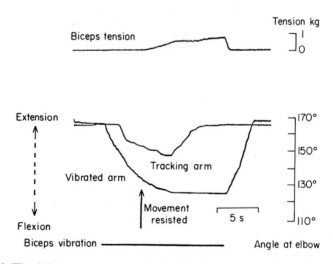

FIG. 8. 20. The right arm was initially supported by the hand lying upon a sandbag so that the subject did not have to exert a voluntary effort to maintain its position. The right biceps was then vibrated so as to produce the usual tonic vibration reflex. After the limb had traversed a certain distance its movement was arrested by the pulling tight of a string which was applied to the hand, which had been made insentient by a prolonged period of anoxia so the subject had no cutaneous clues as to when his arm started and stopped moving. The termination of the tracking movement before the end of the vibration is probably due to the tracking arm then being nearly fully extended. (Goodwin *et al.*, 1972.)

At the arrow the movement was arrested without the subject's knowledge: his hand had been made insentient by anoxia so that he felt no cutaneous or deep sensation when it came up against the stop. Though the elbow-joint was now stationary he signalled that it was extending. The surprised expression of a naive subject when he is allowed to see the final position of his arms is a revealing behavioural test.

If the tonic vibration reflex is imposed on a background of strong isometric voluntary contraction there is no illusion. Goodwin *et al.* suggest that this is due to maximal firing of primary endings of the prime mover's spindles as a result of fusimotor coactivation. But there would also be increased firing of tendon organs, and possibly also of secondary endings; there would also be increased corollary discharge. Whatever the details it seems clear that additional activities associated with strong voluntary contraction can cancel the illusory perception aroused by selective artificial excitation of the spindle primaries.

In view of our interest in the effect of servo-action of feedback on ramp movements (section 8.3.6), the effect of vibration on the performance of a prime-mover muscle engaged in a tracking task, and on the perception of this active movement, is also interesting. Vibration must be expected to disturb the performance by adding to the quantity of input from the coactivated spindle primaries and possibly also by superimposing its artificial rhythm on the natural patterning of the impulses from the spindles. The task was to track the passively imposed flexion and extension of the left arm by voluntary movement of the right arm. On the right of Fig. 8.21, the movement was of isotonic flexion against gravity. When biceps, the prime mover, was vibrated, the movement speeded up, running ahead of the movement it was supposed to be tracking. This would be explained by an increase in servo-action. The subject was unaware of the error: he had

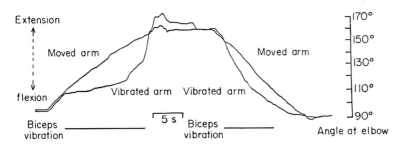

FIG. 8.21. The effect of vibration applied to an arm that the subject was using to make a tracking movement. The left arm was moved by the experimenter and the subject was asked to track it with his right arm. During the periods indicated vibration was applied to the biceps of the right arm which was the one which was being moved voluntarily. The arm was moving in the vertical plane with the upper arm lying horizontal so that the biceps muscle will have been contracting throughout. See text. (Goodwin *et al.*, 1972.)

the illusion that he was tracking correctly. On the left of Fig. 8.21, the movement of extension was effected by gravity, controlled by progressive relaxation of biceps. When vibration was applied, the movement of the tracking arm was slowed so that it lagged behind the 'target' arm. The increased input from the spindle primaries would have reflexly excited the biceps motoneurones and reduced the speed of relaxation of the muscle. Again, the subject was unaware of the error: he had the illusion that the tracking was proceeding at the correct speed and that the tracking arm was at every instant in its correct relation to the target arm. When the vibration was withdrawn he quickly corrected the positional error.

This experiment may be interpreted on the following lines. Consider the right side of Fig. 8.21. The subject was reading the course of the passive flexion of the target limb and issuing a stream of motor commands to the tracking limb, whose active flexion aroused a stream of perceptions which matched the velocity and the successive instantaneous positions of the target limb. The increased input from the spindles of the prime mover, biceps, which was here artificially elicited by vibration, could normally have occurred only if the movement had been resisted. Its function would have been to keep the movement automatically on target by servo-action. It would be essential that the successful load-compensation should not disturb the subject's consciousness that he was still tracking correctly.

When, therefore, the limb was artificially speeded up by vibration and the subject did not perceive that this was happening, this could have been due to the operation of some central nervous 'gate' which prevented the the increased signals from the primary endings of biceps from reaching the sensorium. But it is more likely that conflicting perceptions would have been aroused by the vibrated biceps spindles on the one hand and by the joint receptors and muscle spindles of the antagonist triceps on the other, when the elbow flexion was speeded up, and that these conflicting perceptions would have cancelled algebraically (Fig. 8.22). The reality is likely to be even more complex.

8.5.3.3 *No illusion of movement on attempting to use paralysed muscles*

When movement is paralysed at the periphery in acute experiments, whether by ischaemia by a pressure cuff, by general curarization (cf. Goodwin *et al.*, 1972) or by the elegant method of local curarization of the forearm and hand (McCloskey and Torda, 1975), people know that they cannot move and have no illusions of movements (from internal feedback or sense of effort). Goodwin *et al.* noted that in ischaemic paralysis they had 'all experienced this awareness of an inability to move the moment that one tries to do so; indeed, on the first attempt one is considerably surprised that one does not succeed'. McCloskey's and Torda's subjects

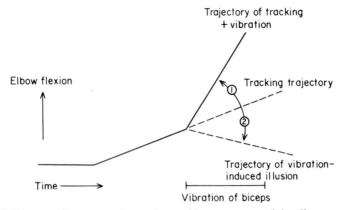

FIG. 8.22. Diagram of response of an active tracking movement of the elbow to vibration of the tendon of the prime mover, biceps (based on Fig. 8.21, inverted for ease of presentation).
1. Perception of accelerated flexion of elbow, signalled by joint receptors and by passive lengthening of muscle spindles of triceps; cancelled algebraically by
2. Vibration-induced illusion that flexion of elbow has decelerated.

'were first asked, with vision excluded, to make attempts to move the paralysed but unanaesthetised digits. All were aware that they could not do so, and were unanimous in their denials of any sensations of movement accompanying their attempts. When movements were achieved by muscle groups which were weakened but not paralysed they were perceived with apparently normal accuracy. Passive "imposed" movements of paralysed joints were accurately perceived.'

8.5.3.4 *Perceived 'movement' of a phantom limb*

The argument for perception of movements of the joints of a phantom limb by internal feedback of sense of effort has been weakened by observations (Henderson and Smyth, reviewed by Goodwin *et al.*) that movements of phantom joints (as distinct from movements of the phantom as a whole with movements of the real joint which moves the stump) are always associated with contraction of muscles within the stump, and are lost if these contractions are abolished by denervation. Presumably such contractions would represent surviving fractions of the complex totality of the muscles that would have taken part in the movement that was willed by the subject, and would provide response feedback which could be interpreted (by some amputees but not by all) as including 'movements' of the phantom joints. Such 'movements' are always limited and poorly graded.

We may conclude, with Goodwin *et al.* (1972), that internal feedback or sense of effort, acting without response feedback, have failed to arouse any perception of active movement in any situation so far investigated; but that correct appreciation of the movements signalled by the primary endings must require calibration of their mixed signal of length and velocity by comparison with the inputs streaming in from the length-measuring spindle secondaries and force-measuring tendon organs of the prime movers and from the spindles of the antagonist muscles. If the sole input were from the primary endings of the prime-mover muscles, kept discharging throughout the movement by coactivation of α and γ moto-neurones, then, on the evidence of vibration, the perceived direction of movement would be diametrically opposite to its actual direction. If it were equally feasible to stimulate the prime mover's secondary endings or tendon organs in isolation, might it be possible to arouse illusions of movement in the other direction? If so, there would be need to resolve the resulting perceptual conflicts, presumably by reference of the conflicting inputs to an efference copy of the demanded movement. As Goodwin *et al.* (1972) concluded: 'There seems, however, to be no tendency to experience illusions of movements under conditions in which spindle firing may be presumed to be increasing as a result of fusimotor activity. This suggests that corollary discharges do exist and serve to modify the kinaesthetic actions of muscle afferent signals in the light of what the motor system is attempting.' The PT collaterals to the dorsal laminae of the spinal cord, to the nuclei of the dorsal columns and to the thalamus are obvious candidates for providing the presumed corollary discharges (efference copy).

8.5.4   THE HAND AS A SENSE ORGAN

The idea of the hand as a sensory surface which actively explores the environment, rather than receiving stimuli passively, is not new. It is explicit in Sherrington's 'Integrative Action of the Nervous System', in passages which we have quoted in Chapter 1. The distinction is analogous to that between looking and merely seeing. The nineteenth-century psychophysicists were interested in active touch, and Sherrington (1900a) took stock of some of their contributions, including those of Lotze, Neissner and Weber. He noted that for judgement of the size and shape of objects by touch, it is necessary to excite 'a certain number of tactual sensations of definite intensities and imbued with "local signs". These component sensations are combined, either (1) simultaneously or (2) successively as well as simultaneously. The successive component sensa-tions can be acquired by *actively moving the tactual surface*, to increase or renew the simultaneously given groups of sensations, and in so doing the muscular sense is combined with the tactual in obtaining criteria for judging the shape and size of the object by the distances moved.' Elsewhere (1900d) he defined 'muscular sense' to include 'all *reactions on sense arising in motor organs and their accessories*'.

Denny-Brown's studies, which we have cited in section 8.4.2, have shown how the hand tends to orientate itself towards a touch stimulus, and how this reaction is lost after section of the PT. We might say that this bringing of a stimulating object into contact with the highly discriminating receptor surface provided by the glabrous skin of the finger-pads and palm is analogous to the act of bringing the image of an object at the periphery of the field of vision on to the fovea centralis. Sherrington (1900c) wrote: 'In the limbs and mobile parts, when a spot of less discriminative sensitivity is touched, instinct moves the member, so that it brings to the object the part where its own sensitivity is delicate, e.g. the finger tips. It is apparent to most of us that if, with closed eyes, we attend to the consciousness of the resting arm, the hand, and especially fingers, are the parts we are most aware of, best outlined, so to say, in consciousness. There arise lines of habitual association between all points of the member and its sensitive tip. James writes: "I think anyone must be aware when he touches a point of his hand or wrist that it is the relation to the finger-tips of which he is usually most conscious." '

In considering the relations between movement and tactile exploration, Sherrington (1900c) identified two extremes: (1) 'the same tactual point' being moved over the explored object: the same touch-sense related to 'a series of "muscular" sensations differing in intensity; "active touch"; (2) An object is allowed to move over a series of tactual points, the tactual surface being held stationary, i.e. one muscular sensation is combined with a series of tactual; "passive touch".' In 'passive touch', successive stimuli are more easily linked and interpreted than simultaneous: 'It is easier to read letters as they are traced on the skin than letters already fully shaped and pressed upon the skin.'

Among the illusions cited in Sherrington's review (1900c), one in particular seems of special interest. 'The points of a pair of compasses, when moved with a sufficient speed over a length of skin, appear to get wider apart as they pass from skin less endowed with local sign to skin more endowed, e.g. from ear to lip (Weber). Moved in the opposite direction, they seem conversely to close together. Moreover, if moved with uniform speed, they appear to travel faster as they pass over the more perceptive region, e.g. towards lip (Vierordt).' It would be specially interesting to compare these perceptions in the hand, to see if the illusions do occur there in passive movement and whether they are modified or do not occur in active movement. And if they *are* so modified, the suggestion will naturally arise that the non-illusory perception in 'active touch' has been corrected by reference to an efference copy of the active movement. The suggestion could be tested in cases of 'pure motor hemiplegia' (Brodal, 1973). If PT collaterals were involved in the efference copy, there might be some persistence of illusion in patients with sufficient motor control of proximal joints to permit them to make the necessary active movement of the sensory surface (e.g. palmar surface of forearm to tip of index finger) across the compass points, for comparison with passive movement of the compass points along the same track at the same speed.

If there were a question of comparison of inputs from the muscles (as Sherrington thought) with inputs from the skin, it might be possible to institute a comparison of the perceptions in experiments in which the fusimotor axons had been blocked by infiltration of the motor points of the muscles with procaine.

Modern writers (Katz, reviewed by Krueger, 1970; Gibson, 1962) have again taken up the question of 'active touch', but do not yet seem to have designed any crucial experiments to define the contribution of its motor component, or to have introduced any novel concepts. Experiments by Gibson (1962), in which one of six small 'cookie cutters' about 2.5 cm across was either pressed on to the subject's open palm by the experimenter, or held above the tips of his upturned fingers so that he could explore its shape with them. He had to state to which one of the six outline drawings within his vision it corresponded. The score by guesswork would have been 17 per cent; for passive touch on the palm there were 49 per cent correct responses, and for active touch by the finger-tips, 95 per cent. There are probably too many factors here to sort out in a single experiment: the difference between discrimination by the skin of the finger-tip and of the palm is admittedly different: the subject is trying to relate the pattern of cutaneous stimuli to pattern of visual stimuli in terms not of receptor surfaces but of identities of specific objects, and such identities are not tied to unique combinations of peripheral or retinal receptors, but are subject to all the complexities subsumed under the terms 'stimulus generalization' and 'the perceptual constancies'. The classical psycho-physicists were aware of the psychological properties of tactual space: 'Tactual space includes the idea of the skin as a *continuous surface*, although its organs are punctiform. This results from infinitely graded muscular sensations accompanying infinitely graded rectilinear movements possible in various directions in a plane.' (Sherrington, 1900c.) Katz (cited by Krueger, 1970) remarked on 'the bridging of the gap between the fingers . . . if you close your eyes, spread your fingers somewhat apart, then draw them over a surface, you will experience the surface as full and as extending into the area between the paths of the fingers'.

Sherrington (1900c) noted: 'Alphabets for the blind have linear or punctate letters. The threshold of space for recognition of line direction is more than twice as high as for successive points. The dimensional distances being the same, the point alphabet is therefore the easier, especially if the points be taken in succession as in the New York horizontal point-letters; the Braille point-letters are vertical.' We have heard it stated that blind readers can read Braille with greater facility if they move their fingers actively across it, than if it is moved passively across their fingers, but we have been unable to find published experimental authority for this statement. Day and Dickinson (1976) compared the rate of learning Braille numerals by naive blindfolded subjects in two conditions: passive, in which the numerals were moved sideways across the pulp of the index finger at about 0.5 cm s^{-1}, and active, in which the sliding carriage to which the index finger was attached was moved sideways by active movement of the subject's arm, at about the same speed, so that the index finger was moved across the numerals. The carriage could only be moved in the forward direction. Day and Dickinson found no difference in the learning between the active and passive conditions. They comment that the subjects might have done better in the active condition if the task had been self-paced—if, that is, the subjects had been allowed to linger on each symbol and then to move quickly on to the next. They thought that experienced Braille readers might have shown differences between the active and passive performances. It might indeed be expected that the active exploratory movements that would be used by an experienced reader of Braille would be more complex than the simple continuous sideways movement: that they would include very small fore-and-aft and oblique movements, small reversals of direction of sideways movement, small tiltings and changes of pressure, etc., which the naive subjects would not have learned to make.

No greater feat of tactile discrimination is known than that which enabled the blind and deaf Helen Keller to receive speech by placing the digit-tips of her left hand on the lips and larynx of whoever she was conversing with, while holding their right hand in hers. It seems that every possible neural resource would have needed to be mobilized for this, and that the resources would have included the integration of efference copy and of muscle-feedback from some extremely delicate exploratory movements with the cutaneous inputs from the sliding and vibratory stimuli to the finger tips. With its known wealth of axon collaterals to relay nuclei it is hard to believe that the PT was not involved.

8.6 Detecting the actions of peripheral inputs and central programmes on PTN

In Chapter 6 we reviewed some of the evidence which indicates external feedback from peripheral receptors in the moving part to output neurones in the motor cortex. This feedback could be involved in the focusing of output on to particular alpha and fusimotor neurones which would reinforce the action producing the output. This function of feedback is stressed by Asanuma (1975). But it is not the only possible one and we have already indicated that many exceptions exist to the precisely organized and limited input–output coupling within cortical columns which provides the general basis for this view of the involvement of peripheral feedback in movement performance.

A possible example of positive reinforcement by peripheral feedback has been described by Lund and Lamarre (1973, 1974). In the special instance of neuronal discharges in the lateral parts of the precentral cortex of monkeys performing rhythmical chewing movements, responses to both active and passive jaw movements were observed; loads that aided jaw opening increased the discharge of units that fired with active jaw opening movements. Some 'jaw closing' cells received inputs from receptors within the mouth and were responsive to pressure on the teeth. These cells were considered as candidates in the control of force of jaw closure when this movement was opposed by a resistance between the teeth. If such cells were involved in the control of force of contraction of jaw closing muscles, elimination of the positive feedback from around the teeth should reduce the force of voluntary biting. This proposal was tested in a group of human subjects whose bite was monitored with a strain gauge between the teeth and with electromyograms. After infiltration of local anaesthetic around the roots of the upper and lower premolar teeth on one side, there was a fall in the voluntary applied force that could be developed in the bite on that side. This recovered as the local anaesthetic effect declined. Control injections round the contralateral teeth did not affect the bite.

It is possible that the peripheral inputs from skin fields (mostly confined to the fingers and hand) which project to some output neurones in the motor cortex of monkeys have a positive feedback role as would be suggested by their position on the advancing surface of the skin. But it is clear that this form of feedback is quantitatively much less evident than feedback from detectors of movement in the monkey. Although in some examples, a clear case can be made for identifying the receptors involved in movement detection as muscle spindles (when the responses to passive stretch, vibration and localized muscle tapping would all be consistent with this), the receptors providing the feedback about movement to the remainder of the sampled output neurones could not be distinguished with certainty. Joint receptors themselves could be involved, giving the localization of the input to a single joint that is so often the case. Consistent with a role for joint receptors would also be the maximum effects with wide angles of movement and near the extremes of joint movement. But responses of other cells over a limited range of movement and responses of most output neurones to only one direction of movement suggest the involvement of receptors other than those from joints. We are quite ignorant about the stream of afferent signals along many parallel paths from muscles, joints, tendons, fascia and skin which enters the central nervous system in response to even such a simple stimulus as passive flexion of a finger. Interactions between a variety of the elements in this totality could easily occur, and the resultant which reaches the output units of the motor cortex may not have its origins in a single receptor population.

Even when the most likely input has been identified as coming from muscle receptors (as is the case for the unit illustrated in Fig. 6.15, p. 250) because a localized responsive point was found over the belly of the muscle, and because stretching this muscle by passive joint movement produced a response whereas relaxing this muscle caused a pause in discharge, some uncertainties remain. The response of the cell during active contraction of the particular muscle in which its receptors seemed to be located could indicate coactivation of fusimotor fibres, but it could conceivably be a response to stretch of antagonist muscles whose spindles were sensitized by fusimotor drive during the active movement. It could also possibly be a response of tendon organs made more sensitive during the active contraction of the muscle but also capable of responding to brief taps to the muscle belly if these were delivered in appropriate relationship to the tendon organ in the fibrous origins of the muscle. The point of all this discussion is to warn against immediate acceptance of the simplistic view that, because for a majority of PTNs examined, active and passive joint movements in the same direction were associated with responses of the neurone, receptors in the joint will be reinforcing the discharges of the PTN during movement and that a tight and precise input–output coupling of these particular receptors to their own output neurones in the cortex exists.

We have shown that output neurones tend to receive more convergent influences than do the input (receiving) neurones in the same region of cortex. Moreover, we have demonstrated that, while a general tendency exists for input and output of local nests of neurones all to be related to the same periphery, there is overlap in these relationships so that in any one nest some units can exist whose peripheral territory is remote from the region to which the others are responsive. This denies the separateness within sharp boundaries of the organized input–output modules which relate to a particular muscle or movement.

While it is clear, from the experiments of Evarts and his colleagues described in Chapter 7, that an appropriate input arriving from peripheral receptors detecting a disturbance of movement can be associated, in an adequately prepared central nervous system which has been instructed to react, with a very short latency movement-response output, the detailed involvement of cortical input–output modules in the cause of this association require further investigation. Moreover, the susceptibility of the output to adequate 'preparation to move' and the influence of instructions about direction of movement all argue for a flexibility in the long-loop reflex which would allow a variety of modes of operation. A given input does not invariably and inevitably lead to a definite, single and stereotyped output. But under appropriate conditions, a long-loop reflex response can be shown to occur.

The anatomical connections of the PT allow for activity in PTNs to influence transmission through afferent relays and these influences have been studied at a number of levels in the central nervous system. It is possible that individual PTNs are so connected to spinal or subcortical relay centres that they can regulate their own input. Suggestions have been made, based on experiments in anaesthetized animals, that PT activity suppresses transmission in afferent systems conveying cutaneous information while selecting kinaesthetic inputs by facilitation of transmission in their pathways (Tsumoto et al., 1975). If these modifications occur in particular input lines during natural activity of PTNs and normal movement, the output elements of the motor cortex could be in control of their own inputs. Some of the different responses of some PTNs during active and passive movements could then be a result of the PTNs own activity in modifying its input. But no tests of the responsiveness of cortical neurones to the same peripheral stimulus have been carried out by delivering that identical stimulus when the receptive zone was moving and when it was still, to assess the influence of movement.

In any case, even though competent long-loop reflexes from peripheral receptors have been demonstrated, most natural activity of output neurones in relation to movement is not generated from this source. In connection with conditioned and voluntary movement large numbers of PTNs begin their discharge and are found to be in action well before the beginning of movement and well ahead of any activation of receptors which could have resulted from the movement or of any facilitated afferent transmission which would have followed the PT activity. Moreover, movement itself may be accomplished and new movement tasks may be learned even after all afferent feedback from the limb has been abolished by dorsal root section (Taub and Berman, 1968; Bossom, 1974). We must seek elsewhere than in peripheral receptors for the determinants of this PT activity in relation to movement performance.

Some information about the potential involvement of different neural sites in the selection of and activation of PTNs in association with movement performance may be obtained by examining the timing of actions in these places in relation to the time of execution of the movement. While the long-loop reflex has been shown to occupy a total stimulus-response time of the order of 30 ms for the monkey's forelimb (and 40 to 50 ms for the human thumb), the reaction time for a movement response to a flash of light is of the order of 300 ms (Evarts, 1966). In this experiment, even in cases of a minimum (180 ms) reaction time, PTNs became active after 100 ms or so (i.e. the reaction to the visual stimulus had a latency of 100 ms) and their responses preceded by 70 to 100 ms the onset of muscle activity. Similarly, in all those cases where voluntary self-paced arm or hand movements have been used as the responses of monkeys, PTN discharge builds up as early as 100 ms before the movement and the activity of even the most closely coupled PTNs precedes muscle contractions by a period of 50 ms or more. Since only 10 ms or thereabouts should be taken up in activation of motoneurones and muscles, the crescendo of PTN discharge well before this cannot be acting as an immediate trigger for movement. Indeed the movement responses would have to be very stereotyped and inflexible if PTNs were coupled to muscular action (via motoneurones) in this rigid 'reflex' manner. The subtle changes in motoneurone output which characterize skilled movements and the enormous variety and flexibility of actions which one associates with voluntary arm and hand movement must suggest other actions for the PTN discharges so long in advance of movement performance.

Indirect evidence for an increase in activity over the motor cortex in man 100 ms or less in advance of voluntary movement suggests that the output from the human cortex also begins long before movement occurs. This activity could be the response in appropriate and selected output modules to elements of the programme for movement located elsewhere. Efforts have been made to examine the timing of neuronal discharges in other situations to decide whether activities at these sites lead or follow the PT activity in relation to movement performance. None of the investigations has given a clear-cut answer.

A brief report by Evarts (1970) indicated that most of 30 neurones in the ventrolateral nucleus of the monkey's thalamus changed their activity as much as 100 ms ahead of brisk movements of the wrist in response to a conditioning stimulus. DeLong and Evarts (1971) reported that neurones in the putamen and globus pallidus also changed their firing in advance of conditioned movements and could have been concerned in influencing the activity of the motor cortex prior to the onset of movement. And Thach (1975) has recorded, on alternate days in the same monkey, the discharges of neurones in the dentate nucleus and in the motor cortex which were associated with prompt arm movements in response to a light signal. In both situations the majority of neurones changed their firing before movement began. Some of the cerebellar neurones began to discharge before some of the cortical neurones. But the distributions of times of onset of firing in relation to movement overlapped so completely for the two populations that it would be quite impossible to conclude either that the cerebellum was influencing the motor cortex or the reverse.

How could this question be resolved? If one wished to demonstrate that a particular neurone, say in VL, was influencing one or many output cells in the motor cortex and in some way commanding or programming their discharge prior to movement, simultaneous recordings from the cell in VL and its influenced output neurones in the motor cortex would be needed. The experiment would be feasible. Weak stimulation at the site of the VL recording should reveal whether or not the VL location projected to the cells under simultaneous study in the motor cortex. If the discharges of the VL neurone and sampled PTNs were correlated, it should be possible to test statistically whether the actions of the VL neurone influenced the probability of firing of the PTN or was influenced by it, and to state what the temporal relationship of this influence might be.

In searching for the 'instructions' which a locus such as VL could transmit to the motor cortex as part of its programme for movement, it will be necessary to consider more subtle and general influences than the simple triggering of cortical neurones to discharge. Some influences must select appropriate cortical outputs, not just those destined to influence motoneurones, but also those preparing subcortical centres and spinal relays for the occurrence of a future movement. These selected neurones must be recruited to the task in correct spatial combinations and temporal sequences. While some are being facilitated, others must be inhibited. Perhaps we have searched only for a 'go' signal in structures which do not specify the beginning of movement but rather some other aspects of its organization.

Given that many structures in the brain, including the motor cortex, contain neurones whose activity changes so long in advance of movement, what action could this changed discharge have in relation to movement performance? We have indicated that particular populations of PTNs are called up ahead of the contractions of particular muscles. We must conclude that these PTNs have influenced the outputs to those muscles in such a way that they (and not others) contract appropriately when the trigger for movement does occur. If we consider that the continuing activity of the PTNs in the 100 ms or so before movement is priming (but not discharging) a particular selection of motoneurones, inhibiting their antagonists, setting to appropriate levels the excitability of a range of subcortical structures, spinal interneurones and afferent relay centres, advising particular neurones in the cerebellar cortex and basal ganglia of its change and so on, then a general increase in excitability of the whole motor apparatus 100 ms later could result in responses only from those structures prepared by the PTN activity. The motoneurones brought close to their firing level by PTN activity would be selectively responsive to a general command to move. Whether this selection, in appropriate sequences, is the function of the PTN responses so far in advance of movement remains to be demonstrated.

The source of the command to move in voluntary self-paced movements must probably be sought other than in the PTNs themselves because movement can still occur in the absence of PTN influences on spinal centres. But development of force of contraction is slowed and the precision of movements is decreased, perhaps because the priming effects on particular motoneurones in their specified sequences is absent. Moreover, the selection of only some motoneurones to fractionate muscle action and perform such delicate movements as independent flexion of an index finger cannot be achieved at all. Now the command to move can only cause flexion of all the digits together.

Brooks (1975) has again revived interest in the view, derived from the observations of Holmes (1917), that the cerebellum might be concerned in the initiation of movement as well as its on-going regulation. He and his colleagues combined the technique of reversible interruption of the outflow of the lateral or intermediate parts of the cerebellum by cooling the dentate or interpositus nucleus with recording of the discharges of individual PTNs. The basic concept underlying these experiments and one which gains some support from the results of the experiments is that 'muscle choice and movement parameters would become "programmed" in the cerebellum with learning, to fashion the motor commands that issue from the motor cortex'. Similar experiments involving cooling of the outflow of the basal ganglia (the globus pallidus) suggest a role for neurones in these structures in the guidance of movement without visual control. It is of great importance to have a theory about nervous involvement in the evolution of movement because this theory will suggest experiments. Concepts of function can be and have been derived from the analysis of the disorders of movement which occur in patients with disease of central nervous structure, where, for example, disease of the lateral cerebellum is associated with disorders of rate, range, direction and coordination of movement (Holmes, 1917).

But it may be helpful to suggest a general framework, based on a set of interlocking control systems, in which aspects of movement are not specified by individual structures (e.g. 'initiation' by the lateral cerebellum) but are derived from the interactions between a large number of neural elements and have available both internal and external feedback (Fig. 8.23). A number of diagrams of the connexions between neural structures, which could provide the basis for such an organization of control systems, have been produced. They point up many of the unanswered questions in relation to control of movement performance. Even at the level of spinal reflex function, where many of the connections have been well described, we are far from a complete understanding of changing activities in neural circuits during the period occupied by even a simple movement of one limb. But within the framework of our concept of the organization of movement performance, it is possible to identify questions which may appropriately be asked and whose solution is technically feasible.

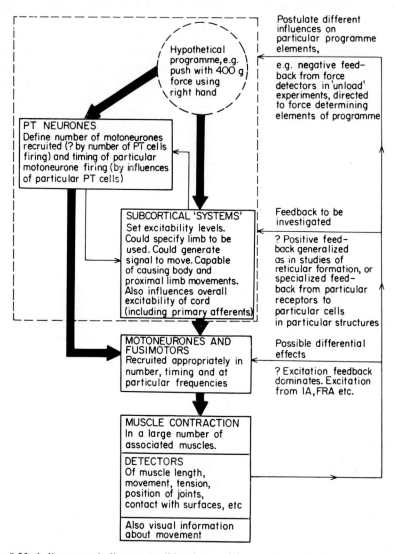

FIG. 8.23. A diagram to indicate a possible scheme of the neural organization of movement performance and to allow identification of questions capable of yielding experimental answers. A programme for movement is conceived as arising within the brain and being generated though a system of interconnected and mutually interacting structures. The effects of this programme will be expressed both through corticospinal and subcorticospinal 'systems', the latter arising from some parts of a subcortical network which must include other interconnected neurones in cerebellum, basal ganglia and thalamus as well as the origins of the conventional vestibulospinal, reticulospinal, rubrospinal, etc. tracts.

In examining those aspects of the study of neural function in control of movement which are within the reach of the experimentalist using methods of study available at the present time, one must still recognize a fundamental and important problem which limits progress in this work. The classical technique of physiologists and psychologists of providing a stimulus whose nature, duration, magnitude and quality may all be controlled and then observing the responses of neurones or subjects to this stimulus allows modification one at a time of aspects of the detail of the stimulus. By this technique it has been possible to understand a great deal about the coding of the analysis of sounds, for example, by the peripheral structures of the auditory apparatus. But no such control of the detailed aspects of movement performances is in the hands of the experimenter. The animal, using his central nervous apparatus in manners both inborn and learned, executes the movements which the physiologist would study. Each performance may vary in subtle ways from all those which have preceded it. The experimenter cannot regulate these variations; he must measure them. Understanding the relationships between changes in neuronal activity in any part of the brain and changes in movement performance therefore involve double sets of measurements, with their own errors and inconsistencies, analysis of the relationship between these and then tests of the significance and meaningfulness of the relationships described.

In all the studies prompted by concepts of the nervous system's role in control of movement the aim must be not simply description of associations but analysis of the mechanisms by which controls operate. It will not be enough to conclude that the PT functions to confer skill and precision of performance on an animal's movements—the challenge is to attempt to understand *how* these special characters of the performance are contributed by the normal functions of the PTNs and how those aspects of the PTNs involvement in movement are themselves specified.

A stage may have been reached at which it would be helpful to set aside the now established division between motor systems and sensory systems and to realize that the processes of central nervous actions involve selection of inputs, evaluation of their significance by comparison with internal information *and* the production of appropriate output responses. The

The output effects of all this activity converge eventually on motor centres in the spinal cord and modify the levels of excitability of interneurones concerned in local reflex function and in afferent transmission. Feedback about movement is theoretically capable of influencing these interacting systems at any level. Questions to be asked involve the nature of the origins of this feedback to any particular station, the direction of the effect produced at that station and the significance of that effect for the output of the station and for movement performance. Some of the matters have been investigated for PTNs. Very little information exists about these matters at other situations.

output responses may produce behaviour. They also contribute to sensation. An example which relates to the field we have been examining is the relationships of neural output to judgements of the heaviness of a load to be lifted—the more neural output involved in the lifting, the more the 'sense of effort' and the heavier the load is judged to be.

8.7 Summary

In Chapter 1 we drew diagrams (Figs 1.2, p. 8 and 1.4, p. 18) to show the intermediate position occupied by the 'motor cortex' (Woolsey's MsI) in relation to the structures which 'command' it from upstream and to the structures which it excites and inhibits in the brainstem and spinal cord. In the following chapters we saw that this cortex is built up of overlapping sub-areas which project to specific targets lying downstream. These sub-areas define the overlapping localization of colonies of PTN which project to specific targets and which are available for selection by 'higher-level' motor programmes—programmes which depend on the integrity of the forebrain and cerebellum. Of these sub-areas, those which project monosynaptically to motoneurones of the hands and feet of primates are the simplest to isolate experimentally. They may serve as a model of the structuring of the other projection areas of which the motor cortex is built up. Our aim in this chapter has been to try to picture the activity of the corticospinal neurones in voluntary movements in man and in learned movements in monkeys: to discover whatever may be possible about the selection of PTN by 'higher-level' programmes, about the selection of spinal outputs by the CST, and about the modification of activity of the PTN by inputs from the moving parts.

The rapid expansion of research on motor control in the last three decades has illuminated the structure of the segmental motor mechanisms, especially in the lumbosacral spinal cord of the cat. The skeletomotor neurones (α motoneurones) are linked up by local networks of interneurones which distribute excitation and inhibition from passively lengthened and actively contracting muscles in reciprocal fashion between the motoneurone pools of agonists and antagonists. The fusimotor neurones (γ motoneurones) provide for servo-excitation of the agonist muscles, and the local interneuronal networks automatically see to the reciprocal inhibition of their antagonists. These segmental arrangements form the structural basis of all movements, whether these are gene-endowed and relatively stereotyped, or acquired by learning and relatively modifiable. Fusimotor and skeletomotor neurones are generally called into action together in movements of all types (Granit's '$\alpha\gamma$ linkage').

Following Hughlings Jackson's thinking, we can arrange movements in hierarchical levels ascending from 'most automatic' to 'least automatic'.

'More automatic' movements would include the relatively stereotyped patterns of flexion and extension which can be evoked by noxious stimulation of the limbs, as in the classical flexion reflex and crossed extensor reflex; these are organized by networks of propriospinal interneurones. More complex intersegmental networks, integrated by structures in the brain stem, control the muscles which are concerned with the special, relatively automatic movements of respiration and four-footed locomotion and with the orientation and postural fixation of the limbs and trunk with respect to gravity. Superimposed on all these are the 'least automatic' movements which are acquired by learning, which are highly developed in the performances of the hands of monkeys and men, and on which our interest has been focused throughout this book. Such 'least automatic' movements compete with the 'more automatic' movements for access to the elemental segmental networks. Their neural apparatus may also engage the interneuronal networks which distribute postural support and ready made flexor and extensor synergies amongst the motoneurones of limbs and trunk.

The fantastic complexity of the processes of selection and combination of motor outputs can be realized only in the context of accurate, concrete descriptions of motor performance. The three-dimensional trajectories and velocities of human voluntary movements can be described only by the detailed analysis of graphic records. Of such recordings ('cyclograms' and 'kymocyclograms') and their analysis N. Bernstein was a pioneer and a master. He found that attempted repetitions of the same movement were never absolutely identical. Since the external force-fields are not always the same, he concluded that the output from the central nervous system to the muscles would have to be different on each attempted repetition. The minimum hierarchy of 'black boxes' would have to include one for the 'motor image' of the movement, *simultaneously* present in its totality, and others for the *successive* engagement of different combinations of muscles during its course. Another box would be needed to compare the actual position of the limb at any instant (Istwert) with its prescribed position at that instant (Sollwert). The output of this box would enable the brain to correct any deviations from the prescribed trajectory and velocity during the further sequencing of the movement. Bernstein found that any movement, such as striking a nail with a hammer, always responded as a whole to a disturbance at any part.

To describe a complex movement accurately is a far cry from being able to describe the exact combinations, quantities and sequencing of the muscular contractions and relaxations which bring it about. The muscles which act on joints which have more than one degree of freedom, or which act across more than one joint, are combined, simultaneously and successively, in ways which are infinitely more complex than the more stereotyped reciprocal relationships between the agonists and antagonists which act at a single hinge joint. The importance of supraspinal switching of the Ia-inhibitory interneurones should here be obvious. The student of motor control cannot afford to neglect what is known of the actions of groups of muscles in producing the various movements at particular joints. Rather little has been added to the classical accounts of muscle-combinations given by Duchenne in 1867 and by Beevor in 1904. These accounts need to be updated by simultaneous electromyography of several muscles, combined with cyclography or kymocyclography of the whole movements.

A start along this road has been made by studies of what may be called 'minimal units of performance': of brief ballistic movements aimed at stationary targets, and of simple ramp movements in pursuit of moving targets. The ramp movements are subject to correction by visual feedback from the moving target and also by feedback from the moving parts. To the extent that the responses are of minimal latency and the movements are limited to minimal fields of distal forelimb musculature, the probability that the CST is involved in the selection of outputs is maximized. The output of the skeletomotor neurones has been recorded by single-fibre and integrated electromyography and correlated with records of the movements made with position-transducers and accelerometers. It has been found that inhibition of antagonist motoneurones precedes excitation of the agonists. In a ballistic movement there is a preprogrammed sequence of 1, agonist excitation; 2, agonist silence and antagonist excitation; 3, antagonist silence and agonist re-excitation. Not until the third stage do the agonist motoneurones become accessible to feedback from the moving parts, as the movement leaves its 'ballistic' and enters its 'ramp' phase. During the ramp phase there is evidence of servo-assistance, involving not only a segmental but also a cerebral (possibly a transcortical) loop. Such servo-assistance is possible only if the spindles of the prime movers discharge continuously throughout the movement. Sampling of single spindle-afferents in human nerves shows that their discharge is indeed sustained throughout a simple voluntary movement. This is proof of $\alpha\gamma$ coactivation in voluntary movement.

It is important to know the extent to which the relatively hard-wired corticomotoneuronal component of the CST is capable of addressing single skeletomotor neurones selectively. The recruitment-order of skeletomotor neurones in voluntary movement follows in general the 'size principle', but in an intrinsic muscle of the human hand, the motor units which are fired at low force-thresholds can be individually selected at will by subjects who have been given a minimal experience of visual and auditory displays of their characteristic action potentials.

To determine the contribution of the CST to the execution of 'minimal units of performance', it would be necessary, in an ideal experiment, to block the PT temporarily and reversibly by cooling and to compare the resulting performance with the normal. Surgical interruption of the PT is less than ideal because its acute effects are complicated by locally spreading oedema and vascular spasm, and its chronic effects are complicated by a reorganization of the functions of the surviving motor outputs to compensate for the deficit. Cooling of the medullary pyramids could not be justified in man. In chronic studies, man has the advantage that he can produce with a normal hand, and attempt with an abnormal hand, performances which a monkey can only give after prolonged and laborious training; but the lesions of the PT can rarely compare, in accuracy of localization, with the artificial lesions which can be placed in monkeys and later defined microanatomically. Nevertheless there is much to be learned by comparing EMG, Ia input, etc. in minimal units of performance executed by the normal and abnormal hand. Above all, it is only in man, and especially in people who have cultivated special manual skills, that an adequate description of disabilities, and of residual abilities, is possible. It is therefore important to obtain detailed neuroanatomical correlation whenever the quality of the clinical study has been high enough to make the enormous labour worth-while. In monkeys, detection of disability demands specially designed and searching tests. Such tests have shown that loss of relatively independent movements of the fingers is permanent, together with difficulty in relaxing the grasp and in correctly orientating the hand to a tactile stimulus. Reaction-time is also lengthened in choice-reaction tasks. After PT section, the 'more automatic' uses of the forelimb in locomotion and climbing are preserved from the outset.

In addition to knowing the effects of disconnecting the spinal segments from the CST, we would like to know the effects of deafferentation of the CST neurones. Cutting the cervical dorsal roots deprives the CNS as a whole, and not only the CST neurones, of all modalities of input from the forelimbs. Monkeys soon learn to reach for food under visual guidance, but the trajectories and velocities of their movements are permanently abnormal. Their abilities in 'minimal units of performance' have yet to be tested. In man, accurate ballistic movements are impossible after lesion of the dorsal columns. Unfortunately, selective deafferentation of the motor cortex, and selective interruption of different modalities of input, can hardly be achieved. Interruption of corticocortical association fibres between the visual and motor areas of monkeys impairs the ability of the contralateral hand and fingers to orientate themselves correctly to a visually presented food target, and to detach from it a food-morsel which is perfectly visible but difficult to locate by 'active touch'.

In man, all inputs from the hand can be blocked by ischaemia without interfering with the inputs from the extrinsic muscles in the forearm; the inputs from hand and forearm can be blocked together and the forearm then allowed to recover while the hand remains blocked. The primary endings of muscle spindles can be selectively excited by vibrating the tendons. Such experiments have thrown light on our perception of active movement. Without feedback from the parts we are moving, we are unaware that we are in fact moving them. 'Corollary discharges' by CST collaterals therefore create no sensation of movement. The attempt to move muscles which have been paralysed by neuromuscular blocking drugs creates no illusion of movement. Vibration of a tendon creates the illusion that a muscle is being lengthened even when it remains stationary. Thus, fusimotor activation of the spindle primaries of a muscle which *flexes* a joint would, if uncorrected by other inputs, create the illusion that the joint was being *extended*. Such correction could be due to joint receptors and spindle secondaries, to the spindles of antagonists, and to corollary discharges of CST collaterals into relay nuclei.

Recordings from antidromically labelled PTN and from adjacent cortical neurones in monkeys can give information about the timing of discharges that are regularly related to a particular movement. A picture of the 'ramp of recruitment' of the population of PTN whose discharges are related to the movement can be built up from records collected successively from individual neurones. The picture reflects the time-course of the command sent to the PTN from the programme upstream. Though the monosynaptic pathway to the motoneurones of forearm muscles can fire the muscle fibres in about 10 ms, the PTN are active as much as 100 ms in advance of the movement. The earliest detectable action on spinal motoneurones is inhibitory. Possibly the PTN are not the final triggers for movement. By a crescendo of patterned discharge, appropriate colonies of PTN may partially depolarize selected motoneurones, facilitate interneurones, and 'set' the excitabilities of afferent relay neurones in preparation for the inputs which the movement is 'expected' to generate.

Thus the provenance and modality of the *peripheral* inputs to those PTN which are related to specific movements at a particular joint, and which would be involved in the governing of the movement throughout its course, are now accessible to detailed mapping; but the location and structure of the 'higher-level' programmes which provide the PTN with their *central* inputs remain elusive. The PTN from which we can record most readily are among the largest. Some of them are connected monosynaptically to the motoneurones of distal muscles: these PTN are situated at one remove only from the neuromuscular junctions. Such directness 'downstream' is a measure of the probable complexity 'upstream'. These PTN are evidently important in the management of the fingers. Blinkered, however, by the limited resolving power of our present techniques, we remain ignorant of the activities and actions of the myriads of smaller PTN which furnish over 90 per cent of the axons of the PT.

Bibliography

The numbers in square brackets refer to the page in the text where mention of a given work is made.

ADAM, J., MARSDEN, C. D., MERTON, P. A. and MORTON, H. B. (1976). The effect of lesions in the internal capsule and the sensorimotor cortex on servo action in the human thumb. *J. Physiol.* **254**, 27–28P.   [368]

ADEY, W. R., CARTER, I. D. and PORTER, R. (1954). Temporal dispersion in cortical response. *J. Neurophysiol.* **17**, 167–182.   [229]

ADRIAN, E. D. (1937). The spread of activity in the cerebral cortex. *J. Physiol.* **88**, 127–161.   [51, 207]

ADRIAN, E. D. (1941). Afferent discharges to the cerebral cortex from peripheral sense organs. *J. Physiol.* **100**, 159–191.   [229]

ADRIAN, E. D. (1943). Afferent areas in the brain of ungulates. *Brain*, **66**, 89–103.   [13]

ADRIAN, E. D. and MORUZZI, G. (1939). Impulses in the pyramidal tract. *J. Physiol.* **97**, 153–199.   [124, 217]

AGNEW, R. F., PRESTON, J. B. and WHITLOCK, D. G. (1963). Patterns of motor cortex effects on ankle flexor and extensor motoneurons in the "pyramidal" cat preparation. *Expl. Neurol.* **8**, 248–263.   [124]

ALBE-FESSARD, D. and BOWSHER, D. (1960). Responses of monkey thalamus to somatic stimuli under chloralose anaesthesia. *Electroen. Neurophysiol.* **19**, 1–15.   [254]

ALBE-FESSARD, D. and LIEBESKIND, J. (1966). Origine des messages somato-sensitifs activant les cellules du cortex moteur chez le singe. *Expl. Brain Res.* **1**, 127–146.   [230, 232, 304]

ALBE-FESSARD, D., LAMARRE, Y. and PIMPANEAU, A. (1966). Sur l'origine fusoriale de certaines efférences somatiques atteignant le cortex moteur du Singe. *J. Physiol., Paris,* **58**, 443–444.   [230]

ALBE-FESSARD, D., ARFEL, G., GUIOT, G., DEROME, P. and GUILBAUD, G. (1967). Thalamic unit activity in man. *Electroen. Neurophysiol. Suppl.* **25**, 132–142.   [255]

ALLEN, G. I. and TSUKAHARA, N. (1974). Cerebrocerebellar Communication Systems. *Physiol. Rev.* **54**, 957–1006.   [117, 215, 217]

ALLEN, G. I., KORN, H. and OSHIMA, T. (1969). Monosynaptic pyramidal activation of pontine cells projecting to the cerebellum. *Brain Res.* **15**, 272–275.   [117]

ALLEN, G. I., OSHIMA, T. and TOYAMA, K. (1971). Unitary components in cortico-pontine activation of the cat. *Brain Res.* **35**, 245–249.   [76]

AMASSIAN, V. E. and BERLIN, L. (1958). Early cortical projection of Group I afferents in the forelimb muscle nerves of cat. *J. Physiol.* **143**, 61P   [222]

AMASSIAN, V. E., WEINER, H. and ROSENBLUM, M. (1972). Neural systems subserving the tactile placing reaction: a model for the study of higher level control of movement. *Brain Res.* **40**, 171–178.   [222]

ANDERSEN, P. and ANDERSSON, S. A. (1968). 'Physiological Basis of the Alpha Rhythm.' Chapter V. Appleton-Century-Crofts, New York.   [62]

ANDERSEN, P., ECCLES, J. C., SCHMIDT, R. F. and YOKOTA, T. (1964a). Slow potential waves produced in the cuneate nucleus by cutaneous volleys and by cortical stimulation. *J. Neurophysiol.* **27**, 78–91.   [112, 123]

ANDERSEN, P., ECCLES, J. C., SCHMIDT, R. F. and YOKOTA, T. (1964b). Depolarization of presynaptic fibers in the cuneate nucleus. *J. Neurophysiol.* **27**, 92–106.
[112, 114, 123]

ANDERSEN, P., ECCLES, J. C., SCHMIDT, R. F. and YOKOTA, T. (1964c). Identification of relay cells and interneurons in the cuneate nucleus. *J. Neurophysiol.* **27**, 1080–1095.
[112, 115]

ANDERSEN, P., ECCLES, J. C., OSHIMA, T. and SCHMIDT, R. F. (1964d). Mechanisms of synaptic transmission in the cuneate nucleus. *J. Neurophysiol.* **27**, 1096–1116.
[114, 115]

ANDERSEN, P., ECCLES, J. C. and SEARS, T. A. (1964e). Cortically evoked depolarization of primary afferent fibers in the spinal cord. *J. Neurophysiol.* **27**, 63–77.
[123]

ANDERSEN, P., HAGAN, P. J., PHILLIPS, C. G. and POWELL, T. P. S. (1975). Mapping by microstimulation of projections from Area 4 to motor units of the baboon's hand. *Proc. R. Soc., London, B.*
[176, 187, 188, 189, 191, 195, 196]

APPLEBAUM, A. E., BEALL, J. E., FOREMAN, R. D. and WILLIS, W. D. (1975). Organization and receptive fields of primate spinothalamic tract neurons. *J. Neurophysiol.* **38**, 572–586.
[254]

ARMSTRONG, D. M. (1965). Synaptic excitation and inhibition of Betz cells by antidromic pyramidal volleys. *J. Physiol.* **178**, 37–38P.
[60, 108, 272]

ARMSTRONG, D. M. and HARVEY, R. J. (1966). Responses in the inferior olive to stimulation of the cerebellar and cerebral cortices in the cat. *J. Physiol.* **187**, 553–574.
[120]

ARMSTRONG, D. M., HARVEY, R. J. and SCHILD, R. F. (1973). The spatial organisation of climbing fibre branching in the cat cerebellum. *Expl. Brain Res.* **18**, 40–58.
[158, 174]

ASANUMA, H. (1975). Recent developments in the study of the columnar arrangement of neurons within the motor cortex. *Physiol. Rev.* **55**, 143–156.
[211, 213, 221, 393]

ASANUMA, H. and ARNOLD, A. P. (1975). Noxious effects of excessive currents used for intracortical stimulation. *Brain Res.* **96**, 103–107.
[186, 197]

ASANUMA, H. and FERNANDEZ, J. J. (1974). Organization of projection from the thalamic relay nuclei to the motor cortex in the cat. *Brain Res.* **71**, 515–522.
[254]

ASANUMA, H. and HUNSPERGER, R. W. (1975). Functional significance of projection from the cerebellar nuclei to the motor cortex in the cat. *Brain Res.* **98**, 73–92.
[225]

ASANUMA, H. and OKAMOTO, K. (1959). Unitary study on evoked activity of callosal neurons and its effect on pyramidal tract cell activity on cats. *Jap. J. Physiol.* **9**, 473–483.
[226]

ASANUMA, H. and OKUDA, O. (1962). Effects of transcallosal volleys on pyramidal tract cell activity of cat. *J. Neurophysiol.* **25**, 198–208.
[226]

ASANUMA, H. and ROSÉN, I. (1972). Topographical organization of cortical efferent zones projecting to distal forelimb muscles in the monkey. *Expl. Brain Res.* **14**, 243–256.
[183, 185, 257]

ASANUMA, H. and ROSÉN, I. (1973). Spread of mono- and poly-synaptic connexions within cat's motor cortex. *Expl. Brain Res.* **16**, 507–520.
[179]

ASANUMA, H. and SAKATA, H. (1967). Functional organization of a cortical efferent system examined with focal depth stimulation in cats. *J. Neurophysiol.* **30**, 35–54.
[173, 198, 200, 221]

ASANUMA, H. and WARD, J. E. (1971). Patterns of contraction of distal forelimb muscles produced by intracortical stimulation in cats. *Brain Res.* **27**, 97–109. [200]

ASANUMA, H., STONEY, S. D. Jr. and ABZUG, C. (1968). Relationship between afferent input and motor outflow in cat motorsensory cortex. *J. Neurophysiol.* **31**, 670–681. [188, 201, 202, 220, 221, 222]

ASANUMA, H., STONEY, S. D. Jr. and THOMPSON, W. D. (1971). Characteristics of cervical interneurones which mediate cortical motor outflow to distal forelimb muscles of cats. *Brain Res.* **27**, 79–95. [200]

ASANUMA, H., FERNANDEZ, J., SCHEIBEL, M. E. and SCHEIBEL, A. B. (1974). Characteristics of projections from the nucleus ventralis lateralis to the motor cortex in cats: an anatomical and physiological study. *Expl. Brain Res.* **20**, 315–330. [216, 225]

ASANUMA, H., ARNOLD, A. and ZARZECKI, P. (1976a). Further study on the excitation of pyramidal tract cells by intracortical microstimulation. *Expl. Brain Res.* **26**, 443–461. [180, 181, 201]

ASANUMA, H., SHINODA, Y., ARNOLD, A. and ZARZECKI, P. (1976b). Re-examination of functional arrangements of pyramidal tract neurons in the motor cortex of the cat. *In* 'Afferent and Intrinsic Organization of Laminated Structures in the Brain' (Ed. O. Creutzfeldt), Suppl. I, *Expl. Brain Res.* In press. [31, 122, 154, 177, 181, 221]

ASANUMA, H., SHINODA, Y. and ZARZECKI, P. (1976c). Branching of cortico-spinal fibres in the monkey. *Neuroscience Abstracts*, **2**, 537. [154]

ATKINSON, D. H., SEQUIN, J. J. and WIESENDANGER, M. (1974). Organization of corticofugal neurones in somatosensory area II of the cat. *J. Physiol.* **236**, 663–679. [99, 219]

BAKER, M. A., TYNER, C. F. and TOWE, A. L. (1971). Observations on single neurons recorded in the sigmoid gyri of awake, nonparalysed cats. *Expl. Neurol.* **32**, 388–403. [219]

BANNISTER, C. M. and PORTER, R. (1967). Effects of limited direct stimulation of the medullary pyramidal tract on spinal motoneurones in the rat. *Expl. Neurol.* **17**, 265–275. [16]

BARD, P. (1938). Studies on the cortical representation of somatic sensibility. *Harvey Lect.* **33**, 143–169. [222]

BARNARD, J. W. and WOOLSEY, C. N. (1956). A study of localization in the cortico-spinal tracts of monkey and rat. *J. comp. Neurol.* **105**, 25–50. [31]

BARRON, D. H. (1934). The results of unilateral pyramidal section in the rat. *J. comp. Neurol.* **60**, 45–56. [360]

BASMAJIAN, J. V. (1963). Control and training of individual motor units. *Science, N.Y.* **141**, 440–441. [346, 347]

BASMAJIAN, J. V., BAEZA, M. and FABRIGAR, C. (1965). Conscious control and training of individual spinal motor neurons in normal human subjects. *J. New Drugs*, **5**, 78–85. [346]

BATES, J. A. V. (1951). Electrical activity of the cortex accompanying movement. *J. Physiol.* **113**, 240–257. [311]

BATES, J. A. V. (1957). Observations on the excitable cortex in man. *In* 'Lectures on the Scientific Basis of Medicine', vol. 5, pp. 333–347. Athlone Press, London. [37, 42]

BATUEV, A. S. and LENKOV, D. A. (1973). Intracellular study of identified cortico-fugal neurons in the cat motor cortex. *Acta biol. med. germ.* **31**, 705–712. [99, 110]

BATUEV, A. S., LENKOV, D. N. and PIRIGOV, A. A. (1974). Postsynaptic responses of motor cortex neurons of cats to sensory stimulation of different modalities. *Acta Neurobiol. Exp.* **34**, 317–321.   [218]

BEEVOR, C. E. (1904). 'The Croonian Lectures on Muscular Movements and their Representation in the Central Nervous System', pp. 84, 86. Adlard, London.   [40, 335, 336]

BEEVOR, C. E. and HORSLEY, V. (1890). A record of the results obtained by electrical excitation of the so-called motor cortex and internal capsule in an Organ-Outan (*Simia satyrus*). *Phil. Trans. R. Soc. Series B.* **181**, 129–158.   [27]

BELL, F. R. and LAWN, A. M. (1956). Delineation of motor areas in the cerebral cortex of the goat. *J. Physiol.* **133**, 159–166.   [13]

BERNARD, C. G. and BOHM, E. (1954). Cortical representation and functional significance of the cortico-motoneuronal system. *Archs. Neurol. Psychiat., Chicago,* **72**, 473–502.   [143]

BERNHARD, C. G., BOHM, E. and PETERSÉN, I. (1953). Investigations on the organization of the corticospinal system in monkeys. (*Macaca Mulatta*). *Acta physiol. scand.* **29**, Suppl. 106, 79–105.   [141, 142, 143, 144]

BERNHARD, C. G., BOHM, E. and PETERSÉN, I. (1955). An analysis of causes of postoperative limb pareses following anterolateral chordotomy. *Acta psychiat. neurol. scand.* **30**, 779–792.   [142]

BERNSTEIN, N. (1967). 'The Coordination and Regulation of Movements'. Pergamon Press, Oxford.   [328, 335, 372, 373]

BERREVOETS, C. E. and KUYPERS, H. G. J. M. (1975). Pericruciate cortical neurons projecting to brainstem reticular formation, dorsal column nuclei and spinal cord in the cat. *Neuroscience Letters,* **1**, 257–262.   [96]

BESSOU, P., LAPORTE, Y. and PAGÈS, B. (1968). Frequencygrams of spindle primary endings elicited by stimulation of static and dynamic fusimotor fibres. *J. Physiol.* **196**, 47–63.   [151]

BETZ, V, (1874) Anatomischer Nachweis sweier Gehirn centra. *Centralblatt f. d. Med. Wissensch,* **12**, 578–595. Cited by A. M. Lassek (1954).   [53]

BEVAN LEWIS, W. (1878). On the comparative structure of the cortex cerebri. *Brain,* **1**, 79–86.   [53]

BISHOP, A. (1964). Use of the hand in lower primates. *In* 'Evolutionary and Genetic Biology of Primates' (Ed. J. Buettner-Janusch), vol. 2, pp. 133–225. Academic Press, New York.   [14]

BISHOP, P. O., JEREMY, D. and LANCE, J. W. (1953). Properties of pyramidal tract. *J. Neurophysiol.* **16**, 537–550.   [58]

BIZZI, E. (1968). Discharge of frontal eye field neurons during saccadic and following eye movements in unanaesthetized monkeys. *Expl. Brain Res.* **6**, 69–80.   [305]

BIZZI, E. and SCHILLER, P. H. (1970). Single unit activity in the frontal eye fields of unanaesthetized monkeys during eye and head movement. *Expl. Brain Res.* **10**, 151–158.   [306]

BOSSOM, J. (1974). Movement without proprioception. *Brain Res.* **71**, 285–296.   [373, 374, 375, 396]

BOYNTON, E. P. and HINES, M. (1933). On the question of threshold in stimulation of the motor cortex. *Am. J. Physiol.* **106**, 175–182.   [45]

BRANCH, C. L. and MARTIN, A. R. (1958). Inhibition of Betz cell activity by thalamac and cortical stimulation. *J. Neurophysiol.* **21**, 380–390.   [216]

BRINDLEY, G. S. and CRAGGS, M. D. (1972). The electrical activity in the motor cortex that accompanies voluntary movement. *J. Physiol.* **223**, 28–29P.   [316]

BRINKMAN, J. and KUYPERS, H. G. J. M. (1973). Cerebral control of contralateral and ipsilateral arm, hand and finger movements in the split-brain rhesus monkey. *Brain*, **96**, 653–674.   [376]

BRINKMAN, J. and PORTER, R. (1976). Activities of cells in the supplementary motor cortex of the monkey during performance of a learned motor task. *Proc. Aust. physiol. pharmacol. Soc.* **7**, 88.   [308]

BRODAL, A. (1973). Self-observations and neuroanatomical considerations after a stroke. *Brain,* **96**, 675–694.   [10, 367, 370, 372, 379, 391]

BRODAL, P., MARŠALA, J. and BRODAL, A. (1967). The cerebral cortical projection to the lateral reticular nucleus in the cat, with special reference to the sensori-motor cortical areas. *Brain Res.* **6**, 252–274.   [119]

BROOKHART, J. M. (1952). A study of corticospinal activation of motorneurons. *Res. Publ. Ass. Res. nerv. ment. Dis.* **30**, 157–173.   [124, 269, 272]

BROOKS, V. B. (1975). Roles of cerebellum and basal ganglia in initiation and control of movements. *Can. J. Neurol. Sci.* **2**, 265–277.   [358, 399]

BROOKS, V. B. and STONEY, S. D. Jr. (1971). Motor mechanisms: the role of the pyramidal system in motor control. *A. Rev. Physiol.* **33**, 337–392. [215, 222, 296]

BROOKS, V. B., RUDOMIN, P. and SLAYMAN, C. L. (1961a). Sensory activation of neurons in the cat's cerebral cortex. *J. Neurophysiol.* **24**, 286–301.
                                                                      [218, 219, 220]

BROOKS, V. B., RUDOMIN, P. and SLAYMAN, C. L. (1961b). Peripheral receptive fields of neurons in the cat's cerebral cortex. *J. Neurophysiol.* **24**, 302–325.
                                                                      [218, 219, 220]

BROOKS, V. B., ADRIEN, J. and DYKES, R. W. (1972). Task-related discharge of neurons in motor cortex and effects of dentate cooling. *Brain Res.* **40**, 85–88.
                                                                             [311]

BROWN, A. G. and GORDON, G. (1977). Subcortical mechanisms concerned in somatic sensation. *Br. med. Bull.* **33**, 121–128.   [376]

BROWN, M. C., ENGBERG, I. and MATTHEWS, P. B. C. (1967). The relative sensitivity to vibration of muscle receptors of the cat. *J. Physiol.* **192**, 773–800. [385]

BROWN, T. Graham (1915a). Studies on the physiology of the nervous system. XXII. On the phenomenon of facilitation. I: Its occurrence in reactions induced by stimulation of the 'motor' cortex of the cerebrum in monkeys. *Q. J. exp. Physiol.* **9**, 81–99.   [34]

BROWN, T. Graham (1915b). XXIII. On the phenomenon of facilitation. 2. Its occurrence in response to subliminal cortical stimuli in monkeys. *Q. J, exp. Physiol.* **9**, 102–116.   [34]

BROWN, T. Graham (1915c). XXIV. On the phenomenon of facilitation. 3. 'Secondary facilitation' and its location in the cortical mechanism itself in monkeys. *Q. J. exp. Physiol.* **9**, 117–130.   [34]

BROWN, T. Graham (1915d). XXV. On the phenomenon of facilitation. 4. Its occurrence in the subcortical mechanism by the activation of which motor effects are produced on artificial stimulation of the 'motor' cortex. *Q. J. exp. Physiol.* **9**, 131–145.   [34]

BROWN, T. Graham (1916a). XXVI. On the phenomenon of facilitation. 5. Additional note on 'secondary facilitation' in the cortical motor mechanism in monkeys. *Q. J. exp. Physiol.* **10**, 97–102.   [34]

BROWN, T. Graham (1916b). XXVII. On the phenomenon of facilitation. 6. The motor activation of parts of the cerebral cortex other than those included in the so-called 'motor' areas in monkeys (excitation of the post-central gyrus); with a note on the theory of cortical localization of function. *Q. J. exp. Physiol.* **10**, 103–143.   [34]

BROWN, T. Graham and SHERRINGTON, C. S. (1912). On the instability of a cortical point. *Proc. R. Soc. B.* **85**, 250–277.   [37]

BROWN, W. J. and FANG, H. C. H. (1961). Spastic hemiplegia in man. Lack of flaccidity in lesion of pyramidal tract. *Neurology, Minneap.* **11**, 829–835.   [365]

BUBNOFF, N. and HEIDENHAIN, R. (1881). Ueber Erregungs-und Hemmungs-vorgänge innerhalb der motorischen Hirncentren. *Arch. ges. Physiol.* **26**, 137–200. (Translation by G. von Bonin and W. S. McCulloch, 1944.) *In* 'The Precentral Motor Cortex' (Ed. P. C. Bucy), pp. 174–210. University of Illinois Press, Urbana.   [38]

BUCY, P. C. (1957). Is there a pyramidal tract? *Brain*, **80**, 376–392.   [365, 367]

BUCY, P. C., KEPLINGER, J. E. and SEQUEIRA, E. B. (1964). Destruction of the 'Pyramidal Tract' in man. *J. Neurosurg.* **21**, 385–398.   [365]

BUCY, P. C., LADPLI, R. and EHRLICH, A. (1966). Destruction of the pyramidal tract in the monkey. *J. Neurosurg.* **25**, 1–20.   [362]

BURGESS, P. R. and CLARK, F. J. (1969). Characteristics of knee joint receptors in the cat. *J. Physiol.* **203**, 317–335.   [249]

BURNS, B. D. (1958). 'The Mammalian Cerebral Cortex'. Arnold, London.   [207]

BUSER, P. (1966). Subcortical controls of pyramidal activity. *In* 'The Thalamus' (Eds. D. P. Purpura and M. D. Yahr), pp. 323–347. Columbia University Press, New York and London.   [217]

BUSER, P. and IMBERT, M. (1961). Sensory projections to the motor cortex in cats: a microelectrode study. *In* 'Sensory Communication' (Ed. W. A. Rosenblith), pp. 607–626. M.I.T. Press, Cambridge, Massachusetts.   [218]

BUXTON, D. F. and GOODMAN, D. C. (1967). Motor function and the cortico-spinal tracts in the dog and raccoon. *J. comp. Neurol.* **129**, 341–360. [16, 112]

CAMPBELL, C. B. G., YASHON, D. and JANE, J. A. (1966). The origin, course and termination of corticospinal fibers in the slow loris, *Nycticebus coucang* (Boddaert). *J. comp. Neurol.* **127**, 101–112.   [15]

CARMICHAEL, E. A. (1947). Myoclonus. *Proc. R. Soc. Med.* **40**, 553–554.   [355]

CARPENTER, M. B. (1971). Central oculomotor pathways. *In* 'The Control of Eye Movements' (Eds P. Bach-y-Rita, C. C. Collins and J. E. Hyde), pp. 67–103. Academic Press, New York and London.   [120]

CARPENTER, D. LUNDBERG, A. and NORRSELL, U. (1963). Primary afferent depolari-zation evoked from the sensorimotor cortex. *Acta physiol. scand.* **59**, 126–142.
                                                                              [123]

CASSELL, K., SHAW, K. and STERN, G. (1973). A computerised tracking technique for the assessment of Parkinsonian motor disabilities. *Brain*, **96**, 815–826. [369]

CHAMBERS, R. A. and GILLIATT, R. W. (1954). The clinical assessment of postural sensation in the fingers. *J. Physiol.* **123**, 42P.   [371, 383]

CHAMBERS, W. W. and LIU, C. N. (1957). Corticospinal tract of the cat. An attempt to correlate the pattern of degeneration with deficits in reflex activity following neocortical lesions. *J. comp. Neurol.* **108**, 23–56.   [121]

CHANG, H-T. (1951). Changes in excitability of the cerebral cortex following a single electric shock applied to the cortical surface. *J. Neurophysiol.* **14**, 95–112.   [62]

CHANG, H-T., RUCH, T. C. and WARD, A. A. Jr. (1947). Topographical representa-tion of muscles in motor cortex in monkeys. *J. Neurophysiol.* **10**, 39–56.   [40]

CHING, J. and HARTRIDGE, H. (1935). The physiology of rapid movements. *J. Physiol.* **83**, 40–42P.   [335]

CLARE, M. H., LANDAU, W. M. and BISHOP, G. H. (1964). Electrophysiological evidence of a collateral pathway from the pyramidal tract to the thalamus in the cat. *Expl Neurol.* **9**, 262–267.   [117]

CLARK, W. E. Le Gros (1962a). 'The Antecedents of Man'. University Press, Edinburgh. [14]

CLARK, W. E. Le Gros (1962b). The sorting principle in sensory analysis as illustrated by the visual pathways. *Ann. R. Coll. Surg.* **30**, 299–308. [208]

CLIFTON, G. L., COGGESHALL, R. E., VANCE, W. H. and WILLIS, W. D. (1976). Receptive fields of unmyelinated ventral root afferent fibres in the cat. *J. Physiol.* **256**, 573–600. [373]

CLOUGH, J. F. and SHERIDAN, J. D. (1968). A fast pathway for cortical influence on cervical gamma motoneurones in the baboon. *J. Physiol.* **195**, 26–27. [150]

CLOUGH, J. F. M., KERNELL, D. and PHILLIPS, C. G. (1968). The distribution of monosynaptic excitation from the pyramidal tract and from primary spindle afferents to motoneurones of the baboon's hand and forearm. *J. Physiol.* **198**, 145–166. [147, 157, 188, 343, 348, 350, 353]

CLOUGH, J. F. M., PHILLIPS, C. G. and SHERIDAN, J. D. (1971). The short-latency projection from the baboon's motor cortex to fusimotor neurones of the forearm and hand. *J. Physiol.* **216**, 257–279. [150, 151]

COGGESHALL, R. E., APPLEBAUM, M. L., FAZEN, M., STUBBS, T. B. and SYKES, M. T. (1975). Unmyelinated axons in human ventral roots, a possible explanation for the failure of dorsal rhizotomy to relieve pain. *Brain,* **98**, 157–166. [373]

COLE, J. D. and GORDON, G. (1976a). Dissimilar timing of corticofugal inhibition of the gracile and cuneate nuclei in cats anaesthetized with pentobarbitone. *J. Physiol.* **256**, 38–39P. [111, 112]

COLE, J. D. and GORDON, G. (1976b). Difference in timing of cortico cuneatend a cortico gracile actions. *In* 'Sensory functions of the Skin' (Ed. Y. Zotterman). Wenner-Gren Center Symposium Series, vol. 27. In press. Pergamon Press, Oxford. [111]

COLONNIER, M. L. (1966). The structural design of the neocortex. *In* 'Brain and Conscious Experience' (Ed. J. C. Eccles), pp. 1–23. Springer-Verlag, Berlin, Heidelberg, New York. [207, 208]

CONRAD, B., MATSUNAMI, K., MEYER-LOHMANN, J., WIESENDANGER, M. and BROOKS, V. B. (1974). Cortical load compensation during voluntary elbow movements. *Brain Res.* **71**, 507–514. [302]

COOPER, S. and DENNY-BROWN, D. E. (1928). Responses to stimulation of the motor area of the cerebral cortex. *Proc. R. Soc. B,* **102**, 222–236. [139]

COQUERY, J-M. and COULMANCE, M. (1971). Variations d'amplitude des réflexes monosynaptiques avant un mouvement volontaire. *Physiol. Behav.* **6**, 65–69. [340]

CORAZZA, R., FADIGA, E. and PARMEGGIANI, P. L. (1963). Patterns of pyramidal activation of cat's motoneurons. *Archs. ital. Biol.* **101**, 337–364. [131, 133]

CORDA, M., EKLUND, G. and EULER, C. von (1965). External intercostal and phrenic α motor responses to changes in respiratory load. *Acta physiol. scand.* **63**, 391–400. [351]

COULTER, J. D., EWING, L. and CARTER, C. (1976). Origin of primary sensorimotor cortical projections to lumbar spinal cord of cat and monkey. *Brain Res.* **103**, 366–372. [96]

CRAGGS, M. D. (1975). Cortical control of motor prostheses; using the cord-transected baboon as the primate model for human paraplegia. *Adv. Neurol.* **10**, 91–101. [317]

CRAGGS, M. D. and RUSHTON, D. N. (1976). The stability of the electrical stimulation map of the motor cortex of the anaesthetized baboon. *Brain,* **99**, 575–600. [42]

CREED, R. S. (1934). Conditioned reflexes. *Nature, Lond.* **134**, 792–793. [4]

CREUTZFELDT, O. D., LUX, H. D. and NACIMIENTO, A. C. (1964). Intracelluläre Reizung corticaler Nervenzellen. *Pflugers Archges. Physiol.* **281**, 129–151. [58]

CREVEL, H. van and VERHAART, W. J. C. (1963a). The rate of secondary degeneration in the central nervous system. 1. The pyramidal tract of the cat. *J. Anat.* **97**, 429–449. [95, 96, 97, 99]

CREVEL, H. van and VERHAART, W. J. C. (1963b). The 'exact' origin of the pyramidal tract. A quantitative study in the cat. *J. Anat.* **97**, 495–515. [95, 98, 99]

CROSS, M. J. and McCLOSKEY, D. I. (1973). Position sense following surgical removal of joints in man. *Brain Res.* **55**, 443–445. [383]

CURTIS, D. R. (1969). Central synaptic transmitters. *In* 'Basic Mechanisms of the Epilepsies' (Eds H. H. Jasper, A. A. Ward Jr. and A. Pope), pp. 105–135. Little, Brown, Boston. [65]

CURTIS, D. R. and CRAWFORD, J. M. (1969). Central synaptic transmission-microelectrophoretic studies. *A. Rev. Pharmac.* **9**, 209–240. [63]

CURTIS, D. R. and FELIX, D. (1971). The effect of bicuculline upon synaptic inhibition in the cerebral and cerebellar cortices of the cat. *Brain Res.* **34**, 301–321. [65]

CUSHING, H. (1909). A note upon the faradic stimulation of the post-central gyrus in conscious patients. *Brain,* **32**, 44–53. [28]

DARIAN-SMITH, I. and YOKOTA, T. (1966a). Cortically evoked depolarization of trigeminal cutaneous afferent fibers in the cat. *J. Neurophysiol.* **29**, 170–184. [116]

DARIAN-SMITH, I. and YOKOTA, T. (1966b). Corticofugal effects on different neuron types within the cat's brain stem activated by tactile stimulation of the face. *J. Neurophysiol.* **29**, 185–206. [116]

DAWSON, G. D. (1947). Cerebral responses to electrical stimulation of peripheral nerve in man. *J. Neurol. Neurosurg. Psychiat.* **10**, 134–140. [311, 355]

DAWSON, G. D. (1950). Cerebral responses to nerve stimulation in man. *Br. med. Bull.* **6**, 326. [311]

DAY, R. H. and DICKINSON, R. G. (1977). Learning to identify Braille numerals with active and passive touch. *Aust. J. Psychol.* Research Note (in press). [393]

DEECKE, L., SCHEID, P. and KORNHUBER, H. H. (1969). Distribution of readiness potential, pre-motion positivity and motor potential of the human cerebral cortex preceding voluntary finger movements. *Expl Brain Res.* **7**, 158–168. [312, 349]

DE GAIL, P., LANCE, J. W. and NEILSON, P. D. (1966). Differential effects on tonic and phasic reflex mechanisms produced by vibration of muscles in man. *J. Neurol. Neurosurg. Psychiat.* **29**, 1–11. [385]

DEJERINE, J. (1901). 'Anatomie des Centres Nerveux', vol. 2, pp. 82–90. Rueff, Paris. [6]

DELONG, M. R. (1971). Activity of pallidal neurons during movement. *J. Neurophysiol.* **34**, 414–427. [9, 310]

DELONG, M. R. and EVARTS, E. V. (1971). Activity of basal ganglia neurons prior to movement. *Fedn Proc.* **30**, 433 (Abstract). [310, 397]

DELONG, M. R. and STRICK, P. L. (1974). Relation of basal ganglia, cerebellum and motor cortex units to ramp and ballistic limb movements. *Brain Res.* **71**, 327–335. [310]

DEMYER, W. (1959). Number of axons and myelin sheaths in the adult human medullary pyramids. Study with silver impregnation and iron hematoxylin staining methods. *Neurology, Minneap.* **9**, 42–47. [136]

DeMYER, W. and RUSSELL, J. R. (1958). The number of axons in the right and left medullary pyramids of *macaca rhesus* and the ratio of axons to myelin sheaths. *Acta morph. neerl.-scand.* 2, 134–139.   [136]

DENNY-BROWN, D. (1950). Disintegration of motor function resulting from cerebral lesions. *J. Nerv. ment. Dis.* 112, no. 1, 1–45.   [4]

DENNY-BROWN, D. (1962). 'The Basal Ganglia and their Relation to Disorders of Movement'. University Press, Oxford.   [9]

DENNY-BROWN, D. (1966). 'The Cerebral Control of Movement'. Liverpool University Press, Liverpool.   [322, 361, 363, 373]

DEVANANDAN, M. S. and HEATH, P. D. (1975). A short latency pathway from forearm nerves to area 4 of the baboon's cerebral cortex. *J. Physiol.* 248, 43–44P.   [251]

DONALDSON, I. M. L. (1973). The properties of some human thalamic units: some new observations and a critical review of the localization of thalamic nuclei. *Brain,* 96, 419–440.   [255]

DUCHENNE de Boulogne, G. B. (1867). 'Physiologie des Mouvements'. Baillière, Paris.   [335, 384]

ECCLES, J. C. (1967). Circuits in the cerebellar control of movement. *Proc. Nat. Acad. Sci., U.S.A.* 58, 336–343.   [322]

ECCLES, J. C., ECCLES, R. M. and LUNDBERG, A. (1957). The convergence of monosynaptic excitatory afferents on to many different species of alpha motoneurones. *J. Physiol.* 137, 22–50.   [350]

ECCLES, J. C., ITO, M. and SZENTÁGOTHAI, J. (1967). 'The Cerebellum as a Neuronal Machine'. Springer-Verlag, New York.   [9, 215, 217]

ELDRED, E., GRANIT, R. and MERTON, P. A. (1953). Supraspinal control of the muscle spindles and its significance. *J. Physiol.* 122, 498–523.   [350]

ELGER, C., SPECKMANN, E.-J. and CASPERS, H. (1974). Monosynaptic responses of cervical motoneurons to cortical stimulation in the rat. *Proc. int. Union Physiol. Sci.* XI: XXVI International Congress, 161.   [16]

ELLIOT-SMITH, G. (1924). 'The Evolution of Man'. Oxford University Press, London.   [14]

ENDO, K., ARAKI, T. and YAGI, N. (1973). The distribution and pattern of axon branching of pyramidal tract cells. *Brain Res.* 57, 484–491.
                                  [103, 104, 109, 110, 112, 117, 119]

EULER, C. von (1966). Proprioceptive control in respiration. *In* 'Muscular Afferents and Motor Control' (Ed. R. Granit), pp. 197–207. Almqvist & Wiksell, Stockholm.   [304]

EVARTS, E. V. (1964). Temporal patterns of discharge of pyramidal tract neurons during sleep and waking in the monkey. *J. Neurophysiol.* 27, 152–171.
                                                        [268, 273, 293]

EVARTS, E. V. (1965a). Relation of cell size to effects of sleep in pyramidal tract neurons. *In* 'Progress in Brain Research' (Eds K. Akert, C. Bally and J. P. Schadé), vol. 18, pp. 81–91. Elsevier, Amsterdam.   [268, 273]

EVARTS, E. V. (1965b). Relation of discharge frequency to conduction velocity in pyramidal tract neurons. *J. Neurophysiol.* 28, 216–228.   [268, 269, 273]

EVARTS, E. V. (1966). Pyramidal tract activity associated with a conditioned hand movement in the monkey. *J. Neurophysiol.* 29, 1011–1027.   [397]

EVARTS, E. V. (1967). Representation of movements and muscles by pyramidal tract neurons of the precentral motor cortex. *In* 'Neurophysiological Basis of Normal and Abnormal Motor Activities' (Eds. M. D. Yahr and D. P. Purpura), pp. 215–253. Raven Press, New York.   [353]

EVARTS, E. V. (1968). Relation of pyramidal tract activity to force exerted during voluntary movement. *J. Neurophysiol.* **31**, 14–27.   [196, 281, 283, 290]

EVARTS, E. V. (1969). Activity of pyramidal tract neurons during postural fixation. *J. Neurophysiol.* **32**, 375–385.   [287]

EVARTS, E. V. (1970). Actitivity of ventralis lateralis neurons prior to movement in the monkey. *The Physiologist,* **13**, no. 3, 191.   [9, 310, 397]

EVARTS, E. V. (1972a). Pre- and post-central neuronal discharge in relation to learned movement. From—Movement and unitary activity in sensorimotor cortex. *In* 'Corticothalamic Projections and Sensorimotor Activities' (Eds T. Frigyesi, E. Rinvik and M. D. Yahr), pp. 449–458. Raven Press, New York.   [277, 307]

EVARTS, E. V. (1972b). Contrasts between activity of precentral and postcentral neurons of cerebral cortex during movement in the monkey. *Brain Res.* **40**, 25–31.   [277, 307]

EVARTS, E. V. (1973). Motor cortex reflexes associated with learned movement. *Science,* **179**, 501–503.   [300, 301, 304, 307, 316]

EVARTS, E. V. and GRANIT, R. (1976). Relations of reflexes and intended movements. *Prog. Brain Res.* **44**, 1–14.   [344]

EVARTS, E. V. and TANJI, J. (1974). Gating of motor cortex reflexes by prior instruction. *Brain Res.* **71**, 479–494.   [256, 302]

EVARTS, E. V. and THACH, W. T. (1969). Motor mechanisms of the CNS: cerebro-cerebellar interrelations. *A. Rev. Physiol.* **31**, 451–498.   [117, 215]

EVARTS, E. V., BIZZI, E., BURKE, R. E., DELONG, M. and THACH, W. T. Jr. (1971). Central control of movement. *Neurosci. Res. Prog. Bull.* **9**, 7–170.   [215, 336]

EYZAGUIRRE, C. and KUFFLER, S. W. (1955). Process of excitation in the dendrites and in the soma of single isolated sensory nerve cells of the lobster and crayfish. *J. gen. Physiol.* **39**, 87–119.   [60]

FELIX, D. and WIESENDANGER, M. (1971). Pyramidal and non-pyramidal motor cortical effects on distal forelimb muscles of monkeys. *Expl. Brain Res.* **12**, 81–91.   [48]

FERRIER, D. (1873). Experimental researches in cerebral physiology and pathology. *West Riding Lunatic Asylum med. Rep.* **3**, 1–50.   [24]

FERRIER, D. (1875). Experiments on the brain of monkeys. *Proc. R. Soc. Lond.* **23**, 409–430.   [22, 24]

FERRIER, D. (1876). 'The Functions of the Brain'. 323 pp. Smith Elder, London.   [24, 36, 45]

FERRIER, D. (1886). 'The Functions of the Brain' (2nd ed.). Smith Elder, London.   [9, 24, 26, 27, 36, 82]

FERRIER, D. (1890). 'The Croonian Lectures on Cerebral Localisation'. Smith Elder, London.   [27, 32]

FERRIER, D. and YEO, G. F. (1884). A record of experiments on the effects of lesion of different regions of the cerebral hemispheres. *Phil. Trans. R. Soc.* Part II, 1884, 479–564.   [27, 93]

FETZ, E. E. and BAKER, M. A. (1969). Response properties of precentral neurons in awake monkeys. *The Physiologist,* **12**, 223P (Abstract).   [237]

FETZ, E. E. and BAKER, M. A. (1973). Operantly conditioned patterns of precentral unit activity and correlated responses in adjacent cells and contralateral muscles. *J. Neurophysiol.* **36**, 179–204.   [304]

FETZ, E. E. and CHENEY, P. D. (1976). Terminal distribution of corticomotoneuronal cells in alert monkeys. *Neurosci. Abst.* **2**, 540.   [295]

FETZ, E. E. and FINOCCHIO, D. V. (1971). Operant conditioning of specific patterns of neural and muscular activity. *Science, N.Y.* **174**, 431–435.   [292]

FETZ, E. E. and FINOCCHIO, D. V. (1972). Operant conditioning of isolated activity in specific muscles and precentral cells. *Brain Res.* **40**, 19–24. [292, 297]

FETZ, E. E. and FINOCCHIO, D. V. (1975). Correlations between activity of motor cortex cells and arm muscles during operantly conditioned response patterns. *Expl. Brain Res.* **23**, 217–240. [273]

FETZ, F. E., BAKER, M. A., FINOCCHIO, D. V. and SOSO, M. J. (1974). Responses of precentral 'motor' cortex cells during passive and active joint movements. *Soc. Neurosci.* 4th Ann. Meet. p. 208. [237]

FETZ, E. E., GERMAN, D. C. and CHENEY, P. D. (1975). Connections between motor cortex cells and motoneurons revealed by correlation techniques in awake monkeys. *Neurosci. Abst.* **1**, 163. [295]

FIDONE, S. J. and PRESTON, J. B. (1969). Patterns of motor cortex control of flexor and extensor fusimotor neurons. *J. Neurophysiol.* **32**, 103–115. [134, 150]

FLOWERS, K. A. (1976). Visual 'closed loop' and 'open loop' characteristics of voluntary movement in patients with Parkinsonism and intention tremor. *Brain,* **99**, 269–310. [369]

FOERSTER, O. (1927). Schlaffe und spastische Lähmung. *In* 'Handbuch der normalen und pathologischen Physiologie' (Eds A. Bethe, G.v. Bergmann, G. Embden and A. Ellinger), vol. 10, pp. 900–901. Springer, Berlin. [382]

FRANCOIS-FRANCK, C. E. (1887). 'Lecons sur les Fonctions Motrices du Cerveau'. Doin, Paris. [5, 27, 36]

FREUND, H.-J., BÜDINGEN, H. J. and DIETZ, V. (1975). Activity of single motor units from human forearm muscles during voluntary isometric contractions. *J. Neurophysiol.* **38**, 933–946. [345]

FRITSCH, G. and HITZIG, E. (1870). Uber die elektrische Erregbarkeit des Grosshirns. *Archs Anat. Physiol. Wiss.* Med. **37**, 300–332. (Translation by Bonin, G. Von. *In* 'The Cerebral Cortex', pp. 73–96. C. C. Thomas, Springfield.) [5, 22, 23, 79, 82]

FULTON, J. F. (1943). 'Physiology of the Nervous System' (2nd ed.), p. 499. Oxford University Press, London. [7]

FULTON, J. F. (1949). 'Functional Localization in the Frontal Lobes and Cerebellum'. Clarendon Press, Oxford. [40, 41]

GELLHORN, E. and HYDE, J. (1953). Influence of proprioception on map of cortical responses. *J. Physiol.* **122**, 371–385. [43]

GERBRANDT, L. K., GOFF, W. R. and SMITH, D. B. (1973). Distribution of the human average movement potential. *Electroen. Neurophysiol.* **34**, 461–474. [313]

GHELARDUCCI, B., ITO, M. and YAGI, N. (1975). Impulse discharges from flocculus Purkinje cells of alert rabbits during visual stimulation combined with horizontal head rotation. *Brain Res.* **87**, 66–72. [226]

GIBSON, J. J. (1962). Observations on active touch. *Psychol. Rev.* **69**, 477–491. [392]

GILDEN, L., VAUGHAN, H. G. Jr. and COSTA, L. D. (1966). Summated human EEG potentials with voluntary movement. *Electroen. Neurophysiol.* **20**, 433–438. [312]

GILMAN, S., CARR, D. and HOLLENBERG, J. (1976). Kinematic effects of deafferentation and cerebellar ablation. *Brain,* **99**, 311–330. [374]

GLEES, P. and COLE, J. (1950). Recovery of skilled motor functions after small repeated lesions of motor cortex in macaque. *J. Neurophysiol.* **13**, 137–148. [31]

GOLDRING, S. and RATCHESON, R. (1972). Human motor cortex: Sensory input data from single neuron recordings. *Science, N.Y.* **175**, 1493–1495. [260, 277, 314]

GOLDRING, S., ARAS, E. and WEBER, P. C. (1970). Comparative study of sensory input to motor cortex in animals and man. *Electroen. Neurophysiol.* **29**, 537–550.   [313]

GONSHOR, A. and MELVILL JONES, G. (1976). Extreme vestibulo-ocular adaptation induced by prolonged optical reversal of vision. *J. Physiol.* **256**, 381–414. [226]

GOODWIN, G. M. and LUSCHEI, E. E. (1975). Discharge of spindle afferents from jaw-closing muscles during chewing in alert monkeys. *J. Neurophysiol.* **38**, 560–571.   [304]

GOODWIN, G. M., McCLOSKEY, D. I. and MATTHEWS, P. B. C. (1972). The contribution of muscle afferents to kinaesthesia shown by vibration-induced illusions of movement and by the effects of paralysing joint afferents. *Brain*, **95**, 705–748.   [380, 381, 383, 386, 388, 389, 390]

GORDON, G. (1968). Recherches sur la fonction des noyaux somesthésiques primaires chez le chat. Actualités Neurophysiologiques, Huitième Série (Ed. A.-M. Monnier), pp. 89–110. Ed. Masson, Paris.   [115]

GORDON, G. and MILLER, R. (1969). Identification of cortical cells projecting to the dorsal column nuclei of the cat. *Q. Jl exp. Physiol.* **54**, 85–98.
                                                                                                        [55, 111, 114]

GOWERS, W. R. (1899). 'A Manual of Diseases of the Nervous System' (Eds W. R. Gowers and J. Taylor), vol. I. Churchill, London.   [379, 381, 382]

GRANIT, R. (1955). 'Receptors and Sensory Perception', p. 268. Yale University Press, New Haven.   [350]

GRANIT, R. (1968). The functional role of the muscle spindle's primary end organs. *Proc. R. Soc. Med.* **61**, 69–78.   [350]

GRANIT, R. (1970). 'The Basis Of Motor Control'. Academic Press, London and New York.   [345]

GRANIT, R. (1973). Demand and accomplishment in voluntary movement. *In* 'Control of Posture and Locomotion' (Eds R. B. Stein, K. B. Pearson, R. S. Smith and J. B. Redford). Plenum Press, New York.   [333]

GRANIT, R. (1975). The functional role of the muscle spindles—facts and hypotheses. *Brain*, **98**, 531–556.   [353, 382]

GRANIT, R. and BURKE, R. E. (1973). The control of movement and posture (Conference report). *Brain Res.* **53**, 1–28.   [347]

GRANIT, R. and KAADA, B. R. (1952). Influence of stimulation of central nervous structures on muscle spindles in cat. *Acta physiol. scand.* **27**, 130–160.   [134]

GRANIT, R. and PHILLIPS, C. G. (1957). Effects on Purkinje cells of surface stimulation of the cerebellum. *J. Physiol.* **135**, 73–92.   [217]

GRANT, G., LANDGREN, S. and SILFVENIUS, H. (1975). Columnar distribution of U-fibres from the postcruciate cerebral projection area of the cat's Group I muscle afferents. *Expl Brain Res.* **24**, 57–74.   [224]

GRAY, E. G. (1959). Axo-somatic and axodendritic synapses of the cerebral cortex: an electron microscope study. *J. Anat.* **93**, 420–433.   [54, 207]

GRAY, E. G. and GUILLERY, R. W. (1966). Synaptic morphology in the normal and degenerating nervous system. *Int. Rev. Cytol.* **19**, 111–182.   [95]

GRIGG, P. and PRESTON, J. B. (1971). Baboon flexor and extensor fusimotor neurons and their modulation by motor cortex. *J. Neurophysiol.* **34**, 428–436.
                                                                                                        [150, 151]

GRILLNER, S. (1970). Is the tonic stretch reflex dependent upon Group II excitation? *Acta physiol. scand.* **78**, 431–432.   [353]

GRIMBY, L. and HANNERZ, J. (1968). Recruitment order of motor units on voluntary contraction: changes induced by proprioceptive afferent activity. *J. Neurol. Neurosurg. Psychiat.* **31**, 565–573.   [346]

GRIMM, R. J. and RUSHMER, D. S. (1974). The activity of dentate neurons during an arm movement sequence. *Brain Res.* **71**, 309–326. [309]

GUSTAFSSON, B. and JANKOWSKA, E. (1976). Direct and indirect activation of nerve cells by electrical pulses applied extracellularly. *J. Physiol.* **258**, 33–61. [181]

HAAXMA, R. and KUYPERS, H. G. J. M. (1975). Intrahemispheric cortical connexions and visual guidance of hand and finger movements in the rhesus monkey. *Brain*, **98**, 239–260. [377, 378]

HAGBARTH, K.-E. and EKLUND, G. (1966). Motor effects of vibratory muscle stimuli in man. *In* 'Muscular Afferents and Motor Control' (Ed. R. Granit), pp. 177–186. Almqvist & Wiksell, Stockholm. [371, 385, 386]

HAGBARTH, K.-E. and VALLBO, Å. B. (1969). Single unit recordings from muscle nerves in human subjects. *Acta physiol. scand.* **76**, 321–334. [337, 351]

HALLETT, M., SHAHANI, B. T. and YOUNG, R. R. (1975a). E.M.G. analysis of stereotyped voluntary movements in man. *J. Neurol. Neurosurg. Psychiat.* **38**, 1154–1162. [337, 340, 341, 344]

HALLETT, M., SHAHANI, B. T. and YOUNG, R. R. (1975b). E.M.G. analysis of patients with cerebellar deficits. *J. Neurol. Neurosurg. Psychiat.* **38**, 1163–1169. [368]

HAMMOND, P. H. (1956). The influence of prior instruction to the subject on an apparently involuntary neuro-muscular response. *J. Physiol.* **132**, 17–18P. [354]

HAMMOND, P. H. (1960). An experimental study of servo action in human muscular control. *Proc. III. Int. Con. Med. Elect.* 190–199. Institution of Electrical Engineers, London. [354]

HAMMOND, P. H., MERTON, P. A. and SUTTON, C. G. (1956). Nervous gradation of muscular contraction. *Br. med. Bull.* **12**, 214–218. [349]

HARVEY, R. J., PORTER, R. and RAWSON, J. A. (1976). Activity related to the performance of a learned motor task in Purkinje cells of the intermediate zone of the monkey cerebellum. *Proc. Aust. Physiol. Pharmacol. Soc.* **7**, 25. [310]

HASSLER, R. and MUHS-CLEMENT, K. (1964). Architektonischer Aufbau des sensomotorischen und parietalen Cortex der Katze. *J. Hirnforsch.* **6**, 377–420. [223]

HEAD, H. (1920). 'Studies in Neurology', vol. II, pp. 605–608. Henry Frowde and Hodder & Stoughton, London. [378]

HEBB, D. O. (1949). 'The Organization of Behavior. A Neuropsychological Theory'. John Wiley, New York. [322]

HENNEMAN, E., SOMJEN, G. and CARPENTER, D. O. (1965). Functional significance of cell size in spinal motoneurons. *J. Neurophysiol.* **28**, 460–580. [345]

HEPP-REYMOND, M.-C. and WIESENDANGER, M. (1972). Unilateral pyramidotomy in monkeys: effect on force and speed of a conditioned precision grip. *Brain Res.* **36**, 117–131. [362]

HEPP-REYMOND, M.-C., TROUCHE, E. and WIESENDANGER, M. (1974). Effects of unilateral and bilateral pyramidotomy on a conditioned rapid precision grip in monkeys (*Macaca fascicularis*). *Expl Brain Res.* **21**, 519–527. [362]

HERN, J. E. C., LANDGREN, S., PHILLIPS, C. G. and PORTER, R. (1962). Selective excitation of corticofugal neurones by surface-anodal stimulation of the baboon's motor cortex. *J. Physiol.* **161**, 73–00. [82, 88]

HERN, J. E. C., PHILLIPS, C. G. and PORTER, R. (1962). Electrical thresholds of unimpaled corticospinal cells in the cat. *Q. Jl exp. Physiol.* **47**, 134–140. [81]

HERRICK, C. J. (1948). 'The Brain of the Tiger-Salamander'. Chicago. [321]

HINES, M. (1944). Significance of the precentral motor cortex. *In* 'The Precentral Motor Cortex' (Ed. P. C. Bucy), pp. 461–494. University of Illinois, Illinois. [40]

HODGKIN, A. L. (1948). The local electric changes associated with repetitive action in a non-medullated axon. *J. Physiol.* **107**, 165–181. [60]

HOFF, E. C. and HOFF, H. E. (1934). Spinal terminations of the projection fibres from the motor cortex of primates. *Brain,* **57**, 454–474. [95]

HOLMES, G. (1917). The symptoms of acute cerebellar injuries due to gunshot injuries. *Brain,* **40**, 461–535. [399]

HOLMES, G. (1927). Local epilepsy. *Lancet,* i, 957–962. [31, 38, 43]

HOLMES, G. (1939). The cerebellum of man. *Brain,* **62**, 1–30. [369]

HOLMES, G. (1946). 'Introduction to Clinical Neurology'. Livingstone, Edinburgh. [379]

HOLMES, G. and MAY, W. P. (1909). On the exact origin of the pyramidal tracts in man and other mammals. *Brain,* **32**, 1–43. [96, 99, 135]

HONGO, T. and JANKOWSKA, E. (1967). Effects from the sensorimotor cortex on the spinal cord in cats with transected pyramids. *Expl Brain Res.* **3**, 117–134. [109]

HONGO, T., JANKOWSKA, E. and LUNDBERG, A. (1969a). The rubrospinal tract. I. Effects of alpha-motoneurones innervating hindlimb muscles in cats. *Expl Brain Res.* **7**, 344–364. [109]

HONGO, T., JANKOWSKA, E. and LUNDBERG, A. (1969b). The rubrospinal tract. II. Facilitation of interneuronal transmission in reflex paths to motoneurones. *Expl Brain Res.* **7**, 365–391. [109, 147]

HORE, J. and PORTER, R. (1971). The role of the pyramidal tract in the production of cortically evoked movement in the brush-tailed possum. (*Trichosurus vulpecula*). *Brain Res.* **30**, 232–234. [47]

HORE, J., PHILLIPS, C. G. and PORTER, R. (1973). The effects of pyramidotomy on motor performance in the brush-tailed possum (*Trichosurus vulpecula*). *Brain Res.* **49**, 181–184. [359]

HORE, J., PRESTON, J. B. DURKOVIC, R. G. and CHENEY, P. D. (1976). Responses of Cortical Neurons (Areas 3a and 4) to Ramp stretch of Hindlimb Muscles in the Baboon. *J. Neurophysiol.* **39**, 484–500. [232]

HORSLEY, V. (1909). The Linacre Lecture on the function of the so-called motor area of the brain. *Br. Med. J.* **2**, 125–132. [28, 32, 372]

HORSLEY, V. and SCHÄFER, E. A. (1888). A record of experiments upon the functions of the cerebral cortex. *Phil. Trans. R. Soc. B.* **179**, 1–45. [27]

HUBEL, D. H. and WIESEL, T. N. (1962). Receptive fields, binocular interaction and functional architecture in the cat's visual cortex. *J. Physiol.* **160**, 106–154. [208]

HUFSCHMIDT, H.-J. and HUFSCHMIDT, T. (1954). Antagonist inhibition as the earliest sign of a sensory-motor reaction. *Nature, Lond.* **174**, 607. [337]

HULTBORN, H., JANKOWSKA, E. and LINDSTRÖM, S. (1971a). Recurrent inhibition from motor axon collaterals of transmission in the Ia inhibitory pathway to motoneurones. *J. Physiol.* **215**, 591–612. [146]

HULTBORN, H., JANKOWSKA, E. and LINDSTRÖM, S. (1971b). Recurrent inhibition of interneurones monosynaptically activated from group Ia afferents. *J. Physiol.* **215**, 613–636. [146]

HUMPHREY, D. R. (1972). Relating motor cortex spike trains to measures of motor performance. *Brain Res.* **40**, 7–18. [287]

HUMPHREY, D. R., SCHMIDT, E. M. and THOMPSON, W. D. (1970). Predicting measures of motor performance from multiple cortical spike trains. *Science,* **179**, 758–762. [288]

ILLERT, M., LUNDBERG, A. and TANAKA, R. (1974). Disynaptic corticospinal effects in forelimb motoneurones in the cat. *Brain Res.* **75**, 312–315. [129, 197, 200]

JACKSON, J. H. (1875). Cases of partial convulsion from organic brain disease, bearing on the experiments of Hitzig and Ferrier. *Medical Times and Gazette*, 1, 578–579. [30]

JACKSON, J. H. (1886). Discussion of brain surgery by V. Horsley. *Br. Med. J.* 2, 674–675. [30]

JACKSON, J. H. (1931). 'Selected Writings of John Hughlings Jackson' (Ed. J. Taylor), vol. I. Hodder & Stoughton, London.
[22, 23, 26, 30, 31, 36, 323, 324, 325, 326, 327]

JACKSON, J. H. (1932). 'Selected Writings of John Hughlings Jackson' (Ed. J. Taylor), vol. II. Hodder & Stoughton, London.
[3, 9, 29, 30, 31, 323, 326, 327]

JANKOWSKA, E., PADEL and TANAKA, R. (1975a). The mode of activation of pyramidal tract cells by intracortical stimuli. *J. Physiol.* 249, 617–636.
[177, 178, 179, 180, 181, 183]

JANKOWSKA, E., PADEL and TANAKA, R. (1975b). Projections of pyramidal tract cells to amotoneurones innervating hind-limb muscles in the monkey. *J. Physiol.* 249, 637–667.
[76, 147, 169, 177, 181, 182, 190, 191, 196, 208, 209, 213]

JANKOWSKA, E. and ROBETSR, W. J. (1972). An electrophysiological demonstration of the axonal projections of single spinal interneurones in the cat. *J. Physiol.* 222, 597–622. [176]

JANKOWSKA, E. and TANAKA, R. (1974). Neuronal mechanism of the disynaptic inhibition evoked in primate spinal motoneurones from the corticospinal tract. *Brain Res.* 75, 163–166. [146, 339]

JANSEN, J. K. S. and RUDJORD, T. (1965). Dorsal spinocerebellar tract: response pattern of nerve fibres to muscle stretch. *Science, N.Y.* 149, 1109–1111. [335]

JASPER, H. H. and BERTRAND, G. (1966). Thalamic units involved in somatic sensation and voluntary and involuntary movements in man. *In* 'The Thalamus' (Eds D. P. Purpura and M. D. Yahr), pp. 365–390. Columbia University Press, New York. [255]

JASPER, H. and PENFIELD, W. (1949). Electrocorticograms in man: effect of voluntary movement upon the electrical activity of the precentral gyrus. *Arch. Psychiat. Nervankh*, 183, 163–174. [311]

JEFFERSON, G. (1953). The prodromes to cortical localization. *J. Neurol. Neurosurg. Psychiat.* 16, 59–72. [6, 93]

JOFFROY, A. J. and LAMARRE, Y. (1974). Single cell activity in the ventral lateral thalamus of the unanaesthetized monkey. *Expl Neurol.* 42, 1–16. [254]

JONES, E. G. (1975). Lamination and differential distribution of thalamic afferents within the sensory-motor cortex of the squirrel monkey. *J. comp. Neurol.* 160, 167–204. [96, 211, 228]

JONES, E. G. and POWELL, T. P. S. (1968). The ipsilateral cortical connexions of the somatic sensory areas in the cat. *Brain Res.* 9, 71–94. [223, 224]

JONES, E. G. and POWELL, T. P. S. (1969). Connexions of the somatic sensory cortex of the rhesus monkey. II. Contralateral cortical connexions. *Brain*, 92, 717–730. [372]

JUNG, R. and DIETZ, V. (1975). Verzögerter Start der Willkürbewegung bei Pyramidenläsionen des Menschen. *Arch. Psychiat. Nervkrankh.* 221, 87–109. [370]

KATO, M. and TANJI, J. (1972). Conscious control of motor units of human finger muscles. *In* 'Neurophysiology Studied in Man' (Ed. G. G. Somjen). Excerpta Medica, Amsterdam. [313, 347]

KAY, R. H. (1964). 'Experimental Biology', pp. 293–304. Reinhold, New York. [115]

KEMP, J. M. and POWELL, T. P. S. (1971). The connexions of the striatum and globus pallidus: synthesis and speculation. *Phil. Trans. R. Soc. B.* **262**, 441–457. [9, 101, 104, 109, 215, 216, 228]

KENNARD, M. A. (1938). Reorganization of motor function in the cerebral cortex of monkeys deprived of motor areas in infancy. *J. Neurophysiol.* **1**, 477–496. [358]

KERNELL, D. (1966a). Input resistance, electrical excitability, and size of ventral horn cells in cat spinal cord. *Science, N.Y.* **152**, 1637–1640. [58, 345]

KERNELL, D. (1966b). The repetitive discharge of motoneurones. *In* 'Muscular Afferents and Motor Control' (Ed. R. Granit), pp. 351–362. Nobel Symposium. I. John Wiley, New York. [59]

KERNELL, D. and Wu Chien-Ping. (1967a). Responses of the pyramidal tract to stimulation of the baboon's motor cortex. *J. Physiol.* **191**, 653–672. [66, 88]

KERNELL, D. and Wu Chien-Ping. (1967b). Post-synaptic effects of cortical stimulation on forelimb motoneurones in the baboon. *J. Physiol.* **191**, 673–690. [67]

KIEVIT, J. and KUYPERS, H. G. J. M. (1975). Subcortical afferents to the frontal lobe in the rhesus monkey studied by means of retrograde horseradish peroxidase transport. *Brain Res.* **85**, 261–266. [228, 254, 255]

KIRKWOOD, P. A. and SEARS, T. A. (1975). Monosynaptic excitation of motoneurones from muscle spindle secondary endings of intercostal and triceps surae muscles in the cat. *J. Physiol.* **245**, 64–66P. [353]

KLEE, M. R. and LUX, H. D. (1962). Intracelluläre Untersuchungen über den Einfluss hemmender potentiale im motorischen Cortex. II. Die Wirkungen elektrischer Reizung des Nucleus caudatus. *Arch. Psychiat. Nervkrankh.* **203**, 667–689. [110, 215]

KNAPP, H. D., TAUB, E. and BERMAN, A. J. (1963). Movements in monkeys with deafferented forelimbs. *Expl Neurol.* **7**, 305–315. [373]

KOEZE, T. H., PHILLIPS, C. G. and SHERIDAN, J. D. (1968). Thresholds of cortical activation of muscle spindles and α motoneurones of the baboon's hand. *J. Physiol.* **195**, 419–449. [151, 353]

KOIKE, H., OKADA, Y. and OSHIMA, T. (1968a). Accommodative properties of fast and slow pyramidal tract cells and their modification by different levels of their membrane potential. *Expl Brain Res.* **5**, 189–201. [58]

KOIKE, H., OKADA, Y., OSHIMA, T. and TAKAHASHI, K. (1968b). Accommodative behavior of cat pyramidal tract cells investigated with intracellular injection of currents. *Expl Brain Res.* **5**, 173–188. [58]

KOIKE, H., MANO, N., OKADA, Y. and OSHIMA, T. (1970). Repetitive impulses generated in fast and slow pyramidal tract cells by intracellularly applied current steps. *Expl Brain Res.* **11**, 263–281. [58, 59]

KOIKE, H., MANO, N., OKADA, Y. and OSHIMA, T. (1972). Activities of the sodium pump in cat pyramidal tract cells investigated with intracellular injection of sodium ions. *Expl Brain Res.* **14**, 449–462. [58]

KORNHUBER, H. H. (1971). Motor functions of cerebellum and basal ganglia: the cerebellocortical saccadic (ballistic) clock, the cerebellonuclear hold regulator, and the basal ganglia ramp (voluntary speed smooth movement) generator. *Kybernetik,* **8**, 157–162. (By Springer-Verlag, 1971.) [310, 344]

KOSTYUK, P. G. and VASILENKO, D. A. (1968). Transformation of cortical motor signals in spinal cord. *Proc. Inst. Elect. Engrs,* **56**, 1049–1058. [129]

KRNJEVIĆ, K. and SCHWARTZ, S. (1967). The action of gamma-aminobutyric acid on cortical neurones. *Expl Brain Res.* **3**, 320–336. [65]

KRUEGER, L. E. (1970). David Katz's Der Aufbau der tastwelt (the world of touch): a synopsis. *Percept. Psychophys.* **7**, 337–341. [392]

KUBOTA, K. and NIKI, H. (1971). Prefrontal cortical unit activity and delayed alteration performance in monkeys. *J. Neurophysiol.* **34**, 337–347. [307]

KUNO, M. and WEAKLY, J. N. (1972). Facilitation of monosynaptic excitatory synaptic potentials in spinal motoneurones evoked by internuncial impulses. *J. Physiol.* **224**, 271–286. [76]

KÜNZLE, H. and WIESENDANGER, M. (1974). Pyramidal connections to the lateral reticular nucleus in the cat: a degeneration study. *Acta anat.* **88**, 105–114. [119]

KUYPERS, H. G. J. M. (1958). An anatomical analysis of cortico-bulbar connexions to the pons and lower brain stem in the cat. *J. Anat.* **92**, 198–218. [101, 119, 120, 121]

KUYPERS, H. G. J. M. (1960). Central cortical projections to motor and somato-sensory cell groups. (An experimental study in the Rhesus monkey). *Brain,* **83**, 161–184. [136]

KUYPERS, H. G. J. M. (1964). The descending pathways to the spinal cord, their anatomy and function. *In* Progress in Brain Research, 'Organization of the Spinal Cord' (Eds J. C. Eccles and J. P. Schadé), vol. 11, pp. 178–202. Elsevier, Amsterdam. [15, 137]

KUYPERS, H. G. J. M. and TUERK, J. D. (1964). The distribution of the cortical fibres within the nuclei cuneatus and gracilis in the cat. *J. Anat.* **98**, 143–162. [115]

LANCE, J. W. (1954). Pyramidal tract in spinal cord of cat. *J. Neurophysiol.* **17**, 253–270. [58]

LANCE, J. W. and MANNING, R. L. (1954). Origin of the pyramidal tract in the cat. *J. Physiol.* **124**, 385–399. [58, 97, 99]

LANDAU, W. M., BISHOP, G. H. and CLARE, M. H. (1965). Site of excitation in stimulation of the motor cortex. *J. Neurophysiol.* **28**, 1206–1222. [85]

LANDGREN, S. and SILFVENIUS, H. (1968). Cortical projections of Group I muscle afferents from the hindlimb. *Acta physiol. scand.* **73**, 14A–15A. [223]

LANDGREN, S. and SILFVENIUS, H. (1969). Projection to cerebral cortex of Group 1 muscle afferents from the cat's hindlimb. *J. Physiol.* **200**, 353–372. [223]

LANDGREN, S. and SILFVENIUS, H. (1971). Nucleus Z, the medullary relay in the projection path to the cerebral cortex of Group I muscle afferents from the cat's hindlimb. *J. Physiol.* **218**, 551–571. [223]

LANDGREN, S., PHILLIPS, C. G. and PORTER, R. (1962a). Minimal synaptic actions of pyramidal impulses on some alpha motoneurones of the baboon's hand and forearm. *J. Physiol.* **161**, 91–111. [65, 145]

LANDGREN, S., PHILLIPS, C. G. and PORTER, R. (1962b). Cortical fields of origin of the monosynaptic pyramidal pathways to some alpha motoneurones of the baboon's hand and forearm. *J. Physiol.* **161**, 112–125. [88, 155, 160, 163, 168, 170, 171, 172, 195]

LASHLEY, K. S. (1950). In search of the engram. *In* Symp. Soc. exp. Biol. no. 4, pp. 454–483, Cambridge University Press, Cambridge. [9, 205, 329, 364]

LASSEK, A. M. (1948). The pyramidal tract: basic considerations of corticospinal neurons. *Res. Publs Ass. nerv. ment. Dis.* **27**, 106–128. [10, 95, 135]

LASSEK, A. M. and KARLSBERG, P. (1956). The pyramidal tract of an aquatic carnivore. *J. comp. Neurol.* **106**, 425–531. [13]

LAURSEN, A. M. (1970). Selective increase in choice latency after transection of a pyramidal tract in monkeys. *Brain Res.* **24**, 544–545. [363]

LAURSEN, A. M. and WIESENDANGER, M. (1966). Motor deficits after transection of a bulbar pyramid in the cat. *Acta physiol. scand.* **68**, 118–126. [360]

LAURSEN, A. M. and WIESENDANGER, M. (1967). The effect of pyramidal lesions on response latency in cats. *Brain Res.* **5**, 207–220.   [360, 363]

LAWRENCE, D. G. and HOPKINS, D. A. (1976). The development of motor control in the rhesus monkey: evidence concerning the role of corticomotoneuronal connections. *Brain,* **99**, 235–254.   [362]

LAWRENCE, D. G. and KUYPERS, H. G. J. M. (1968). The functional organization of the motor system in the monkey. I. The effects of bilateral pyramidal lesions. *Brain,* **91**, 1–14.   [290, 361, 362, 366]

LEMON, R. N., HANBY, J. A. and PORTER, R. (1976). Relationship between the activity of precentral neurones during active and passive movements in conscious monkeys. *Proc. R. Soc. B.* **194**, 341–373.   [237, 258, 273, 277]

LEMON, R. N. and PORTER, R. (1976). Afferent input to movement-related precentral neurones in conscious monkeys. *Proc. R. Soc. B.* **194**, 313–339.
                                      [196, 214, 241, 245, 249, 251, 304]

LE VAY, S., HUBEL, D. H. and WIESEL, T. N. (1975). The pattern of ocular dominance columns in macaque visual cortex revealed by a reduced silver stain. *J. comp. Neurol.* **159**, 559–576.   [209]

LEWIS, M. McD. (1974). Pyramidal Tract Discharge Related to Voluntary Movement Performance: Ph.D. Thesis, Monash University.   [268]

LEWIS, R. and BRINDLEY, G. S. (1965). The extrapyramidal cortical motor map. *Brain,* **88**, part II, 397–406.   [48]

LEWIS, M. McD. and PORTER, R. (1974). Pyramidal tract discharge in relation to movement performance in monkeys with partial anaesthesia of the moving hand. *Brain Res.* **71**, 245–251.   [286, 299, 300]

LEYTON, A. S. F. and SHERRINGTON, C. S. (1917). Observations on the excitable cortex of the chimpanzee, orang-utan and gorilla. *Q. Jl exp. Physiol.* **11**, 135–222.   [28, 31, 32, 37, 38, 79, 138, 336, 364]

LI, C-L. and TEW, J. M. Jr. (1964). Reciprocal activation and inhibition of cortical neurones and voluntary movements in man: cortical cell activity and muscle movement. *Nature, Lond.* **203**, 264–265.   [314]

LIDDELL, E. G. T. (1960). 'The Discovery of Reflexes'. Clarendon Press, Oxford.
                                                          [5, 7, 21, 93]

LIDDELL, E. G. T. and PHILLIPS, C. G. (1944). Pyramidal section in the cat. *Brain,* **67**, 1–00.   [360]

LIDDELL, E. G. T. and PHILLIPS, C. G. (1950). Thresholds of cortical representation. *Brain,* **73**, 125–140.   [45]

LIU, C. N. and CHAMBERS, W. W. (1964). An experimental study of the corticospinal system in the monkey (*Macaca mulatta*). (The spinal pathway and preterminal distribution of degenerating fibres following discrete lesions of the pre- and postcentral gyri and bulbar pyramid.) *J. comp. Neurol.* **123**, 257–284.   [15]

LIVINGSTON, A. and PHILLIPS, C. G. (1957). Maps and thresholds for the sensorimotor cortex of the cat. *Q. Jl exp. Physiol.* **42**, 190–205.   [79]

LLOYD, D. P. C. (1941). The spinal mechanism of the pyramidal system in cats. *J. Neurophysiol.* **4**, 525–546.   [124]

LONG, C. and BROWN, M. E. (1964). Electromyographic kinesiology of the hand: muscles moving the long finger. *J. Bone Jt Surg.* **46A**, 1683–1706.   [336]

LORENTE DE NÓ, R. (1938). Cerebral cortex: architecture, intracortical connexions, motor projections. *In* 'Physiology of the Nervous System' (Ed. J. F. Fulton), Oxford University Press, London.   [208]

LUCIER, G. E., RÜEGG, D. C. and WIESENDANGER, M. (1975). Responses of neurones in the motor cortex and in area 3a to controlled stretches of forelimb muscles in cebus monkeys. *J. Physiol.* **251**, 833–853. [232, 233]

LUND, J. P. and LAMARRE, Y. (1973). The importance of positive feedback from periodontal pressoreceptors during voluntary isometric contraction of jaw closing muscles in man. *J. biol. Buccale,* **1**, 345–351. [394]

LUND, J. P. and LAMARRE, Y. (1974). Activity of neurons in the lower precentral cortex during voluntary and rhythmical jaw movements in the monkey. *Expl Brain Res.* **19**, 282–299. [394]

LUNDBERG, A. (1959). Integrative significance of patterns of connections made by muscle afferents in the spinal cord. XXI Congreso Internacional de Ciencias Fisiologicas, Buenos Aires 9–15 Aug. pp. 100–105. [350]

LUNDBERG, A. (1964). Supraspinal control of transmission in reflex paths to motoneurones and primary afferents. *In* 'Progress in Brain Research', vol. 12, pp. 197–221. Elsevier, Amsterdam, London, New York. [76]

LUNDBERG, A. and VOORHOEVE, P. (1962). Effects from the pyramidal tract on spinal reflex arcs. *Acta physiol. scand.* **56**, 201–219. [128]

LUNDBERG, A., NORRSELL, U. and VOORHOEVE, P. (1962). Pyramidal effects on lumbo-sacral interneurones activated by somatic afferents. *Acta physiol. scand.* **56**, 220–229. [128]

LUSCHEI, E. S., GARTHWAITE, C. R. and ARMSTRONG, M. E. (1971). Relationship of firing patterns of units in face area of monkey precentral cortex to conditioned jaw movements. *J. Neurophysiol.* **34**, 552–562. [306]

LUX, H. D. and KLEE, M. R. (1962). Intracelluläre Untersuchungen uber den Einfluss hemmender Potentiale im motorischen cortex. I. Die Wirkung elektrischer Reizung unspezifischer Thalamuskerne. *Arch. Psychiat. Nervkrankh* **203**, 648–666. [215]

McCLOSKEY, D. I. (1973). Differences between the senses of movement and position shown by the effects of loading and vibration of muscles in man. *Brain Res.* **61**, 119–131. [386]

McCLOSKEY, D. I. and TORDA, T. A. G. (1975). Corollary motor discharges and kinaesthesia. *Brain Res.* **100**, 467–470. [388]

McCLOSKEY, D. I., EBELING, P. and GOODWIN, G. M. (1974). Estimation of weights and tensions and apparent involvement of a 'sense of effort'. *Expl Neurol.* **42**, 220–332. [380]

MAGNI, F., MELZACK, R., MORUZZI, G. and SMITH, C. J. (1959). Direct pyramidal influences on the dorsal-column nuclei. *Archs ital. Biol.* **97**, 357–377. [112]

MAGNI, R. and WILLIS, W. D. (1964a). Subcortical and peripheral control of brain stem reticular neurons. *Archs. ital. Biol.* **102**, 434–448. [76, 110]

MAGNI, F. and WILLIS, W. D. (1964b). Afferent connections to reticulo-spinal neurons. *In* 'Progress in Brain Research: Physiology of Spinal Neurons' (Eds J. C. Eccles and J. P. Schadé), vol. 12, pp. 246–258. Elsevier, Amsterdam, London, New York. [76, 110]

MALIS, L. I., PRIBRAM, K. H. and KRUGER, L. (1953). Action potentials in 'motor' cortex evoked by peripheral nerve stimulation. *J. Neurophysiol.* **16**, 161–167. [229, 254]

MARSDEN, C. D., MERTON, P. A. and MORTON, H. B. (1972). Servo action in human voluntary movement. *Nature, Lond.* **238**, 140–143. [304, 315, 354, 355]

MARSDEN, C. D., MERTON, P. A. and MORTON, H. B. (1973). Is the human stretch reflex cortical rather than spinal? *Lancet,* **i**, 759–761. [368]

RSDEN, C. D., MERTON, P. A., MORTON, H. B., HALLETT, M., ADAM, J. and
RUSHTON, D. N. (1977). Disorders of movement in cerebellar disease in man.
In 'The Physiological Aspect of Clinical Neurology' (Ed. F. Clifford Rose),
pp. 179–199. Blackwells, Oxford.   [338, 342, 344, 356, 368]

MARSHALL, C. (1934). Experimental lesions of the pyramidal tract. *Archs Neurol.
Psychiat., Chicago,* **32**, 778–796.   [360]

MARSHALL, C. (1936). The functions of the pyramidal tracts. *Q. Rev. Biol.* **11**,
35–56.   [106]

MASSION, J. (1973). Le mouvement et son organisation centrale. *Archs ital. Biol.*
111, 481–492.   [4, 215]

MASSION, J. and PAILLARD, J. (1974) (eds). Motor aspects of behaviour and programmed nervous activities. Colloques Internationaux du CNRS No. 226,
Brain Res. **71**, 189–575.   [215]

MATTHEWS, P. B. C. (1964). Muscle spindles and their motor control. *Physiol. Rev.*
44, 219–288.   [135, 350]

MATTHEWS, P. B. C. (1969). Evidence that the secondary as well as the primary
endings of the muscle spindles may be responsible for the tonic stretch reflex
of the decerebrate cat. *J. Physiol.* **204**, 365–393.   [353]

MATTHEWS, P. B. C. (1970). A reply to criticism of the hypothesis that the group II
afferents contribute excitation to the stretch reflex. *Acta physiol. scand.* **79**,
431–433.   [353]

MATTHEWS, P. B. C. (1972). 'Mammalian Muscle Receptors and their Central
Actions'. Arnold, London.   [132, 135, 233, 350]

MATTHEWS, P. B. C. and SIMMONDS, A. (1974). Sensations of finger movement
elicited by pulling upon flexor tendons in man. *J. Physiol.* **239**, 27–28P.   [383]

MEGAW, E. D. (1974). Possible modification to a rapid on-going programmed
manual response. *Brain Res.* **71**, 425–441.   [334, 341]

MEGIRIAN, D. and TROTH, R. (1964). Vestibular and muscle nerve connections
to pyramidal tract neurons of cat. *J. Neurophysiol.* **27**, 481–492.   [218]

MERTON, P. A. (1953). Speculations on the servo-control of movement. Ciba
Foundation symposium on the spinal cord (Eds J. L. Malcolm and J. A. B.
Gray), pp. 247–255. Churchill, London.   [349, 350, 356]

MERTON, P. A. (1964). Human position sense and sense of effort. Symposia of the
Society for Experimental Biology, **18**, 387–400.   [383]

METTLER, F. A., ADES, H. W., LIPMAN, E. and CULLER, E. A. (1939). The extrapyramidal system: an experimental demonstration of function. *Arch. Neurol.
Psychiat.* **41**, 984–995.   [215]

MEYER, J. S. and HERNDON, R. M. (1962). Bilateral infarction of the pyramidal
tracts in man. *Neurology, Minneap.* **12**, 637–642.   [365]

MILLS, C. K. (1888). Cerebral localization in its practical relations. *Trans. Congress,
Amer. Phys. and Surg. I,* 184–284, p. 237.   [29]

MILNER-BROWN, H. S., STEIN, R. B. and YEMM, R. (1973). The orderly recruitment
of human motor units during voluntary isometric contractions. *J. Physiol.*
230, 359–370.   [345]

MORUZZI, G. (1950). 'Problems in Cerebellar Physiology'. Thomas, Springfield.
                                                                    [216]

MOTT, F. W. and SHERRINGTON, C. S. (1895). Experiments upon the influence of
sensory nerves upon movement and nutrition of the limbs. *Proc. R. Soc.* **57**,
481–488.   [296, 373]

MOUNTCASTLE, V. B. (1957). Modality and topographic properties of single
neurons of cat's somatic sensory cortex. *J. Neurophysiol.* **20**, 408–434.
                                                                [208, 218]

MOUNTCASTLE, V. B. and POWELL, T. P. S. (1959). Neural mechanisms subserving cutaneous sensibility, with special reference to the role of afferent inhibition in sensory perception and discrimination. *Bull. Johns Hopkins Hosp.* **105**, 201–232. [253]

MOUNTCASTLE, V. B., COVIAN, M. R. and HARRISON, C. R. (1952). The central representation of some forms of deep sensibility. *Res. Publs Ass. Res. nerv. ment. Dis.* **30**, 339–370. [222]

MOUNTCASTLE, V. B., LYNCH, J. C., GEORGOPOULOS, A., SAKATA, H. and ACUNA, C. (1975). Posterior parietal association cortex of the monkey: command functions for operations within extrapersonal space. *J. Neurophysiol.* **38**, 871–908. [209, 308]

MUIR, R. B. (1973). A model of cortico-motoneuronal synaptic action. *Proc. Aust. Physiol. Pharmacol. Soc.* **4**, no. 1, 70. [75]

MUIR, R. B. (1975). The role of corticomotoneuronal synapses in the control of movement. Ph.D. Thesis, Monash University. [70, 295]

MUIR, R. B. and PORTER, R. (1973). The effect of a preceding stimulus on temporal facilitation at corticomotoneuronal synapses. *J. Physiol.* **228**, 749–763. [70, 71]

MURPHY, J. T., WONG, Y. C. and KWAN, H. C. (1975). Afferent-efferent linkages in motor cortex for single forelimb muscles. *J. Neurophysiol.* **38**, 990–1014 [223, 225, 226]

NAPIER, J. R. (1956). The prehensile movements of the human hand. *J. Bone Jt Surg.* **38B**, 902–913. [15, 362]

NAPIER, J. R. (1960). Studies of the hands of living primates. *Proc. zool. soc. Lond.* **134**, 647–657. [362]

NAPIER J. R. (1961). Prehensility and oposability in the hand of primates. *Symp. Zool. Soc. Lond.* **5**, 115–132. [14]

NAPIER, J. R. and NAPIER, P. H. (1967). 'A Handbook of Living Primates: Morphology, Ecology and Behaviour of Nonhuman Primates.' Academic Press, London and New York. [268]

NATHAN, P. and SEARS, T. A. (1960). Effects of posterior root section on the activity of some muscles in man. *J. Neurol. Neurosurg. Psychiat.* **23**, 10–122. [373]

NICHOLS, T. R. and HOUK, J. C. (1973). Reflex compensation for variations in the mechanical properties of muscle. *Science, N.Y.* **181**, 182–184. [328]

NYBERG-HANSEN, R. and BRODAL, A. (1963). Sites of termination of corticospinal fibers in the cat. An experimental study with silver impregnation methods. *J. comp. Neurol.* **120**, 369–391. [121]

NYBERG-HANSEN, R. and BRODAL, A. (1964). Sites and modes of termination of rubrospinal fibres in the cat. An experimental study with silver impregnation methods. *J. Anat.* **98**, 235–253. [109]

NYQUIST, J. K. (1975). Somatosensory properties of neurons of thalamic nucleus ventralis lateralis. *Expl Neurol.* **48**, 123–135. [216, 225]

OSCARSSON, O. (1965). Functional organization of the spino- and cuneo-cerebellar tracts. *Physiol. Rev.* **45**, 495–522. [124, 335]

OSCARSSON, O. (1971). *In* 'Central Control of Movement' (Eds E. V. Evarts, E. Bizzi, R. E. Burke, M. DeLong and W. T. Thach Jr.). *Neuro. Res. Prog. Bull.* **9**, 7–170. [330]

OSCARSSON, O. and ROSÉN, I. (1963). Projection to cerebral cortex of large muscle-spindle afferents in forelimb nerves of the cat. *J. Physiol.* **169**, 924–945. [222]

OSCARSSON, O. and ROSÉN, I. (1966). Short-latency projections to the cat's cerebral cortex from skin and muscle afferents in the contralateral forelimb. *J. Physiol.* **182**, 164–184. [222]

OSCARSSON, O., ROSÉN, I. and SULG, I. (1966). Organization of neurones in the cat cerebral cortex that are influenced from Group I muscle afferents. *J. Physiol.* **183**, 189–210.   [223]

PAILLARD, J. (1960). The patterning of skilled movements. *In* 'Handbook of Physiology: Neurophysiology III' (Eds J. Field, H. W. Magoun and V. E. Hall), pp. 1679–1708. American Physiological Society, Washington.   [329]

PAILLARD, J. and BROUCHON, M. (1968). Active and passive movements in the calibration of position sense. *In* 'The Neuropsychology of spatially oriented Behavior' (Ed. S. J. Freedman), pp. 37–55. Dorsey Press, Homewood, Illinois.   [379]

PANDYA, D. N. and KUYPERS, H. G. J. M. (1969). Cortico-cortical connections in the rhesus monkey. *Brain Res.* **13**, 13–36.   [228]

PATTON, H. D. and AMASSIAN, V. E. (1954). Single- and multiple-unit analysis of cortical stage of pyramidal tract activation. *J. Neurophysiol.* **17**, 345–363.
                                                                        [66, 77]

PATTON, H. D. and AMASSIAN, V. E. (1960). The pyramidal tract: its excitation and functions. *In* 'Handbook of Physiology—Neurophysiology' (Ed. J. Field), vol. 2, pp. 837–861. American Physiological Society, Washington. [89, 219]

PATTON, H. D., TOWE, A. L. and KENNEDY, T. T. (1962). Activation of pyramidal tract neurons by ipsilateral cutaneous stimuli. *J. Neurophysiol.* **25**, 501–524. [219]

PENFIELD, W. (1954). Mechanisms of voluntary movement. *Brain,* **77**, 1–17.   [9]

PENFIELD, W. (1958). 'The Excitable Cortex in Conscious Man'. Liverpool University Press, Liverpool.   [37, 326]

PENFIELD, W. and BOLDREY, E. (1937). Somatic motor and sensory representation in the cerebral cortex of man as studied by electrical stimulation. *Brain,* **60**, 389–443.   [43, 45]

PENFIELD, W. and JASPER, H. H. (1954). 'Epilepsy and the Functional Anatomy of the Human Brain'. Churchill, London.   [43]

PENFIELD, W. and RASMUSSEN, A. T. (1950). 'Cerebral Cortex of Man. A Clinical Study of Localisation of Function'. Macmillan, New York.   [43]

PETRAS, J. M. (1966). Corticospinal fiber connexions in spider and rhesus monkeys, gibbon and chimpanzee; some preliminary notes. *Anat. Rec.* **154**, 402.
                                                                        [15, 138]

PETRAS, J. M. (1968). Corticospinal fibers in new world and old world simians. *Brain Res.* **8**, 206–208.   [15]

PETRAS, J. M. and LEHMAN, R. A. W. (1966). Corticospinal fibers in the racoon. *Brain Res.* **3**, 195–197.   [16, 122]

PHILLIPS, C. G. (1956a). Intracellular records from Betz cells in the cat. *Q. Jl exp. Physiol.* **41**, 58–69.   [61]

PHILLIPS, C. G. (1956b). Cortical motor threshold and the thresholds and distribution of excited Betz cells in the cat. *Q. Jl exp. Physiol.* **41**, 70–84.   [62, 79]

PHILLIPS, C. G. (1959). Actions of antidromic pyramidal volleys on single Betz cells in the cat. *Q. Jl exp. Physiol.* **44**, 1–25.   [62, 108]

PHILLIPS, C. G. (1961). Some properties of pyramidal neurones of the motor cortex. Ciba Foundation Symposium on 'The Nature of Sleep' (Eds G. E. W. Wolstenholme and Maeve O'Connor). *Q. Jl exp. Physiol.* pp. 4–24. Churchill, London.   [60, 62, 108]

PHILLIPS, C. G. (1966). Changing concepts of the precentral motor area. *In* 'Brain and Conscious Experience' (Ed. J. C. Eccles), pp. 389–421. Springer-Verlag, New York.   [30, 36, 347]

PHILLIPS, C. G. (1967). Corticomotoneuronal organization. Projection from the arm area of the baboon's motor cortex. *Arch. Neurol.* **17**, 188–195. [164, 165]

PHILLIPS, C. G. (1969). Motor apparatus of the baboon's hand. *Proc. R. Soc. B.* **173**, 141–174.   [304, 353]

PHILLIPS, C. G. (1971). Evolution of the corticospinal tract in primates with special reference to the hand. Proc. 3rd Int. Congr. Primat. Zurich, 1970, vol. 2, pp. 2–23. Karger, Basel.   [15, 272, 364]

PHILLIPS, C. G. (1973). Cortical localization and 'sensorimotor processes' at the 'middle level' in primates—Hughlings Jackson Lecture. *Proc. R. Soc. Med.* V. 66, Section of Neurology, pp. 987–1002, Oct. 1973.   [21, 29, 36, 323]

PHILLIPS, C. G. (1975). Laying the ghost of 'Muscles versus Movements'. *Can. J. Neurol. Sci.* **2**, 209–218.   [36, 40]

PHILLIPS, C. G. and PORTER, R. (1962). Unifocal and bifocal stimulation of the motor cortex. *J. Physiol.* **162**, 532–538.   [83, 160]

PHILLIPS, C. G. and PORTER, R. (1964). The pyramidal projection to motoneurones of some muscle groups of the baboon's forelimb. *In* 'Progress in Brain Research: Physiology of Spinal Neurones' (Eds J. C. Eccles and J. P. Schadé), vol. 12, pp. 222–242. Elsevier, Amsterdam.   [68, 71, 147, 157, 161, 164]

PHILLIPS, C. G., POWELL, T. P. S. and WIESENDANGER, M. (1971). Projection from low-threshold muscle afferents of hand and forearm to area 3a of baboon's cortex. *J. Physiol.* **217**, 419–446.   [230, 231, 251]

POLANYI, M. (1968). Life's irreducible structure. *Science, N.Y.* **160**, 1308–1312.   [322]

PORTER, R. (1967). Cortical actions on hypoglossal motoneurones in cats: a proposed role for a common internuncial cell. *J. Physiol.* **193**, 295–308.   [120]

PORTER, R. (1970). Early facilitation at corticomotoneuronal synapses. *J. Physiol.* **207**, 733–745.   [69, 70, 75]

PORTER, R. (1972). Relationship of the discharges of cortical neurones to movement in free-to-move monkeys. *Brain Res.* **40**, 39–43.   [290]

PORTER, R. and HORE, J. (1969). The time course of minimal corticomotoneuronal excitatory postsynaptic potentials in lumbar motoneurones of the monkey. *J. Neurophysiol.* **32**, 443–451.   [69, 76]

PORTER, R. and LEWIS, M. McD. (1975). Relationship of neuronal discharges in the precentral gyrus of monkeys to the performance of arm movements. *Brain Res.* **98**, 21–36.   [294]

PORTER, R. and MUIR, R. (1971). The meaning for motoneurones of the temporal pattern of natural activity in pyramidal tract neurones of conscious monkeys. *Brain Res.* **34**, 127–142.   [75]

PORTER, R. and RACK, P. M. H. (1976). Timing of the response in the motor cortex of monkeys to an unexpected disturbance of finger position. *Brain Res.* **103**, 201–213.   [301, 304, 316]

PRESTON, J. B., SHENDE, M. C. and UEMURA, K. (1967). The motor cortex-pyramidal system: patterns of facilitation and inhibition on motoneurons innervating limb musculature of cat and baboon and their possible adaptive significance. *In* 'Neurophysiological Basis of Normal and Abnormal Motor Activities' (Eds M. D. Yahr and D. P. Purpura), pp. 61–72. Raven Press, New York.   [131, 149]

PRESTON, J. B. and WHITLOCK, D. G. (1960). Precentral facilitation and inhibition of spinal motoneurons. *J. Neurophysiol.* **23**, 154–170.   [144]

PRESTON, J. B. and WHITLOCK, D. G. (1961). Intracellular potentials recorded from motoneurons following precentral gyrus stimulation in primate. *J. Neurophysiol.* **24**, 91–100.   [144, 145]

PURPURA, D. P., SHOFER, R. J. and MUSGRAVE, F. S. (1964). Cortical intracellular
potentials during augmenting and recruiting responses. II. Patterns of
synaptic activities in pyramidal and nonpyramidal tract neurons. *J. Neurophysiol.* **27**, 133–151.   [216]
PURPURA, D. P. and YAHR, M. D. (1966) (Eds.) 'The Thalamus'. Columbia Univer-
sity Press, New York and London.   [215]
RAMÓN y CAJAL, S. (1909). 'Histologie du Système Nerveux de l'Homme et des
Vertébrés', vol. 1, Maloine, Paris.   [11, 94, 321]
RAMÓN y CAJAL, S. (1911). 'Histologie du Système Nerveux de l'Homme et des
Vertébrés', vol. 2. Maloine, Paris.   [108, 321]
RAMÓN y CAJAL, S. (1937). 'Recollections of my Life'. Translation E. Horne
Craigie and J. Cano. Memoirs of the American Philosophical Society, vol. 8,
pts 1 and 2.   [54]
REXED, B. (1964). Some aspects of the cytoarchitectonics and synaptology of the
spinal cord. *Prog. Brain Res.* **11**, 58–90.   [121]
RINVIK, E. and WALBERG, F. (1963). Demonstration of a somatotopically arranged
corticorubral projection in the cat. *J. comp. Neurol.* **120**, 393–407.   [109]
RISPAL-PADEL, L. and LATREILLE, J. (1974). The organization of projections from
the cerebellar nuclei to the contralateral motor cortex in the cat. *Expl Brain
Res.* **19**, 36–60.   [217]
RISPAL-PADEL, L., MASSION, J. and GRANGETTO, A. (1973). Relations between
the ventrolateral thalamic nucleus and motor cortex and their possible role
in the central organization of motor control. *Brain Res.* **60**, 1–20.   [216]
ROBERTS, W. J. and SMITH, D. O. (1973). Analysis of threshold current during
microstimulation of fibres in the spinal cord. *Acta physiol. scand.* **89**, 384–394.
                                                                                               [175]
ROSÉN, I. and ASANUMA, H. (1972). Peripheral afferent inputs to the forelimb area
of the monkey motor cortex: Input-output relations. *Expl Brain Res.* **14**,
257–273.   [234, 257, 262, 304]
RUSSELL, J. R. and DEMYER, W. (1961). The quantitative cortical origin of pyrami-
dal axons of Macaca rhesus, with some remarks on the slow rate of axolysis.
Neurology, Minneap. **11**, 96–108.   [135]
RUSSELL, W. R. and WHITTY, C. W. M. (1953). Studies in traumatic epilepsy. 2.
Focal motor and somatic sensory fits: a study of 85 cases. *J. Neurol. Neuro-
surg. Psychiat.* **16**, 73–97.   [367]
SAKATA, H. and MIYAMOTO, J. (1968). Topographic relationship between the
receptive fields of neurons in the motor cortex and the movements elicited
by focal stimulation in freely moving cats. *Jap. J. Physiol.* **18**, 489–507.   [222]
SAWA, M., MARUYAMA, N. and KAJI, S. (1963). Intracellular potential during
electrically induced seizures. *Electroenceph. clin. Neurophysiol.* **15**, 209–220.   [62]
SCHÄFER, E. A. (1900). The Cerebral Cortex. *In* 'Textbook of Physiology' (Ed.
E. A. Schäfer), vol. 2, pp. 697–782. Young J. Pentland, Edinburgh and
London.   [7, 21, 27, 31, 36]
SCHMIDT, E. M., JOST, R. G. and DAVIS, K. K. (1974). Plasticity of cortical cell
firing patterns after load changes. *Brain Res.* **73**, 540–544.   [294]
SCHMIDT, E. M., JOST, R. G. and DAVIS, K. K. (1975). Reexamination of the force
relationship of cortical cell discharge patterns with conditioned wrist move-
ments. *Brain Res.* **83**, 213–223.
SCHOEN, J. H. R. (1964). Comparative aspects of the descending fibre systems in
the spinal cord. *In* 'Progress in Brain Research: Organization of the Spinal
Cord' (Eds J. C. Eccles and J. P. Schadé), vol. 11, pp. 203–222. Elsevier,
Amsterdam.   [12, 138]

SCHULTZ, A. H. (1961). Some factors influencing the social life of primates in general and of early man in particular. *In* 'Social Life of Early Man' (Ed. S. L. Washburn), pp. 58–90. Aldine, Chicago. [15]

SCHULTZ, A. H. (1968). Form und Funktion der Primatenhände. *In* 'Handgebrauche und Verständigung bei Affen und Frühmenschen' (Ed. B. Rensch), pp. 9–25. Huber, Bern. [14]

SEVERIN, F. V., ORLOVSKY, G. N. and SHIK, M. L. (1967). Work of the muscle receptors during controlled locomotion. *Biofizika,* **12**, 502–511. (English translation, pp. 575–586.) [304]

SHAPOVALOV, A. I. (1975). Neuronal organization and synaptic mechanisms of supraspinal motor control in vertebrates. *Rev. Physiol. Biochem. Pharmacol.* **72**, 1–54. [16]

SHAPOVALOV, A. I., KARAMJAN, O. A., KURCHAVYI, C. G. and REPINA, Z. A. (1971). Synaptic actions evoked from the red nucleus on the spinal alphamotoneurons in the rhesus monkey. *Brain Res.* **32**, 325–348. [76]

SHERRINGTON, C. S. (1885). On secondary and tertiary degenerations in the spinal cord of the dog. *J. Physiol.* **6**, 177–191. [5, 93]

SHERRINGTON, C. S. (1889). On nerve-tracts degenerating secondarily to lesions of cortex cerebri. *J. Physiol.* **10**, 429–432. [30]

SHERRINGTON, C. S. (1899). Relation between structure and function as examined in the arm. *Trans. Liv. Biol. Soc.* **13**, 1–20. [42]

SHERRINGTON, C. S. (1900a). The spinal cord. *In* 'Textbook of Physiology' (Ed. E. A. Schäfer), vol. 2, pp. 783–883. Young J. Pentland, Edinburgh and London. [11, 36]

SHERRINGTON, C. S. (1900b). The parts of the brain below cerebral cortex, viz. medulla oblongata, pons, cerebellum, corpora quadrigemina, and region of thalamus. *In* 'Textbook of Physiology' (Ed. E. A. Schäfer), vol. 2, pp. 884–919. Young J. Pentland, Edinburgh and London. [46]

SHERRINGTON, C. S. (1900c). Cutaneous sensations. *In* 'Textbook of Physiology' (Ed. E. A. Schäfer), vol. 2, pp. 920–1001. Young J. Pentland, Edinburgh and London. [390, 391, 392]

SHERRINGTON, C. S. (1900d). The muscular sense. *In* 'Textbook of Physiology' (Ed. E. A. Schäfer), vol. 2, pp. 1002–1025. Young J. Pentland, Edinburgh and London. [390]

SHERRINGTON, C. S. (1906). 'The Integrative Action of the Nervous System'. Scribners, New York. 2nd edn. 1947, Cambridge University Press, pp. 290–291. [2, 3, 28, 37, 38, 39, 131, 144]

SHERRINGTON, C. S. (1931). Quantitative management of contraction in lowest level co-ordination. *Brain,* **54**, 1–28. [141, 154, 373]

SHIMAZU, H., YANAGISAWA, N. and GAROUTTE, B. (1965). Cortico-pyramidal influences on thalamic somatosensory transmission in the cat. *Jap. J. Physiol.* **15**, 101–124. [116]

SHOLL, D. A. (1956). 'The Organization of the Cerebral Cortex'. Methuen, London. [209]

SINGER, W., TRETTER, F. and CYNADER, M. (1975). Organization of cat striate cortex: a correlation of receptive-field properties with afferent and efferent connections. *J. Neurophysiol.* **38**, 1080–1098. [209]

SKOGLUND, S. (1956). Anatomical and physiological studies of knee joint innervation in the cat. *Acta physiol. scand.* **36**, suppl. 124. [249]

SLOPER, J. J. (1973). An electron microscope study of the termination of afferent connections to the primate motor cortex. *J. Neurocytol.* **2**, 361–368. [207, 209]

SMITH, A. M., HEPP-REYMOND, M.-C. and WYSS, U. R. (1975). Relation of activity in precentral cortical neurons to force and rate of force change during isometric contractions of finger muscles. *Expl Brain Res.* **23**, 315–332. [286]

SOMJEN, G. G. (1972). *In* 'Neurophysiology Studied in Man' (Ed. G. G. Somjen), p. 343. Excerpta Medica, Amsterdam.   [348]

STEFANIS, C. and JASPER, H. (1964). Recurrent collateral inhibition in pyramidal tract neurons. *J. Neurophysiol.* **27**, 855–877.   [109]

STEIN, J. F. (1976). The effect of cooling parietal lobe areas 5 and 7 upon voluntary movement in awake rhesus monkeys. *J. Physiol.* **258**, 62–63P.   [359]

STEIN, R. B. (1974). Peripheral control of movement. *Physiol. Rev.* **54**, 215–243.
                                                                                                         [350]

STONEY, S. D. Jr., THOMPSON, W. D. and ASANUMA, H. (1968). Excitation of pyramidal tract cells by intracortical microstimulation: effective extent of stimulating current. *J. Neurophysiol.* **31**, 659–669.
                                                 [173, 175, 176, 177, 181, 183, 184, 196]

STRICK, P. L. (1973). Light microscopic analysis of the cortical projection of the thalamic ventrolateral nucleus in the cat. *Brain Res.* **55**, 1–24.   [216]

STRICK, P. L. (1975). Multiple sources of thalamic input to the primate motor cortex. *Brain Res.* **88**, 372–377.   [96, 228, 254, 255]

SWETT, J. E. and BOURASSA, C. M. (1967). Short latency activation of pyramidal tract cells by group I afferent volleys in the cat. *J. Physiol.* **189**, 101–117. [223]

SZENTÁGOTHAI, J. (1969). Architecture of the cerebral cortex. *In* 'Basic Mechanisms of the Epilepsies' (Eds H. H. Jasper, A. A. Ward and A. Pope), pp. 13–28. Churchill, London.   [179, 206, 207, 208]

TAKAHASHI, K. (1965). Slow and fast groups of pyramidal tract cells and their respective membrane properties. *J. Neurophysiol.* **28**, 908–924.   [57]

TAKAHASHI, K., KUBOTA, K. and UNO, M. (1967). Recurrent facilitation in cat pyramidal tract cells. *J. Neurophysiol.* **30**, 22–34.   [60, 108, 272]

TANAKA, R. (1972). Activation of reciprocal Ia inhibitory pathway during voluntary motor performance in man. *Brain Res.* **43**, 649–652.   [146, 339]

TANJI, J. and EVARTS, E. V. (1976). Anticipatory activity of motor cortex neurons in relation to direction of intended movement. *J. Neurophysiol.* **39**, 1062–1068.
                                                                                                         [317]

TAUB, E. and BERMAN, A. J. (1968). Movement and learning in the absence of sensory feedback. *In* 'The Neuropsychology of Spatially Oriented Behavior' (Ed. S. J. Freedman), pp. 173–192. Dorsey Press, Homewood, Illinois.
                                                                                                    [374, 396]

TAYLOR, A. and CODY, F. W. J. (1974). Jaw muscle spindle activity in the cat during normal movements of eating and drinking. *Brain Res.* **71**, 523–530.
                                                                                                         [304]

TAYLOR, A. and DAVEY, M. R. (1968). Behaviour of the jaw muscle stretch receptors during active and passive movements in cats. *Nature, Lond.* **220**, 301–302.
                                                                                                         [304]

THACH, W. T. (1970a). Discharge of cerebellar neurons related to two maintained postures and two prompt movements. I. Nuclear cell output. *J. Neurophysiol.* **33**, 527–536.   [9, 309]

THACH, W. T. (1970b). Discharge of cerebellar neurons related to two maintained postures and two prompt movements. II. Purkinje cell output and input. *J. Neurophysiol.* **33**, 537–547.   [9, 309]

THACH, W. T. (1975). Timing of activity in cerebellar dentate nucleus and cerebral motor cortex during prompt volitional movement. *Brain Res.* **88**, 233–241.
                                                                                                    [310, 397]

THOMPSON, F. J. and FERNANDEZ, J. J. (1975). Patterns of cortical projection to hindlimb muscle motoneurone pools. *Brain Res.* **97**, 33–46.   [221]

THOMPSON, F. J., FERNANDEZ, J., ASANUMA, H. and KUBOTA, K. (1973). Relationship between 3a sensory cortex and motor cortex in the cat. *Fedn Proc. Fedn Am. Socs exp. Biol.* **32**, Ab. 699.   [225]

THOMPSON, W. D., STONEY, S. D. Jr. and ASANUMA, H. (1970). Characteristics of projections from primary sensory cortex to motosensory cortex in cats. *Brain Res.* **22**, 15–27.   [225]

TOWE, A. L. (1973). Relative numbers of pyramidal tract neurons in mammals of different sizes. *Brain, Beh. Evol.* **7**, 1–17.   [12, 89]

TOWE, A. L., PATTON, H. D. and KENNEDY, T. T. (1964). Response properties of neurons in the pericruciate cortex of the cat following electrical stimulation of the appendages. *Expl Neurol.* **10**, 325–344.   [218]

TOWER, S. S. (1935). The dissociation of cortical excitation from cortical inhibition by pyramid section, and the syndrome of that lesion in the cat. *Brain,* **58** 238–255.   [360]

TOWER, S. S. (1940). Pyramidal lesion in the monkey. *Brain,* **63**, 36–90.
                                                              [361, 362, 363]

TOWER, S. S. (1944). The pyramidal tract. *In* 'The Precentral Motor Cortex' (Ed. P. C. Bucy), pp. 151–172. University of Illinois Press, Urbana.   [48]

TROTTER, W. (1934). A landmark in modern neurology. *Lancet,* **227**, 1207–1210.
                                                                         [26]

TSUKAHARA, N. and KOSAKA, K. (1968). The mode of cerebral excitation of red nucleus neurons. *Expl Brain Res.* **5**, 102–117.   [109, 110]

TSUKAHARA, N., FULLER, D. R. G. and BROOKS, V. B. (1968). Collateral pyramidal influences on the corticorubrospinal system. *J. Neurophysiol.* **31**,457–484.
                                                             [103, 109, 110]

TSUMOTO, T., NAKUMURA, S. and IWAMA, K. (1975). Pyramidal tract control over cutaneous and kinaesthetic sensory transmission in the cat thalamus. *Expl Brain Res.* **22**, 281–294.   [116, 396]

TUTTLE, R. H. (1969). Qualitative and functional studies on the hands of the Anthropoidea. I. The Hominoidea. *J. Morph.* **128**, 309–363.   [15]

UCHIZONO, K. (1965). Characteristics of excitatory and inhibitory synapses in the central nervous system of the cat. *Nature, Lond.* **207**, 642–643.   [207]

VALLBO, Å. B. (1970). Slowly adapting muscle receptors in man. *Acta physiol. scand.* **78**, 315–333.   [304, 351]

VALLBO, Å. B. (1971). Muscle spindle response at the onset of isometric voluntary contractions in man. Time difference between fusimotor and skeleto-motor effects. *J. Physiol.* **218**, 405–431.   [351]

VALLBO, Å. B. (1973). Muscle spindle afferent discharge from resting and contracting muscles in normal human subjects. *In* 'New Developments in Electromyography and Clinical Neurophysiology' (Ed. J. E. Desmedt), vol. 3, pp. 251–262, Karger, Basel.   [351]

VALLBO, Å. B. (1974). Afferent discharge from human muscle spindles in non-contracting muscles. Steady state impulse frequency as a function of joint angle. *Acta physiol. scand.* **90**, 303–318.   [379]

VAUGHAN, H. G. Jr., GROSS, E. G. and BOSSOM, J. (1970). Cortical motor potential in monkeys before and after upper limb deafferentation. *Expl Neurol.* **26**, 253–262.   [315]

VEDEL, J. P. (1966). Mise en évidence d'un contróle cortical de l'activité des fibres fusimotrices dynamiques chez le chat par la voie pyramidale. *C. r. Seanc. Acad. Sci.* **262**, 908–911.   [135]

VERHAART, W. J. C. (1948). The pes pedunculi and pyramid. *J. comp. Neurol.* **88**, 139–155.   [268]

WALBERG, F. (1957). Do the motor nuclei of the cranial nerves receive corticofugal fibers? An experimental study in the cat. *Brain,* **80**, 597–605.   [120]

WALBERG, F. (1958). On the termination of the rubro-bulbar fibers. Experimental observations in the cat. *J. comp. Neurol.* **110**, 65–73.   [120]

WALL, P. D., RÉMOND, A. G. and DOBSON, R. L. (1953). Studies on the mechanisms of the action of visual afferents on motor cortex excitability. *Electroenceph. clin. Neurophysiol.* **5**, 385–393.   [218]

WALSHE, F. M. R. (1943). On the mode of representation of movements in the motor cortex, with special reference to 'convulsions beginning unilaterally' (Jackson). *Brain,* **66**, 104–139.   [31, 45]

WALSHE, F. M. R. (1953). Some problems of method in neurology. *Can. med. Ass. J.* **68**, 21–29.   [326]

WALSHE, F. M. R. (1973). 'Diseases of the Nervous System' (11th Edition). Churchill, Livingstone, Edinburgh and London.   [367]

WELFORD, A. T. (1974). On the sequencing of action. *Brain Res.* **71**, 381–392.
                                                                                            [333, 334, 335]

WELT, C., ASCHOFF, J. C., KAMEDA, K. and BROOKS, V. B. (1967). Intracortical organization of cat's motosensory neurons. *In* 'Neurophysiological Basis of Normal and Abnormal Motor Activities' (Eds M. D. Yahr and D. P. Purpura), pp. 255–293. Raven Press, New York.   [219, 220, 221]

WETTSTEIN, A. and HANDWERKER, H. O. (1970). Afferente Verbindungen zu schnell- und langsamleitenden Pyramidenbahnneuronen der Katze. *Pflugers Arch. ges. Physiol.* **320**, 247–260.   [218]

WHITTAKER, V. P. (1964). Investigations on the storage sites of biogenic amines in the central nervous system. *Prog. Brain Res.* **8**, 90–117.   [64]

WIESENDANGER, M. (1969). The pyramidal tract. Recent investigations on its morphology and function. *Ergebn. Physiol.* **61**, 72–136.   [135, 215]

WIESENDANGER, M. (1973). Input from muscle and cutaneous nerves of the hand and forearm to neurones of the precentral gyrus of baboons and monkeys. *J. Physiol.* **228**, 203–219.   [219, 231, 304]

WILLIS, W. D., TATE, G. W., ASHWORTH, R. D. and WILLIS, J. C. (1966). Monosynaptic excitation of motoneurons of individual forelimb muscles. *J. Neurophysiol.* **29**, 410–424.   [131]

WILLIS, W. D., TREVINO, D. L., COULTER, J. D. and MAUNZ, R. A. (1974). Responses of primate spinothalamic tract neurons to natural stimulation of the hindlimb. *J. Neurophysiol.* **37**, 358–372.   [254]

WILSON, S. A. K. (1914). An experimental research into the anatomy and physiology of the corpus striatum. *Brain,* **36**, 427–492.   [7]

WIRTH, F. P., O'LEARY, J. L., SMITH, J. M. and JENNY, A. B. (1974). Monosynaptic corticospinal-motoneuron path in the raccoon. *Brain Res.* **77**, 344–348.   [16, 122]

WOOLSEY, C. N. (1958). Organization of somatic sensory and motor areas of the cerebral cortex. *In* Biological and Biochemical Bases of Behavior' (Eds H. F. Harlow and C. N. Woolsey), pp. 63–81. The University of Wisconsin Press, Madison.   [28, 46]

WOOLSEY, C. N. (1964). Cortical localization as defined by evoked potential and electrical stimulation studies. *In* 'Cerebral Localization and Organization' (Eds G. Schaltenbrand and C. N. Woolsey). The University of Wisconsin Press, Madison.   [28]

Woolsey, C. N. and Chang, H. T. (1948). Activation of the cerebral cortex by antidromic volleys in the pyramidal tract. *A.R.N.M.D.* **27**, 146–161. (*Res. Publs Ass. nerv. ment. Dis.*)   [97, 135]

Woolsey, T. A. and Van Der Loos, H. (1970). The structural organization of layer IV in the somatosensory region (S1) of mouse cerebral cortex. *Brain Res.* **17**, 205–242.   [209]

Woolsey, C. N., Settlage, P. H., Meyer, D. R., Sencer, W., Hamuy, T. P. and Travis, A. M. (1952). Patterns of localization in precentral and 'supplementary' motor areas and their relation to the concept of a premotor area. *Res. Publs Ass. nerv. ment. Dis.* **30**, 238–264.   [34, 43, 45, 149]

Woolsey, C. N., Gorska, T., Wetzel, A., Erickson, T. C., Earls, F. J. and Allman, J. M. (1972). Compete unilateral section of the pyramidal tract at the medullary level in *Macaca mulatta*. *Brain Res.* **40**, 119–124. [51, 290]

Yokota, T. and Voorhoeve, P. E. (1969). Pyramidal control of fusimotor neurons supplying extensor muscles in the cat's forelimb. *Expl Brain Res.* **9**, 96–115.   [135]

Yoshida, M., Yajima, K. and Uno, M. (1966). Different activation of the two types of the pyramidal tract neurones through the cerebello-thalamo-cortical pathway. *Experientia*, **22**, 331–332.   [216]

Yumiya, H., Kubota, K. and Asanuma, H. (1974). Activities of neurons in area 3a of the cerebral cortex during voluntary movements in the monkey. *Brain Res.* **78**, 169–177.   [307]

Zangger, P. and Wiesendanger, M. (1973). Excitation of lateral reticular nucleus neurones by collaterals of the pyramidal tract. *Expl Brain Res.* **17**, 144–151.   [119]

Zuckerman, S. and Fulton, J. F. (1941). The motor cortex in Galago and Perodicticus. *J. Anat.* **75**, 447–456.   [15]

Index

This index should be used in conjunction with the table of contents.

022321